"This is a fantastic resource that provides a
for practitioners who see children and adol
conditions along with expectations for poten

"This is a well written and clinically practical volume that provides essential information needed to guide differential diagnosis, assessment, and intervention approaches. An essential and hands-on resource for all levels of applied practice!"

Elaine Fletcher-Janzen, *Ed.D., NCSP, ABPdN*

Understanding and Managing Neurodevelopmental Disorders in Children and Adolescents

Children are being identified with more neurodevelopmental disorders than in previous decades and understanding these medically complex disorders has become critical as more children are living with these disorders.

This pediatric treatment guide provides cutting-edge research and intervention recommendations for professionals working with children and adolescents. A team of contributors with diverse experience portray medically complex information and neurodevelopmental disorders in an accessible manner. Chapters include information on a range of disorders, such as: cystic fibrosis, diabetes, epilepsy, meningitis, chronic fatigue, and more. Each disorder's physical and neurological manifestations are explored, as well as how the disorder is diagnosed and treated, and information regarding appropriate assessment and intervention. A list of further resources is included at the end of most chapters.

This book is essential for practitioners working with children, including clinical psychologists, school psychologists, child neuropsychologists, clinical and school social workers, school nurses, pediatricians, and graduate students in training within various pediatric specialties.

Denise E. Maricle, Ph.D., LP-MN, NCSP, ABSNP retired from academia in 2023. Over the past 30+ years Dr. Maricle has practiced as a psychologist, school psychologist, pediatric/school neuropsychologist, and an academician and researcher. She currently engages in writing, training, and consultancy work.

Christopher L. Bedford, Ph.D., LP, ABSNP is the executive director of the American Board of School Neuropsychology. Working as a psychologist for more than 15 years, Dr. Bedford currently operates a private practice in Minnesota.

Julie A. Gettman, Ph.D., NCSP, ABSNP is the executive director of the School Neuropsychology Institute. She owns and operates Mindworks

Assessment, a private practice and consulting company specializing in comprehensive neurocognitive assessment for children and adolescents.

Daniel C. Miller, Ph.D., ABPP, ABSNP is the founder of the School Neuropsychology Institute, president of KIDS, Inc., and founder of Report Insights LLC. He has more than 35+ years of experience in school psychology and school neuropsychology. He is the executive director of the Woodcock Institute for Neurocognitive Research and Applied Practice.

Wendi L. Johnson, Ph.D., LP, NCSP, LSSP is an associate professor at Texas Woman's University, and the assistant executive director of the Woodcock Institute for Neurocognitive Research and Applied Practice. Dr. Johnson currently serves as director of the Woodcock Autism Assessment Clinic (WAAC).

Understanding and Managing Neurodevelopmental Disorders in Children and Adolescents

A Pediatric Treatment Guide

Edited by
Denise E. Maricle, Christopher L. Bedford, Julie A. Gettman, Daniel C. Miller and Wendi L. Johnson

Routledge
Taylor & Francis Group
NEW YORK AND LONDON

Designed cover image: Getty Images

First published 2025
by Routledge
605 Third Avenue, New York, NY 10158

and by Routledge
4 Park Square, Milton Park, Abingdon, Oxon OX14 4RN

Routledge is an imprint of the Taylor & Francis Group, an informa business

Library of Congress Cataloging-in-Publication Data
A catalog record for this title has been requested

ISBN: 978-1-032-68447-5 (hbk)
ISBN: 978-1-032-70395-4 (pbk)
ISBN: 978-1-032-70392-3 (ebk)

DOI: 10.4324/9781032703923

Typeset in Times New Roman
by Taylor & Francis Books

Neurodiversity is normative, neurodevelopmental disorders are common, and my family is no exception. Many individuals within my family are living with the various neurodevelopmental disorders described within this text. My beloved family is filled with unique perspectives, vibrant minds, boundless creativity, and unyielding spirits that inspire me daily. I want you each to know that your strength, resilience, and authenticity have shaped my understanding of neurodevelopment and how to effectively brave the challenges that need to be faced even when one is a child. Thank you for being my guiding lights.

Denise E. Maricle

I have had the privilege and pleasure of working with a wide variety of children, adolescents, and adults in my time as a psychologist. Each individual client has taught me something I didn't know and made me a better practitioner for those who came after them. I wouldn't be the psychologist I am today without the experience of working with each of you. Thank you for the faith you placed in me and for trusting me with your care. I hope this text will provide other practitioners with some of the same insights that I learned from you.

Christopher L. Bedford

To Chris, my life and work partner—thank you for your unwavering support, constant collaboration, and encouragement in every step of this journey. And to the dedicated practitioners that participate in the School Neuropsychology Institute's programs: your expertise, compassion, and drive to serve children with unique needs have been some of my greatest teachers. It is a privilege to learn from your dedication to helping children with neurodevelopmental disorders thrive and learn. You inspire me every day to continue growing and striving for excellence.

Julie A. Gettman

This book is dedicated to Dr. Richard W. Woodcock, a friend, colleague, and mentor, who passed away in early 2024 as we were working on this book. His legacy will live on for generations to come. He had a profound influence on both my professional and personal life.

Daniel C. Miller

To my four incredible children, who fill our lives with chaos, laughter, and endless wonder. For the love that stretches beyond biology and embraces every part of who you are. Each of you teaches us resilience, patience, and boundless love. Your unique personalities and incredible journeys continue to teach us every day. This book is dedicated to Isaac, Levi, Ethan, and Ana, as well as those working with or parenting neurodiverse children—may it serve as a guide with support, strength, and inspiration on your path.

Wendi L. Johnson

Contents

Illustrations

Tables

Boxes

About The Editors

Denise E. Maricle, Ph.D., LP-MN, NCSP, ABSNP retired as full professor from Texas Woman's University, Denton, Texas in 2023. While at TWU Dr. Maricle served for over ten years as the program director and APA clinical training director for the program in School Psychology. Dr. Maricle is a Nationally Certified School Psychologist (NCSP), a Licensed Psychologist (MN), and holds the Diplomate in School Neuropsychology from the American Board of School Neuropsychology. Over the past 30+ years Dr. Maricle has practiced as a psychologist at both the non-doctoral and doctoral levels, as a school psychologist, as a pediatric/school neuropsychologist, and as an academician and researcher. She currently serves as a psychological consultant, author, speaker, and trainer for school and pediatric neuropsychology. She has authored and co-authored numerous books, journals, articles, and chapters. Previous books include *Evidence-Based Selective Assessment for Academic Disorders* (2017), *Essentials of School Neuropsychological Assessment*, Third Edition (2019), and *Best Practices in School Neuropsychology: Guidelines for Effective Practice, Assessment, and Evidenced Based Intervention*, Second Edition (2022).

Christopher L. Bedford, Ph.D., LP, ABSNP is the executive director of the American Board of School Neuropsychology. He has been working with children, adolescents, and adults for more than 15 years. His work in psychology began as a therapist in college counseling centers, and he developed expertise in neurocognitive assessment in his post-doctoral training after earning his Ph.D. from the University of Minnesota. Since becoming a licensed psychologist in Minnesota, Dr. Bedford has earned a post-doctoral master's degree in clinical psychopharmacology and was awarded Diplomate status in School Neuropsychology from the American Board of School Neuropsychology. He is the author or co-author of several journal articles and chapters and was co-editor of the *Best Practices in School Neuropsychology: Guidelines for Effective Practice, Assessment, and Evidenced Based Intervention*, Second Edition (2022). Dr. Bedford currently operates a private practice in St. Paul, Minnesota.

Julie A. Gettman, Ph.D., NCSP, ABSNP is the Executive Director of the School Neuropsychology Institute. She is a Licensed School Psychologist, Nationally Certified School Psychologist, and Diplomate in School Neuropsychology from the American Board of School Neuropsychology. Dr. Gettman received her bachelor's degree in psychology at the University of Colorado, Boulder, and her master's degree in educational psychology and doctorate in school psychology at the University of Denver. She has 28 years of experience as a practitioner in public school, university, test publishing, private practice, and forensic settings. She has presented at the district, state, and national level; collaborated with psychology thought leaders and test authors; and is a co-editor of the *Best Practices in School Neuropsychology: Guidelines for Effective Practice, Assessment and Evidenced Based Intervention*, Second Edition (2022). Dr. Gettman owns and operates Mindworks Assessment, a private practice and consulting company specializing in comprehensive neurocognitive assessment for children and adolescents.

Daniel C. Miller, Ph.D., ABPP, ABSNP, NCSP-retired is the Founder of the School Neuropsychology Institute, President of KIDS, Inc., and founder of Report Insights LLC, which produces the PsychWriter Pro, an online automated report generation program. He has more than 40 years of experience in school psychology and more than 35 years of experience in school neuropsychology. Dr. Miller received a doctoral degree from The Ohio State University in 1989. His doctoral studies were a unique blend between school psychology, neuropsychology, and electrophysiology. Dr. Miller is a Retired Licensed Psychologist (OH) and holds the Diplomate in School Psychology from the American Board of Professional Psychology and the Diplomate in School Neuropsychology from the American Board of School Neuropsychology. He is also a Fellow with the National Academy of Neuropsychology. Dr. Miller is a Professor Emeritus in the Department of Social Work, Psychology and Philosophy at Texas Woman's University (TWU). He is currently the Executive Director of the Woodcock Institute for Neurocognitive Research and Applied Practice, which is housed at TWU. Dr. Miller served as the President of NASP in 2003–04 and has been an active leader and presenter in state and national school psychology associations since 1992. He has written numerous journal articles, chapters, and books, including the *Essentials of School Neuropsychology* (2007; 2013; 2019), *Best Practices in School Neuropsychology: Guidelines for Effective Practice, Assessment and Evidenced Based Intervention*, Second Edition (2009; 2022), *Evidence-Based Selective Assessment for Academic Disorders* (2017).

Wendi L. Johnson, Ph.D., LP, NCSP, LSSP is an associate professor at Texas Woman's University, and the Assistant Executive Director of the Woodcock Institute for Neurocognitive Research and Applied Practice in Denton, TX. Dr. Johnson is also the founder and current director of the Woodcock Autism Assessment Clinic (WAAC). In the school psychology program at TWU, Dr. Johnson teaches classes in school neuropsychological assessment, direct behavior interventions, pediatric trauma, and autism/low incident assessment. Dr. Johnson's research team, entitled the B.R.A.I.N. team (**B**ehavior, **R**esearch, **A**ssessment, and **I**ntervention in **N**eurodevelopment), has various projects examining early interventions and best practices in the assessment of autism, supporting families of neurodiverse children and foster/adoptive families, as well as on-going work looking at the experiences of mothers in academia. Prior to academia, Dr. Johnson worked as a school psychologist in North Carolina, Louisiana, and Texas. She continues supporting schools and the practice of school psychology by providing training, consultative support, and supervising graduate practicum experiences.

Contributors

Antshel, Kevin M. Ph.D., ABPP Syracuse University, New York https://orcid.org0000-0002-1139-7790

Bindrich, Cortney Ed.D. Loyola University Chicago, Illinois

Bridges, Rachel M. Ph.D. The University of Texas at Austin, Texas https://orcid.org0009-0002-5702-9587

Canas, Angela Ph.D., ABPP NCSP Children's Medical Center Dallas and University of Texas Southwestern Medical Center, Texas

Cassill, Carolyn Ph.D. Massachusetts General Hospital and Harvard Medical School, Massachusetts https://orcid.org0000-0001-7484-4378

Escalante, Natalie PsyD. Children's Medical Center Dallas, Texas https://orcid.org0009-0007-6423-1392

Goh, Hazel Q. LSSP NCSP Doctoral Student, School Psychology Texas Woman's University, Texas https://orcid.org0009-0000-5098-7200

Hamad, Ruba Doctoral Student Loyola University Chicago, Illinois

Hamilton, Kendra A. Ph.D., LSSP NCSP Baylor University, Texas https://orcid.org0009-0008-0621-1577

Hammer, Jasmine G. Ph.D. Scottish Rite for Children, Texas

Hao, Shania C. BA University of California-Los Angeles Neuropsychology Services, California

Hoskinson, Kristen R. Ph.D. Abigail Wexner Research Institute at Nationwide Children's Hospital, Ohio

Hutaff-Lee, Christa Ph.D., ABPP-CN Children's Hospital Colorado University of Colorado School of Medicine, Colorado https://orcid.org0009-0000-4591-1025

Jones, Alicia M. Ph.D., LSSP NCSP Private Practice, Texas https://orcid.org0000-0002-1226-0809

Joseph, Tessah M.S. Institute for Social and Applied Neuroscience (ISAN), OR

Kokorelis, Christina MD Johns Hopkins University, Maryland

Koterba, Christine Ph.D., ABPP Nationwide Children's Hospital, Ohio

Leonard-Zabel, Ann Marie Ed.D., ABSNP LEP NCSP NEALAC (Private Practice); Curry College, Massachusetts https://orcid.org0009-0002-6180-1429

Longoria, Jennifer N. Ph.D., ABPP-CN St. Jude Children's Research Hospital, Tennessee https://orcid.org0000-0003-0621-6438

Lumas, Allante Ph.D., LSSP Private Practice, Texas

Machado, Brandy B.A. Institute for Social and Applied Neuroscience (ISAN), OR

Mucci, Grace A. Ph.D., MS ABPdN ABPP The Chicago School Anaheim and UCLA Neuropsychological Services, California https://orcid.org0000–0002–9993–959x

Ndip, Nadine E. Ph.D., LP Life Stance Health, Texas

Nelson, Stephanie Ph.D., ABPP ABPdN Private Practice, Washington

Ng, Rowena Ph.D. Center for Neuropsychological and Psychological Assessment Kennedy Krieger Institute, and Johns Hopkins University School of Medicine, Maryland https://orcid.org0000-0001-7193-4300

Nguyen-Martinez, Ashley Psy.D. Children's Hospital Colorado University of Colorado School of Medicine, Colorado

Orantes, Destiny M.S. Doctoral Candidate, Clinical Psychology Syracuse University, New York

Pearce, Elizabeth B.A. University of California Los Angeles Neuropsychological Services, California

Roberts, Heather Ph.D., OTR Texas Woman's University, Texas

Shierk, Angela Ph.D., OTR Scottish Rite for Children, Texas

Schiros, Ashley, M.S. Syracuse University, New York

Schwartz, David D. Ph.D., ABPP Baylor College of Medicine-Houston, Texas

Skinner, Amy Ph.D., LSSP NCSP Harris County Juvenile Probation, Texas

Vargas, Gray Ph.D., ABPP-CN Center for Neuropsychological and Psychological Assessment, Kennedy Krieger Institute, Maryland

Webb, Nadia PsyD., MP FACPN ABPdN Institute for Social and Applied Neuroscience (ISAN) Portugal and USA

Wierzchowski, Andrea Ph.D., LP Private Practice; Scottish Rite for Children, Texas

Wilkinson-Smith, Alison Ph.D., ABPP Children's Medical Center Dallas and University of Texas Southwestern Medical School, Texas https://orcid.org0000-0001-8282-7586

Section I

Neurodevelopmental Disorders: An Introduction

1 Advancing Practice in Neurodevelopment

Denise E. Maricle, Christopher L. Bedford, Julie A. Gettman, Daniel C. Miller and Wendi L. Johnson

Introduction

When proposing a book to a potential publisher, authors are often asked, "why this book?" Our purpose in writing this book was to produce a comprehensive resource about neurodevelopmental disorders in children and adolescents for pediatric professionals. Such a text is essential for addressing the growing complexity and prevalence of these conditions in today's society. As our understanding of pediatric neurodevelopment and neurodevelopmental disorders evolves, there is an increased need for a resource that synthesizes the latest research, highlights assessment techniques, provides evidence-based interventions, and offers practical insights for parents, educators, and healthcare professionals. We hope our book can serve as a valuable guide, offering a nuanced exploration of various neurodevelopmental disorders. By providing a well-rounded perspective, the book empowers readers with the knowledge to recognize early signs, navigate the diagnostic process, and implement effective strategies to support children with neurodevelopmental challenges. Furthermore, fostering awareness and understanding through a dedicated resource can contribute to reducing stigma and promoting inclusivity, ultimately improving the overall well-being and quality of life for children and families facing these disorders.

Professionals such as school psychologists, clinical psychologists, pediatric neuropsychologists, nurses, pediatricians, neurologists, social workers, speech and language pathologists, occupational and physical therapists, and teachers need a solid understanding of neurodevelopmental disorders in children and adolescents due to the pivotal role they play in assessing, diagnosing, and supporting the well-being of young people. Comprehensive knowledge of these disorders allows those working with children to recognize early signs and symptoms, enabling timely intervention and support. Moreover, understanding the neurobiological underpinnings of conditions is crucial for tailoring effective therapeutic approaches. Additionally, professionals working with children and adolescents in hospitals, clinics, or rehabilitation and treatment center settings can enhance a child's progress when there is a deeper understanding of the services and

DOI: 10.4324/9781032703923-2

treatment options available in educational settings. By integrating neurodevelopmental perspectives into practice, pediatric professionals can develop more targeted and evidence-based interventions, fostering optimal cognitive, emotional, and social development in children. This knowledge is essential for all who work with children and adolescents regardless of setting, as it enables them to collaborate more effectively with parents and other professionals to create supportive home and school environments for youth with neurodevelopmental challenges. Well-rounded knowledge and understanding of neurodevelopmental disorders equips pediatric professionals with the tools necessary to make informed assessments, deliver precise interventions, and contribute significantly to the overall well-being of the children under their care.

Tremendous advances in our knowledge of how the brain works have made neuroscience a dominant influence within many fields, including psychology. The neurosciences are intersecting with medicine, psychology, education, economics, social and political policy, law, and gender and diversity. Most of what we know about brain functioning has been learned during the last 10–20 years due to improved technology to study the brain, but the vast majority of this knowledge and research has been acquired by studying adults. Pediatric neuroscience, including pediatric neuropsychology or school neuropsychology, is still an emerging field of interest, knowledge, and research (Miller et al., 2022). For brain science to be translated more quickly into practice there needs to be more information, expanded research, and additional training opportunities for practitioners and practitioners-in-training. The American Psychological Association (APA) has long recognized the relevance of the neurosciences to the various specialty areas within psychology, requiring that accredited programs incorporate the biological and neurological sciences into their programs and training. Additionally, APA has emphasized "Health Psychology" as the primary focus of practitioner training in the field of psychology, and the *Standards of Accreditation for Health Service Psychology and Accreditation Operating Procedures* (SoA-AOP, APA, 2019) require standard training opportunities for all psychologists in foundational areas of psychology, including the biological bases of behavior. A broad knowledge and understanding of common and low incidence disorders, as well as their neurological correlates is important for all psychologists, but more specifically for those practicing with pediatric populations.

Neurodevelopment is a term that denotes development of neurological pathways in the brain that influence performance or functioning. It is often used to refer to conditions (e.g., neurodevelopmental disorders) where the integrity and function of the nervous system is damaged during critical periods of brain development. The development of the human central nervous system is stringently regulated and timed. Any significant deviation from the typical developmental trajectory early in life can result in missing or aberrant neuronal architecture or connectivity. Neurodevelopment is influenced by both genetics and environment.

Neurodevelopmental disorders are a heterogeneous group of multifaceted conditions characterized by impairments in cognition, communication, motor skills, or behavior resulting from disrupted brain development. There are numerous neurodevelopmental disorders that impact individuals, families, and society, many of which will be discussed in the following chapters. Neurodevelopmental disorders are usually characterized by the developmental deficits or delays demonstrated, which usually show up early in the child's development and can persist throughout their lifetime. Children and adolescents with neurodevelopmental disorders may exhibit a wide range of symptoms, such as reduced emotional regulation, motor control issues, problems with social integration, reduced learning ability, or difficulties with attention. Neurodevelopmental disorders are commonly classified along a spectrum of severity, ranging from mild to severe.

There is a plethora of resources available for the common neurodevelopmental disorders, such as autism spectrum disorder (ASD), attention deficit hyperactivity disorder (ADHD), specific learning disabilities (SLD) and even traumatic brain injury (TBI). Yet there is limited information on less common neurodevelopmental disorders or disorders not typically encountered by the average psychologist or pediatric professional. However, these less common disorders are now being seen at higher rates than previously, and practitioners need to increase their knowledge and expertise, so they are prepared when they encounter them in practice. Additionally, it can be challenging to find information on a specific disorder in one place, and the practitioner is often forced to collate and create a repository of numerous resources to gain knowledge about one specific disorder.

The National Organization for Rare Disorders (NORD) indicates that over 6800 rare disorders have now been identified, with 72% of them being genetic disorders and over 70% of them showing initial symptoms beginning during childhood. The editors of this text faced the challenge of selecting a limited number of neurodevelopmental disorders to feature, recognizing that it is impossible to cover all disorders comprehensively in one volume. The selected disorders were chosen to be representative of specific categories or to reflect disorders being seen more frequently than during previous years. Due to page limitations, disorders seen less often could not be discussed. However, as editors and practitioners understanding the difficulty researching less encountered disorders, we have included resources assisting practitioners seeking more information at the end of this chapter and others in this book.

The book is divided into sections, with disorders selected to best exemplify each section. The three chapters in Section I introduce the text, focus on general information needed in practice with neurodevelopmental disorders (Chapter 2), and review issues related to prematurity and problematic birth (Chapter 3).

Section II, encompassing chapters four through twelve, focuses on metabolic, toxic, and inflammatory disorders commonly affecting children and adolescents. These conditions can profoundly affect a child's cognitive, emotional, and behavioral development. Metabolic and toxic disorders, such as those involving metabolic imbalances or exposure to harmful substances, can lead to significant neurodevelopmental issues, while inflammatory disorders often permanently impact brain function and behavior. Understanding these conditions provides pediatric professionals with comprehensive knowledge for accurate diagnosis, targeted intervention, and effective treatment planning, ultimately enhancing outcomes for children facing these complex challenges.

In **Chapter 4**: *Inflammation of the Brain: Pediatric Encephalitis and Meningitis*, the chapter authors draw on their work as pediatric neuropsychologists practicing in a large children's hospital to provide a thorough grounding in two common conditions considered to be global public health threats. Two case studies (autoimmune encephalitis; viral meningitis) are provided to exemplify the real world neurodevelopmental and neuropsychological implications of these disorders.

Chapter 5: *Neonatal Abstinence Syndrome (NAS)* and **Chapter 6**: *Fetal Alcohol Spectrum Disorders (FASD)* address the impact of prenatal ingestion of drugs and alcohol on the developing brain and child. Prenatal exposure to drugs and alcohol is associated with physical, cognitive, neuropsychological, and behavioral problems across the exposed child's life span. Our understanding of prenatal substance exposure is evolving quickly as research advances and new data emerges. For example, Fetal Fentanyl Syndrome (FFS) has recently (2023) entered the professional lexicon as a syndrome separate from NAS and FASD. FFS is associated with specific birth defects (cleft palate, microcephaly, drooping eyelids, webbed toes, and underdeveloped joints), and found to resemble a condition known as Smith-Lemli-Opitz (SLO). SLO is a genetic condition affecting how fetuses make cholesterol, which is critical to early brain development. Fentanyl has been found to interfere with cholesterol metabolism and its use is a significant risk factor for preterm or still birth. Chapters 5 and 6 are complemented by **Chapter 7**: *Neurotoxins and Pediatric Poisoning*, which covers the impact of common toxins and poisons on the developing child's brain, neuropsychological functioning, and everyday behavior.

Chapter 8: *Viral Infections* and **Chapter 9**: *COVID-19 and Long COVID in Children* were inspired by the recent pandemic and the rise of infectious diseases such as Lyme Disease or Zika in children and adolescents. Viral infections have been associated with neurological disorders for years, but the recent SARS-CoV-2 pandemic has brought greater awareness to their impact. Estimates suggest that approximately 1.6 million viruses are circulating world-wide with about half capable of infecting humans. Some of the most common neuro-related diseases caused by viral infections include measles, mumps, meningitis, post-infectious encephalomyelitis, subacute sclerosing panencephalitis, chickenpox, and polio. Chapter 8 addresses the epidemiology, clinical presentation, diagnosis, treatment, and intervention for some common viral infections in pediatric populations, while Chapter 9 focuses solely on COVID-19 and Long COVID.

The final three chapters in this section, **Chapter 10**: *Autoimmune Disorders: Pediatric Myalgic Encephalomyelitis/Chronic Fatigue (ME/CFS), Pediatric Gillian Barré Syndrome (GBS), and Juvenile Primary Fibromyalgia Syndrome (JPFS)*; **Chapter 11**: *Juvenile Arthritis*; and **Chapter 12**: *Postural Orthostatic Tachycardia Syndrome (POTS) and Ehlers Danlos Syndrome (EDS) in Pediatric Patients* share commonalities in that they are all chronic conditions that significantly impact daily functioning and quality of life. These disorders involve complex, multi-system symptoms that lead to overlapping issues such as widespread pain, fatigue, and autonomic dysfunction. Additionally, they frequently present with symptoms that can be challenging to diagnose and manage, and they may affect multiple body systems, making a comprehensive, multidisciplinary approach essential for treatment and care.

Chronic health conditions (e.g., Diabetes, Asthma, Obesity, Colitis, Irritable Bowel Syndrome, etc.) have been increasing steadily over the past 50 years in children and adolescents worldwide. Although scant, epidemiological studies suggest that 1 in 4 children have a chronic disease. Prevalence estimates typically range from 10% to 30% depending on the criteria used (Cortes et al., 2020). In the United States, estimates vary significantly with some sources suggesting 40% of school-aged children and adolescents have at least one chronic health condition. The CDC proposes that about 27% of children in the United States have a chronic condition, and 1 in 15 have multiple chronic conditions (MCCs). Three common medically complex neurodevelopmental disorders impacting children and adolescents are featured in Section III: **Chapter 13**: *Epilepsy and Seizures in Children and Adolescents*, **Chapter 14**: *Evaluation and Management of Neurocognitive Dysfunction in Children and Adolescents with Type 1 Diabetes*, and **Chapter 15**: *Pediatric Stroke and Cerebral Vascular Accident (CVA)*.

The World Health Organization (WHO) reports that genetic disorders and congenital abnormalities occur in about 2% to 5% of all live births and account for up to 30% of pediatric hospital admissions and about 50% of childhood deaths in industrialized countries. Innovative technologies, such as genome sequencing, microarrays, and gene panels, have helped to increase the identification of genetic disorders, improved the diagnosis of rare diseases, and allowed for the identification of the molecular cause of many previously undiagnosed diseases. Section IV features genetic and chromosomal disorders frequently encountered by pediatric specialists. **Chapter 18**: *Genetic Disorders Impacting Cognition* and **Chapter 19**: *Deletion Disorders* review several genetic and chromosomal disorders impacting neurocognitive functioning. **Chapter 16**: *Sickle Cell Disease (SCD)*, **Chapter 17**: *Cystic Fibrosis*, and **Chapter 20**: *Neurofibromatosis Type 1 and Type 2-Related Schwannomatosis* address specific disorders encompassing disorders of the blood, respiratory system, or peripheral nervous system (PNS).

Congenital malformations are estimated to occur in approximately 2% of human births. Generally, CNS anomalies are grouped into several types including neural tube defects and associated spinal cord malformations (myelomeningocele, meningocele, encephalocele), disorders of structural specifications, disorders of posterior fossa, brain stem, and cerebellum, disorders of brain growth and size, and disorders of skull growth and shape. Information on disorders that might be classified as congenital malformations of the CNS, brain and spine, or muscular-skeletal systems is provided in Section V. **Chapter 21**: *Spina Bifida* and **Chapter 23**: *Cerebral Palsy* elucidate two common spinal and muscular-skeletal disorders. **Chapter 22**: *Chiari Malformation* discusses brain and spinal cord malformations common to children and adolescents, and **Chapter 24**: *Demyelinating Disorders* provides information on demyelinating disorders seen in pediatric populations.

The editors' aim was to highlight disorders that are increasingly prevalent and frequently encountered in pediatric practice. Our goal was to offer pertinent, practical, and useful information for a diverse range of pediatric professionals. We recognize the frustration of researching conditions only to encounter overly technical or complex medical information. We hope that the content in this book is more accessible, allowing practitioners to effectively support their clinical work without the need for an advanced medical degree. We are grateful to our chapter authors for their willingness to share their vast expertise and variety of practice experiences. Chapter authors include practitioners encountering children and adolescents in a variety of environments, including hospitals, medical centers, private practice, and educational settings, as well as those serving in academia providing training to the practitioners of the future and conducting research to better inform practice.

In summation, while a child's neurodevelopmental disorder, medical condition, or diagnosis does not define them, it does influence their success at home, school, and in their community. Pediatric professionals need to familiarize themselves with the variety of disorders that may be encountered when working with children or adolescents in various pediatric settings to ensure effective and appropriate assessment, diagnosis, or intervention and accommodation so that they can maximize their potential.

Resources

National Organization for Rare Disease (NORD): rarediseases.org

Has a database on rare diseases with information sources and resources.

National Institute of Health: rarediseases.info.nih.gov

Rare Share: rareshare.org

A global platform for connecting rare disease patients

Rare Genomics: raregenomics.org

Provides a rare diseases list, with information and links to other relevant websites that offer addition information or support

Journal of Neurodevelopment Disorders: https://jneurodevdisorders.biomedcentral.com

Orphanet Journal of Rare Diseases: https://ojrd.biomedcentral.com

World Health Organization (WHO) and United Nations Children's Fund (UNICEF). 2023. Global report on children with developmental disabilities: From the margins to the mainstream. Available at https://www.unicef.org/media/145016/file/Global-report-on-children-with-developmental-disabilities-2023.pdf

References

Cortes, J. B., Fernández, C. S., Bandeira de Oliveira, M. B., Lagos C. M., Martínez, M. T. B., Hernández, C. L., & del Cura González, I. (2020). Chronic diseases in the paediatric population: Comorbidities and use of primary care services. *Anales de Pediatría* (English Edition), *93*(3), 183–193. https://doi.org/10.1016/j.anpede.2019.12.006.

Miller, D. C., Maricle, D. E., Bedford, C. L., & Gettman, J. A. (2022). *Best practices in school neuropsychology: Guidelines for effective practice, assessment, and evidence-based intervention*. Wiley.

2 School Integration for Children with Medical/Physical Disorders and Complex Medical Needs

Julie A. Gettman, Denise E. Maricle, Wendi L. Johnson, Daniel C. Miller and Christopher L. Bedford

Introduction

Children and adolescents spend a significant proportion of their youth in educational settings. Conservatively in the USA, children spend approximately 6–6 ½ hours a day for an average of 180 days per year for 13 years (National Center for Education Statistics [NCES], 2020). The Organization for Economic Cooperation and Development (OECD, 2021) estimated that 8,903 hours were spent in school during the first nine years of education (K-8th). When considering the total years spent in school during childhood (K through 12th grade) and including structured prekindergarten for some students, it translates into a significant percentage of a child's life. Time spent in educational settings places heavy demands on a child's cognitive and emotional resources, and even more so when the child or adolescent has an acute or chronic health condition. Studies show that for some children, chronic health conditions are associated with lower academic achievement and school functioning (Center for Disease Control and Prevention [CDC], 2017). Furthermore, many of these children and their families rely on professionals within the educational setting to help them manage these conditions, increasing the need to thoughtfully develop services and interventions for children with complex medical conditions.

Students who face complications from chronic health conditions may need supportive considerations to optimize their functioning in the school setting. However, research indicates that there is a lack of direct collaboration between outside medical, psychological, and treatment professionals with school districts regarding special education referrals (Norman, 2023). This limited interaction impedes effective coordination and support for students with special needs. Families are often used as intermediaries between community professionals and schools, but they may struggle to accurately convey school concerns to their outside specialists, thus interfering with obtaining appropriate referrals to community professionals. Conversely, schools may not receive complete or accurate information from families who act as intermediaries, resulting in

DOI: 10.4324/9781032703923-3

incomplete care plans in school settings. When schools do not have complete data, they may deny evaluations, causing frustration for families who are struggling to find appropriate services and assistance for their child in school. Effective and accurate communication among all stakeholders is essential to ensure that everyone is informed and aligned in their efforts, so the student is supported.

To facilitate effective coordination with families and schools, professionals outside school settings need a basic understanding of the fundamental legal structure surrounding special education and the management of school records. This includes knowing the legal processes that enable children to access educational services, as well as understanding what health services and accommodations are applicable in school settings (Pierson et al., 2018). It is equally important for school personnel to understand how to support students with chronic medical conditions and know their legal and ethical obligations. This includes understanding the healthcare requirements of these students, how medical information is shared within the boundary of privacy laws, as well as the importance of working together with healthcare providers to ensure that students receive both the necessary medical care and appropriate educational accommodations. This dual understanding fosters a collaborative approach, ensuring that students receive comprehensive support that addresses both their educational and health-related needs.

Individuals with Disabilities Education Act

Child Find

For many children with complex medical needs, support services begin before school entry through birth-to-age-3 programs. These services are often initiated by a pediatrician, child development specialist, or social worker. These programs are part of the Child Find requirements under Part C of the Individuals with Disabilities Education Act (IDEA) and the latest set of amendments titled the Individuals with Disabilities Education Improvement Act (IDEIA, 2004) which mandates the identification and evaluation of children with disabilities, including those with medical conditions, to determine eligibility for special education services. Eligible infants and toddlers receive an Individualized Family Support Plan (IFSP) developed in collaboration with the local education agency and the child's parent or guardian.

Part C of IDEA, specifically under 34 CFR § 303.1 (IDEIA, 2004), focuses on the Early Intervention Program for Infants and Toddlers with Disabilities. This program plays a crucial role in supporting families whose children have complex medical needs by ensuring early identification and intervention services that are tailored to address both medical conditions and developmental delays, thus providing a comprehensive approach to the child's care. Family involvement is emphasized, with resources and guidance provided to help families as they navigate the medical and educational systems. A service coordinator is appointed to assist in accessing and coordinating services and linking families to necessary medical, educational, and community resources. These services are designed to help children meet developmental milestones, which are especially important for those with complex medical needs.

Child Find for school-age students (ages 3 to 21) is covered in Part B of IDEA, which focuses on identifying students who may need special education services once they enter school, whether at the preschool, elementary, or secondary level. For school-age students, including students already in school as well as those who are not yet enrolled, Child Find requires schools to actively seek out and evaluate children who may have disabilities, including those with complex medical needs. By ensuring that children with complex medical conditions are evaluated for potential eligibility for special education services and related supports, Child Find helps prevent educational neglect. This is crucial for children who may otherwise fall behind due to their medical needs and for families who might struggle to secure appropriate educational services on their own. Child Find helps bridge gaps between educational and medical support, ensuring that children with complex medical needs receive the comprehensive services they need to succeed in school.

Eligibility and Classification

Children that are found eligible for special education services in accordance with Child Find are provided with access to specialized educational services and accommodations. This includes tailored Individualized Education Programs (IEPs) that address both their medical and educational needs, which can significantly improve their academic and social outcomes. As a special education law, IDEA provides funding designed to support implementation of the IEP, including necessary specialized instruction and related services designed to provide the student with access to a free and appropriate education (FAPE) (IDEIA, 2004; Pierson et al., 2018). To qualify for an IEP, students must meet criteria for one of 13 distinct eligibility categories under IDEA classification.

Students with chronic health conditions and complex medical needs are most often evaluated for possible eligibility under the special education category of other health impairment (OHI), which is designed for students who have a chronic or acute health condition that adversely affects their educational performance. This category encompasses a wide range of medical conditions that may limit a child's strength, energy, or alertness, including heightened or suppressed responses to environmental stimuli, which can impede their ability to participate fully in the classroom. The eligibility category of OHI includes a variety of chronic or acute medical conditions such as asthma, diabetes, epilepsy, attention deficit hyperactivity disorder (ADHD), heart conditions, hemophilia, leukemia, sickle cell anemia, and Tourette syndrome, among others. To qualify for special education services under OHI, not only must documentation of the health condition be provided to the school, but the condition must also significantly interfere with the child's ability to succeed in the educational environment. Common symptoms of complex medical conditions that can hinder academic progress and classroom participation include fatigue, difficulty concentrating and maintaining stamina throughout the school day, inconsistent energy levels, and side effects of medication.

Children with chronic illnesses often experience interruptions in their schooling due to frequent hospitalizations or medical treatments. This can lead to missing academic instruction necessary for adequate academic progress and fewer opportunities to interact with peers and adults throughout the school day, which can negatively impact social-emotional and behavioral learning. While medical advancements have enabled many of these students to return to school after extended absences, their academic and social progress may still be impacted by the time away from the classroom. By classifying these students under OHI, schools can provide tailored support to help manage the health-related challenges that may otherwise hinder the child's educational progress. This ensures that students with chronic medical conditions receive the necessary interventions to participate in and benefit from their education.

Children with chronic health conditions may also qualify under one of the other distinct eligibility categories under IDEA classification. For instance, a chromosomal disorder that presents with common autism spectrum disorder characteristics may qualify under the autism label, or a diagnosis of hypoxic ischemic encephalopathy that presents with an expressive language disorder may qualify under the classification of speech-language impairment. According to IDEA law, educational goals, services, and accommodations are designed to meet individual needs regardless of the eligibility category. It is important to understand that after a child is found eligible under IDEA for special education services as a child with a disability, and educational need is determined, then those supports and services must be designed to address their unique individual needs. These supports cannot be based solely on the special education classification, disability, or LRE (least restrictive environment) placement. For example, a child being deemed ineligible for specialized instruction in reading because their eligibility is Emotional Disturbance versus a Specific Learning Disability (SLD), or alternatively a child who needs a paraprofessional assistant but is refused the service as the district's policy is to only provide paraprofessional support in self-contained special education classrooms. Once qualified, the IEP and its supports and services should be based on what that child needs to access educational opportunities and make adequate progress in school.

The legal requirements for an Individualized Education Program (IEP) include several key components (Office of Special Education and Rehabilitative Services U.S. Department of Education, 2020). First, the IEP must detail the child's current performance levels, including how their disability impacts their ability to engage with and progress through the general curriculum. This information is derived from evaluations, classroom assessments, and observations by various stakeholders. Next, the IEP must set measurable annual goals that the child should achieve within a year, with these goals addressing academic, social, behavioral, physical, or other educational needs and broken down into short-term objectives. The plan must also specify the special education and related services to be provided, including any supplementary aids, accommodations, modifications to the program, and supports for school staff. Additionally, the IEP must describe the extent to which the child will participate with nondisabled peers in regular classes and school activities. It must outline the accommodations or modifications both in the classroom as well as what is needed for state and district-wide tests or provide reasons why certain tests are not appropriate along with alternative assessment methods. Finally, the IEP must detail how the child's progress will be measured and how parents will be kept informed about this progress.

Public school officials are required to schedule and conduct IEP meetings regularly (at least once every 12 months) to review each child's IEP. These meetings are essential to assess whether the child is meeting the annual goals and to make any necessary revisions to the IEP. While the school is responsible for setting the timing of these meetings, parents of a child with a disability have the right to request an IEP meeting at any time. For instance, if parents believe that their child is not making adequate progress or if they have concerns about the current IEP, they can request a meeting to address these issues (deBettencourt, 2002). Children and adolescents with chronic or complex medical conditions, and those experiencing an acute medical condition or crisis, may need frequent reviews and short-term IEPs.

Section 504 of the Rehabilitation Act of 1973

A student with a chronic medical condition may qualify for accommodations under Section 504 of the Rehabilitation Act of 1973 rather than an Individualized Education Program (IEP) under IDEA when their condition does not require specialized instruction but still significantly impacts one or more major life activities, including learning. A Section 504 plan is generally considered appropriate when the child's chronic medical condition has a lesser impact on their academic performance, but symptoms require accommodations to participate in the regular education environment.

The Rehabilitation Act was originally signed into law in 1973 and was designed as anti-discrimination legislation to protect individuals with disabilities (Pierson et al., 2018). Given that it is a civil rights statute rather than a federal education statute, the federal government does not provide additional funding for students with Section 504 plans in the same way that it does for students with IEPs (National Association of School Psychologists, 2023). To determine eligibility for services under Section 504, school teams must first confirm that a student has a disability as defined by the law. This includes physical or mental impairments that limit major life activities such as walking, seeing, or learning, which encompasses thinking, concentrating, and/or reading (National Association of School Psychologists). A diagnosis alone does not guarantee eligibility, and the impairment must substantially restrict the student's ability to perform these activities. Guidance from the Office of Civil Rights (OCR) suggests that "substantially limits" be broadly construed, in other words there does not need to be a significant restriction of a major life activity, only a substantial impact. This substantial impact does not need to be severe, long-term, or permanent, and the mediating impact of treatment, medication, or other measures to lessen or compensate for symptoms does not need to be considered. Section 504 also covers students who have a history of, or are perceived to have, a disability, ensuring protection against discrimination. For a student to receive accommodations, the impairment must impact their access to school programs or activities, thereby requiring the school to provide necessary support to ensure equal participation and access.

Section 504 plans focus on the accommodations the student needs to have equitable access to public education, rather than providing specialized instruction and measurable goals included in IEPs. Accommodations may include specific strategies and tools that help the student access the general education curriculum (e.g., extended time on tests, preferential seating, modified assignments, or the use of assistive technology); environmental accommodations that include adjustments to the classroom or school environment (e.g., reducing distractions, modifying physical spaces, or providing special equipment); and/or health-related accommodations that include provisions for managing the student's medical needs (e.g., allowing frequent breaks, access to medication, permission to visit the nurse as needed, or implementing an emergency action plan).

Compared to special education services under IDEA, Section 504 is broader and less regulated. Section 504 has fewer specific procedural requirements for school personnel, which may result in less support and monitoring due to the lack of detailed regulations (deBettencourt, 2002). In contrast, IDEA provides specific criteria for eligibility and imposes stricter regulations regarding timelines, parental involvement, and documentation (deBettencourt). While IDEA focuses on special education for students with disabilities, Section 504 ensures protections across a wider range of areas such as access to activities in community settings.

Related Services

An IEP or 504 Accommodation Plan (AP) not only outlines accommodations and modifications for children with complex medical needs but also includes related services essential for the child to access and benefit from their education. IDEA 34 CFR § 300.34 (IDEIA, 2004) defines related services as developmental, corrective, and supportive services necessary for a child with a disability to benefit from special education. These services cover a broad range, including speech-language therapy, audiology, interpretative services, therapeutic recreation, orientation and mobility services, psychological services, physical and occupational therapy, counseling, and transportation (deBettencourt, 2002). Additional services such as school health, social work, parent counseling, and training ensure the child's educational needs are fully met. The law excludes services related to surgically implanted devices or medical device optimization, maintenance, or replacement. These services can also be part of a 504 plan (U.S. Department of Education, n.d.b.).

Individualized Health Care Plans

Understanding how students with complex medical needs are accommodated and supported through IEPs and 504 plans is crucial, but equally important is how their ongoing health and educational requirements are managed on a day-to-day basis. School nurses play a critical role in managing the health needs of students with chronic conditions. Their responsibilities extend beyond basic first aid; they are central to the care coordination process, ensuring that students receive the necessary medical attention and that their health status is consistently monitored throughout the school day.

An Individualized Health Plan (IHP), Education Health Care Plan (EHCP) or Emergency Procedures Plan (EPP) is a critical tool used in schools to manage the healthcare needs of students with chronic or acute health conditions that may impact their attendance or academic performance (National Association of School Nurses, 2020). Usually created and maintained by the school nurse, the IHP outlines the care required for each student, ensuring consistent and effective health management. The IHP details the relevant knowledge and actions needed by school personnel to support the student's access to a free and appropriate education. By integrating health needs into students' educational plans, the plan ensures that all staff members are informed about how to accommodate and support students' health requirements within the academic setting. Additionally, the IHP provides a systematic and organized approach to addressing specific health needs and facilitating effective coordination of care among the school's multidisciplinary team. It includes guidance on how to respond to medical emergencies, support the health components of the student's educational plan, and maintain a focus on the student's overall success. Overall, the IHP serves as a comprehensive guide for managing student-specific healthcare needs, supporting their academic and personal development, and ensuring continuity of care throughout their school experience. There are numerous templates available online, but three possible sources include the National Institutes of Health (NIH; www.nih.gov), the Exceptional Children's Assistance Center (www.ecac-parentcenter.org), and Families Together, Inc (www.familiestogether.org>forms). Templates are also often provided by various state education agencies or may be available from school nursing forums as well.

Family Educational Rights and Privacy Act (FERPA)

Once a student's eligibility for special education services or accommodations is determined, it is crucial to understand how their educational and medical information is managed. This is where privacy regulations come into play, ensuring that student records are handled appropriately and confidentially. Medical professionals must comply with the Health Insurance Portability and Accountability Act (HIPAA), which regulates the privacy and security of protected health information (PHI). However, schools are governed by the Family Educational Rights and Privacy Act (FERPA), which oversees the privacy of student education records. FERPA applies to educational institutions receiving federal funding, including public and private schools, colleges, and universities (HealthPRO Heritage, 2024; U.S. Department of Education, n.d.a.). Under FERPA, protected information includes educational records such as grades, transcripts, class lists, student schedules, and disciplinary records. Parents and eligible students (those over 18 years old) have the right to access, review, and request amendments to their education records. FERPA regulates the disclosure of these records and requires written consent before they can be shared. If medical professionals or other outside practitioners want access to school records, including special education records, a release of information must be signed by the parent and provided to the school, or the parent must request the records themselves and then provide them to the outside agency. If the parent of a child with complex medical needs does not consent to the sharing of records, FERPA does permit schools to disclose records without consent to appropriate officials in the event of a health or safety emergency (U.S. Department of Education).

Collaboration and Coordination with School Nurses, Medical Personnel, and Other Providers

Effective interdisciplinary collaboration is crucial for addressing the needs of students with chronic health conditions. Educating these students involves more than just academic instruction; it requires a team approach that integrates the expertise of school personnel, medical professionals, and families. Strong partnerships between educators and medical professionals can lead to better health outcomes, higher rates of school attendance, and improved academic achievement (Centers for Disease Control and Prevention, 2017). Healthcare professionals often concentrate on the medical needs of children with chronic illnesses and may be unfamiliar with educational policies and laws, while educators may feel unprepared to provide adequate academic support due to limited experience with chronic illness in the school population (Moore et al., 2009; Thompson et al., 2015; Wikel & Markelz, 2023). Additionally, the traditional medical model, which focuses on symptom management and diagnosis, can sometimes conflict with the educational model that addresses academic and social functioning (HealthPRO Heritage, 2024). However, integrating these models can create a more supportive environment for students. By bridging the gap between medical and educational approaches, schools can offer a more inclusive and effective learning environment, promoting the overall health and academic success of students with complex needs. Educators and support staff, empowered with knowledge and tools from both perspectives become more effective advocates and collaborators, actively participating in the care and education of students with complex needs.

To achieve this integration, schools must establish coordinated systems that ensure comprehensive care for students with complex health conditions. The Centers for Disease Control and Prevention (2017) recommends strategies for schools to address the needs of students with chronic health conditions, such as developing interdisciplinary teams, providing school-based health services and care coordination, offering specific education to improve self-management, delivering professional development for staff, providing counseling and psychological services, and ensuring a safe physical environment. Appointing a district and school leader to coordinate a student's care is paramount. Clear and consistent communication among educators, medical personnel, families, and students themselves is essential for ensuring that everyone is on the same page and that students' needs are met holistically. However, research indicates that communication and coordination of care between healthcare providers and school personnel are often insufficient (Schwartz, 2024). To address this gap, schools should implement structured communication protocols and multidisciplinary teams that include both healthcare and educational professionals, ensuring that care plans are effectively integrated and tailored to each student's unique needs. Regular training and collaboration opportunities can further enhance these efforts, leading to more seamless coordination and better outcomes for students with complex health conditions. In addition, students with chronic health conditions often face increased risks for mental health issues such as depression and suicidal ideation (Canavera & Johnson, 2020; Greydanus et al., 2010). Subsequently, integrating mental health services into their care plans is crucial. Given that access to these services is often limited, especially for children with medically complex conditions, schools must work to bridge this gap, providing or referring students to appropriate mental health resources.

Reintegrating students with chronic health conditions back into the school environment after a period of illness or hospitalization poses another challenge. School re-entry programs are essential in easing this transition, providing support not only for students but also for teachers and classmates. Studies have demonstrated that when coordinated school re-entry plans are developed collaboratively with families, school staff, and medical professionals, students with chronic illnesses experience more positive outcomes, including decreased absenteeism and stronger social connections with classmates (Wikel & Markelz, 2023). These programs also facilitate a more supportive and informed school environment through increasing illness-specific knowledge among both educators and peers as well as decreasing anxiety, worry, and other negative emotions, ultimately facilitating smoother transitions and better outcomes for the returning student (Canter & Roberts, 2012).

School re-entry programs are designed to support students with chronic illnesses through three main approaches: peer education, school personnel workshops, and comprehensive student programs (Prevatt et al., 2000; Wikel & Markelz, 2023). Peer education programs involve educational sessions for classmates of students with chronic illnesses. Their goal is to enhance peer understanding and acceptance of these students. School personnel workshops educate school staff about chronic illnesses and their impact on students. The aim is to improve educators' knowledge regarding the specific academic and social needs of these students. Comprehensive student programs offer individualized support to students with chronic illnesses, including tailored academic and social services. All three types of school re-entry programs have demonstrated success in achieving targeted outcomes, such as enhanced participant knowledge about chronic illnesses and improvements in addressing the academic and social needs of students with chronic conditions (Wikel & Markelz).

Deconstructing Medical Charts and Understanding Medical Jargon

In today's educational landscape, schools are increasingly serving students with diverse and complex needs, many of whom have medical diagnoses that significantly impact their learning and development. Conditions such as metabolic, toxic, and inflammatory disorders, medically complex disorders, and genetic and chromosomal disorders present unique challenges that require a nuanced understanding of both medical and educational perspectives. For these students, it is critical that school personnel navigate medical charts and interpret medical jargon in order to provide effective and personalized support.

However, most educational professionals, including classroom teachers, special education teachers, school psychologists, guidance counselors, and school and district administrators, often lack the background knowledge necessary to fully understand and apply medical information in an educational context. Additionally, while related service providers such as speech-language pathologists, occupational therapists, and physical therapists may have knowledge of medically related terminology unique to their fields, their broader medical knowledge, especially regarding rare diseases or disorders, may be limited. As a result, much of the specialized language used in medical records may be entirely unfamiliar to those working in schools.

Moreover, the medical landscape is continually evolving, making it impossible for any single resource to be updated frequently enough to cover all the necessary medical terminology needed for educators to interpret the complex and often rare diagnoses found in student medical records. As a result, educators often need to seek out and integrate multiple sources to understand medical jargon and apply that knowledge effectively in the school setting. Educators can enlist the assistance of the school nurse or utilize reputable online resources (see University of Arkansas, Fort Smith (n.d.) Medical Terminology: Web Resources available from https://library.uafs.edu/c.php?g=1000576&p=7246083) that help support their understanding of medical terminology. Forming collaborative teams with medical professions that can provide meaningful explanations of conditions and including their input will streamline the process and promote meeting the individual needs of the student.

Assessment Recommendations

Completing assessments with children and adolescents with chronic or complex medical conditions often looks different than typical psychoeducational or psychological assessments. They usually require more detailed or different types of assessments, and assessments may be lengthier and more elaborate. Extremely detailed developmental histories and clinical interviews are often a critical component of these types of evaluations. Additionally, it may be beneficial to the assessment process to collect progress monitoring data in short intervals following a child's return to school after an acute medical incident or a diagnosis of a chronic medical condition. For instance, a child who enters school following a left hemisphere stroke that affected language and reading skills may benefit from short, frequent, curriculum-based reading assessment so recovery rate can be closely tracked, and instructional level can be more closely matched to recovery rate.

Evaluation of neuropsychological functions may require the use of specialized assessment instruments outside the main repertoire of the school or clinical psychologist, and if specialized assessment professionals are not available in the school setting, a referral to an external neuropsychologist or clinician may be necessary. Assessment of children with complex medical needs requires collaboration and consultation with various professionals from other disciplines (e.g., speech-language, occupational and physical therapy, medical professionals, rehabilitation specialists) or outside entities.

Assessment professionals should be familiar with methods to modify presentation of assessment materials to accommodate symptomology (e.g., enlarging images, altering how directions are provided, etc.) to allow for access to the assessment materials and accommodate needs. The assessment professional also needs an in-depth understanding of how interpretation is impacted when standardized administration is altered. This section could be an entire book in and of itself. Thankfully, some excellent resources exist for practitioners to reference and use. A classic, but still relevant guide to interviewing is Sattler's (1998) *Clinical and Forensic Interviewing of Children and Families: Guidelines for Mental Health, Education, Pediatric and Child Maltreatment Fields.* Resources for pediatric and school neuropsychological assessment include Miller and Maricle (2019) *Essentials of School Neuropsychological Assessment*, 3rd Edition and Miller, Maricle, Bedford, and Gettman (2022) *Best Practices in School Neuropsychology: Guidelines for Effective Practice, Assessment and Evidenced Based Intervention*, 2nd Edition. Another excellent resource is Baron's (2018) *Neuropsychological Evaluation of the Child: Domains, Methods, & Case Studies*, 2nd Edition.

Conclusion

Improvements in modern medicine have enhanced the survival rates of children who experience complex medical needs, although they may continue to deal with long-term effects from their health conditions. Research indicates that chronic health conditions can be linked to lower academic performance in some students, although the impact can differ depending on the specific condition and other influencing factors (Centers for Disease Control and Prevention, 2017). Schools are vital in managing these conditions, as they often provide essential clinical services and supports for students with chronic health conditions. Similarly, medical professionals play a crucial role by offering specialized care and guidance that can help manage these conditions effectively outside the school setting. Therefore, it is essential for educators and medical professionals to collaborate effectively and understand needs in settings outside their own. By focusing on communication and alignment, they can integrate students with complex medical needs into classrooms and school communities more effectively, ensuring that strategies and tools are consistent with legal requirements and tailored to students' unique needs to support their academic progress.

References

Canavera, K. & Johnson, L. M. (2020). Integrating mental health care for medically complex children. *Pediatrics*, 146(2). e20190898. https://doi.org/10.1542/peds.2019-0898 https://publications.aap.org/pediatrics/article/146/2/e20190898/36864/Integrating-Mental-Health-Care-for-Medically?autologincheck=redirected.

Canter, K. S. & Roberts, M. C. (2012). A systematic and quantitative review of interventions to facilitate school reentry for children with chronic health conditions. *Journal of Pediatric Psychology*, 37(10), 1065–1075. https://doi.org/10.1093/jpepsy/jss071.

Centers for Disease Control and Prevention (CDC, 2017). *Research brief addressing the needs of students with chronic health conditions: Strategies for schools.* Available from: https://www.cdc.gov/healthyschools/chronic_conditions/pdfs/2017_02_15-how-schools-can-students-with-chc_final_508.pdf.

deBettencourt, L. U. (2002). Understanding the differences between IDEA and Section 504. *Teaching Exceptional Children, 34*(3), 16–23. https://doi.org/10.1177/004005990203400302.

Family Educational Rights and Privacy Act (FERPA). 20 U.S.C. § 1232g.

Greydanus, D., Patel, D., & Pratt, H. (2010). Suicide risk in adolescents with chronic illness: Implications for primary care and specialty pediatric practice: A review. *Developmental Medicine and Child Neurology*, 52(12), 1083–1087. https://doi.org/10.1111/j.1469-8749.2010.03771.x.

HealthPRO Heritage (2024). Educational model vs. medical model: What's the difference?HealthPRO Heritage. https://www.healthpro-heritage.com/blog/educational-model-vs-medical-model.

Individuals with Disabilities Education Improvement Act of 2004 (IDEIA). Pub. L. No. 108–446, 118, Stat. 2647.

Moore, J. B., Kaffenberger, C., Goldberg, P., Oh, K. M., & Hudspeth, R. (2009). School reentry for children with cancer: Perceptions of nurses, school personnel, and parents. *Journal of Pediatric Oncology Nursing*, 26(2), 86–99. https://doi.org/10.1177%2F1043454208328765.

National Association of School Nurses (2020). *Use of individualized healthcare plans to support school health services* (Position Statement). Silver Spring, MD: Author. ED605759.pdf

National Association of School Psychologists (2023). *Section 504: A guide for parents and educators* [handout].

National Center for Education Statistics (NCES, 2020). *Schools and Staffing Survey (SASS)*. Available from: https://nces.ed.gov/surveys/sass/tables/sass0708_035_s1s.asp.

Norman, C. L. (2023). *Child find: Improving the referral process between physicians and the local education agency.* (Doctoral dissertation, University of Dayton).

Organization for Economic Cooperation and Development (OCED, 2021). *Education at a glance 2021*. Available from: https://www.oecd.org/en/publications/education-at-a-glance-2021_b35a14e5-en.html.

Office of Special Education and Rehabilitative Services U.S. Department of Education (2000). *A guide to the Individualized Education Program.* iepguide.pdf (ed.gov)

Pierson, E. E., Callan, G. L., & Pierson, S. K. (2018). An overview of special education law, 504, FERPA, and issues relevant for pediatric neuropsychologists. *Journal of Pediatric Neuropsychology*, 4, 27–36. doi:10.1007/s40817-017-0039-y.

Prevatt, R. F., Heffer, R. W., & Lowe, P. A. (2000). A review of school reintegration programs for children with cancer. *Journal of School Psychology*, 38(5), 447–467 https://doi.org/10.1016/S0022-4405(00)46–47.

Schwartz, K. (2024). *Medically complex child: Best practice toolkit for improving coordination of care between parents, providers, and support systems.* [Doctoral project, University of St Augustine, or Health Sciences]. SOAR @ USA: Student Scholarly Projects Collection. https://doi.org/10.46409/sr.XSFK8878.

Thompson, A. L., Christiansen, H. L., Elam, M., Hoag, J., Irwin, M. K., Pao, M., Voll, M., Noll, R.B., & Kelly, K. P. (2015). Academic continuity and school reentry support as a standard of care in pediatric oncology. *Journal of Pediatric Blood and Cancer*, 62, 805–817. https://doi.org/10.1002/pbc.25760.

University of Arkansas, Fort Smith (n.d.). *Medical terminology: Web resources* https://library.uafs.edu/c.php?g=1000576&p=7246083.

U.S. Department of Education (n.d.a.). *Family educational rights and privacy act.* https://www2.ed.gov/policy/gen/guid/fpco/ferpa/index.html.

U.S. Department of Education (n.d.b.). *Protecting students with disabilities: Frequently asked questions about Section 504 and the education of children with disabilities.* https://www2.ed.gov/about/offices/list/ocr/504faq.html.

Wikel, K. & Markelz, A. M. (2023). School reentry plans for students with chronic illness: A literature review. *Research, Advocacy, and Practice for Complex and Chronic Conditions*, 41(1), 22–44. doi:10.14434/rapcc.v41i1.31767 https://scholarworks.iu.edu/journals/index.php/pders/article/view/31767/38895.

3 Prematurity and Related Complications

Wendi L. Johnson, Denise E. Maricle and Hazel Q. Goh

Introduction

Premature birth is a significant international public health concern (Walani, 2020). Globally, every year nearly 15 million infants experience premature birth. The incidence rate of premature birth continues to show an upward trend as a result of substantially enhanced survival rates in Western nations, which is primarily due to advancements in medical care (World Health Organization, 2023). A considerable portion of prematurely born infants necessitate specialized care in neonatal intensive care units (NICUs). Despite notable improvements in NICU treatments, leading to a reduction in preterm neonatal mortality, the incidence of neurodevelopmental morbidities remains substantial. New research shows that for infants born even a few weeks early the risk of learning and behavioral challenges increases in later childhood and adolescence (World Health Organization). Consequently, prematurity stands as a prominent contributor to neurodevelopmental disability worldwide.

Definition of Prematurity

Prematurity or preterm birth are terms for a broad category of infants born at less than a gestational age of 37 weeks. An average-term pregnancy is approximately 40 weeks. Subdivisions of prematurity by gestational age are moderate to late preterm (32 to <37 weeks), very preterm (28 to <32 weeks), and extremely preterm (<28 weeks) (Quinn et al., 2016). Earliest viability is considered 24 weeks, which is when infants have at least a 50% chance of survival. In developed countries with adequate maternal care, at less than 22 weeks survivability is 0%; at 22 weeks it is 10%; at 24 weeks it is 55% to 60%; and at 31 weeks it is about 95%. Of children born prior to 31 weeks, 46% have moderate to severe disabilities, 34% have mild disabilities, and about 20% evidence no disability. Prematurity is also defined by birth weight, with low birth weight (LBW) considered to be <2500 grams (5.8 lbs.), very low birth weight (VLB) <1500 grams (3.3 lbs.) and extremely low birth weight (ELBW) <1000 grams (2.2 lbs.). Using birthweight, one in 10 births is

DOI: 10.4324/9781032703923-4

classified as premature (Walani, 2020). Prior to the advent of the NICU and sophisticated medical techniques, the survival of premature infants weighing less than 1500 grams was an exception. Today, the majority of babies weighing less than 750 grams (1.6 lbs.) or with gestational ages >24 weeks are surviving. Survivability depends on where in the world a child is born, and that survival may come with significant costs (World Health Organization, 2023). Most suffer severe cognitive, neurological, or physical deficits, and the price of treatment and care is often in the millions of dollars.

Prenatal Development

The past 20 years have seen extraordinary progress in understanding how the brain develops and functions. Human brain development has a lengthy trajectory, beginning a few days after conception and continuing through young adulthood. Prematurity means that the infant brain develops outside the protective uterine environment, at a time when the brain is growing more rapidly than at any other time in life (National Research Council, 2000). Neonates born extremely preterm (i.e., <28 weeks) in the second trimester have brains that are not completely developed structurally or functionally as the second trimester is when the human cortex is forming. At around 24 weeks of gestation, the brain is just beginning to exhibit coordinated brain activity necessary for consciousness. At 28 weeks of gestation (beginning of the 3rd trimester) the brain and its nervous system is considered fully formed and functioning; in that fetal brainwave activity can be measured. During the last 3 months of gestation, the human brain is undergoing rapid maturational changes for neuronal processing and connectivity as this time period is characterized by increasing neuronal differentiation, cellular metabolism, and cortical folding. Studies of brain growth in the 3rd trimester show a fourfold increase in gray matter at 29 to 42 weeks and a fivefold increase in white matter between 35 and 41 weeks of gestation (De Asis-Cruz et al., 2022; Lanphear, 2015).

Etiology of Prematurity

The causes of preterm birth are varied and complex with a significant number of unknown factors. Maternal, fetal, and predisposing factors have been acknowledged including antepartum hemorrhage, uterine overdistension, cervical incompetence, hormonal changes, and bacterial infection or inflammation (Quinn et al., 2016). Other risk factors include previous preterm delivery, fertility treatments, multiple births, placental and uterine abnormalities, pre-eclampsia, maternal diabetes, poor nutrition, low socioeconomic status (SES), and use of toxic substances (nicotine, alcohol, legal and illicit drugs). Maternal factors such as over- or underweight, short stature, or maternal age of less than 17 or more than 35 years have also been identified through epidemiological studies.

Potential Implications of Prematurity

Prematurity and LBW are best conceptualized as an index of biological risk as this is a heterogeneous population with variable developmental outcomes. Prematurity is a risk factor for short-term complications occurring in the first days of life such as neonatal respiratory conditions, necrotizing enterocolitis, sepsis, and neurological conditions such as periventricular leukomalacia, intraventricular hemorrhage, hypoxic-ischemic encephalopathy, cerebral palsy, seizures, feeding difficulties, and visual or hearing problems. Premature birth is also related to altered neurodevelopmental outcomes with some developing significant and long-lasting neurological sequelae. Additionally, the NICU environment, which is very different from the intrauterine one, enhances risks for long-term cognitive and behavioral effects. Research on early environments and long-term outcomes of preterm infants show that stimuli such as noise and pain, as well as environmental variables such as nutrition and bonding or attachment delays, impact neurodevelopmental outcomes in some children (Cheong et al., 2020). Despite concerted endeavors to positively enhance the neurological well-being and developmental outcomes of prematurely born children, there exists significant variability in functional disabilities among infants born at the same gestational age. Overall, preterm infants are more likely to develop physical disabilities, require more sophisticated medical care and present a higher risk of behavioral, social–emotional, and learning difficulties in childhood compared to full-term newborns.

Neurological Implications of Prematurity

Because neurodevelopmental outcomes after preterm birth are complex, understanding the neurobiological mechanisms that support brain development is crucial. Studies have shown that preterm children have decreased cerebral volumes at 7–15 years of age, and that cortical gray matter, cortical white matter, the basal ganglia, and the cerebellum have smaller volumes in preterm children (Ment & Vohr, 2008; Thompson et al., 2020). Furthermore, there is evidence to suggest that neurological impact differs between male and female preterm children. Frontotemporal and hippocampal regions seem to be most vulnerable to volumetric changes, the left hemisphere is more often affected than the right, and premature males are more likely to experience white matter abnormalities than females (Vasileiadis et al., 2009). In general, more males are born premature than females.

Functional consequences of perinatal injury to the developing brain potentially impact several domains including motor, cognition, language, behavior, and vision or hearing. For example, severe white matter injury (WMI), such as cystic periventricular leukomalacia (PVL), usually results in spastic diplegic cerebral palsy (CP) and visual dysfunction, often with deficits in cognition and learning. Cognitive deficits can occur in the absence of significant motor impairments. For example, in preterm children with measured cognition in the average range, processing deficits include problems in attention and executive functions (i.e., cognitive flexibility, inhibitory control, and working memory), visually based information processing, and language. Importantly, cognitive and behavior problems are likely to persist through young adulthood. These prevalent neurocognitive impairments point to widely distributed brain abnormalities or problems with brain connectivity related to premature birth.

Specific Medical Sequelae Associated with Prematurity

Prematurity should be acknowledged as a risk factor for both immediate and prolonged complications. While some preterm infants typically exhibit favorable neuropsychological development, many experience significant and enduring neurological sequelae. Premature birth is almost always associated with altered neurodevelopmental outcomes. The following section will highlight the most common potential complications associated with prematurity.

Neonatal Respiratory Challenges – RDS/HMD and BPD

The National Heart, Lung and Blood Institute (2018) lists post prematurity respiratory disease (PRD) as a major complication of preterm birth. PRD includes respiratory distress syndrome (RDS)/hyaline membrane disease (HMD) and bronchopulmonary dysplasia (BPD), but also encompasses prolonged symptoms such as intermittent or chronic wheezing, cough without cold, apnea, cyanosis, and chronic lower respiratory tract infection.

Respiratory Distress Syndrome (RDS)/Hyaline Membrane Disease (HMD)

A diagnosis of RDS/HMD results from immature lung development and is caused by a surfactant deficiency (surfactant is the foamy substance coating the alveoli of the lungs that keeps them fully expanded so newborns can breathe). The lungs of a fetus start making surfactant during the third trimester, so babies born prior to 26 weeks are likely to develop RDS/HMD. Management involves respiratory support such as nasal continuous positive airway pressure (nCPAP) or noninvasive positive pressure ventilation (NIPPV), surfactant replacement therapy, and mechanical ventilation. Babies who require surfactant replacement therapy and ventilation are likely to also develop BPD.

Infants who develop RDS/HMD exhibit a high prevalence of cognitive impairment with concomitant impaired functional status and quality of life. It is important to note that mechanical ventilation is independently associated with persistent cognitive deficits; with visuo-constructive, visual memory, psychomotor speed, and verbal fluency most impacted (Sasannejad et al., 2019). Thus, it is difficult to determine if the cognitive impacts are the result of the disease process or the treatment.

Bronchopulmonary Dysplasia (BPD)

This chronic respiratory disease is typically seen in babies born <28 weeks. BPD is one of the most common serious complications in premature infants (Islam et al., 2015) and is related to RDS, especially when associated with mechanical ventilation and oxygenation. The risk of developing BPD is directly related to the infant's gestational age and birth weight, the severity of the initial lung disease, and the duration of mechanical ventilation (Davidson & Berkelhamer, 2017). BPD can cause swelling and scarring in the lungs predisposing the individual to chronic respiratory diseases such as pneumonia, asthma, or chronic obstructive pulmonary disease (COPD) with long-term effects (Manti et al., 2021).

These types of prematurity respiratory diseases (PRD, i.e., RDS/HMD and BPD) often result in long-term complications for children and adolescents, including asthma-like symptoms, exercise intolerance, abnormal ventilatory responses, pulmonary hypertension, and increased risk of severe respiratory infection (Davidson & Berkelhamer, 2017). The cognitive deficits associated with PRD appear to be linked to poor oxygenation of the brain. Inadequate oxygenation compromises neural activity leading to impairments in memory, attention, and overall cognitive performance.

Gastrointestinal Challenges – Sepsis and NEC

The gastrointestinal (GI) tract is fully formed at 20 weeks' gestation (i.e., the stomach, small and large intestines, colon), but does not become fully functional until about the 29th week. The more premature, the greater the likelihood of gastrointestinal challenges such as sepsis or necrotizing enterocolitis (NEC).

Sepsis

Neonatal sepsis results from an infection in the bloodstream or cerebrospinal fluid typically caused by bacteria such as E coli, listeria, or streptococcus. It is divided into early-onset sepsis (EOS) or late-onset sepsis (LOS), based on the age of presentation (e.g., within 72 hours of birth or 7 days after birth). EOS is generally caused by the transmission of pathogens from the female genitourinary system to the fetus and LOS results from the transmission of pathogens from the environment after delivery (i.e., contact from healthcare workers or caregivers). The immature immune system of the premature infant is the major contributing factor for susceptibility to sepsis (Sewell et al., 2021). Neonatal sepsis has a high mortality rate (up to 54%) despite modern treatment strategies. Adverse outcomes have been reported among survivors of EOS with about 6.3% having long-term hearing loss or seizures. LOS is associated with systemic infections, hemodynamic instability, adverse inflammatory responses, and generalized neuropsychological difficulties (Sewell et al.).

Necrotizing Enterocolitis (NEC)

This disorder of the intestines and digestive system typically develops two to six weeks after birth. Inflammation of the intestine leads to bacterial infection which causes cellular damage to the gastrointestinal organs and results in necrosis of the colon and intestines. This is associated with severe sepsis, intestinal perforation, and significant morbidity and mortality (as high as 50%). Several risk factors have been identified, but prematurity and low birth weight have been identified as primary risks. Genetic factors may also play a role. Worldwide incidence varies between 0.3 to 2.4 infants per 1000 live births and almost 70% of these cases occur in premature infants born before 36 weeks (Gregory et al., 2011). Overall, mortality ranges from 10% to 50%, but in the most severe cases involving perforation, peritonitis, and sepsis, mortality approaches 100%. The prognosis for NEC depends on the severity of the condition when it is recognized, and treatment begins.

Symptoms of NEC are non-specific and include poor feeding, vomiting, lethargy, and abdominal tenderness. In some babies, NEC is mild whereas others may experience severe or life-threatening symptoms. NEC poses both short- and long-term GI issues (Canvasser et al., 2022). In mild cases of NEC, the symptoms resolve, but others may have ongoing intestinal problems including scarring or blockage of the intestine. For example, due to dysfunction or absence of the bowel after surgical removal of necrotic intestine, infants face clinical problems associated with short bowel syndrome including malabsorption and failure to thrive. Approximately 25% of patients with NEC experience some degree of short bowel syndrome resulting in difficulties absorbing nutrients from food and ongoing challenges with elimination (Gregory et al., 2011). Neurodevelopmental and growth delays in children with NEC have been well documented. A clear association exists between NEC and neurodevelopmental impairment including cerebral palsy or other psychomotor impairments, visual or hearing deficiencies, and cognitive impairments (Gregory et al.).

Neurological Challenges in Prematurity-HIE, PVL, and NBH

Neurological disorders involve abnormalities in the structure or function of the brain, spinal cord, and nervous system. Neurological disorders can manifest in different ways affecting movement, sensation, cognition, or behavior. While a full review of neurological disorders associated with prematurity is outside the scope of this text, the chapter will highlight the most common including hypoxic-ischemic encephalopathy (HIE), periventricular leukomalacia (PVL), and neonatal brain hemorrhage (NBH).

Hypoxic-ischemic Encephalopathy (HIE)

This type of brain damage is caused by lack of oxygen to the brain prior to or shortly after birth. Most pathologic events associated with HIE are the result of impaired blood flow and oxygen delivery in the brain. This occurs globally in 1 to 6 out of 1000 live births (Ristovska et al., 2022). The exact cause of HIE is unknown, as many factors can contribute to its development. However, the most common causes are uterine rupture, placental abruption, prolapse of umbilical cord, a cardiovascular compromise with the mother, or fetal-placental hemorrhage. Symptoms of HIE range from mild to severe. Of affected infants, 15% to 20% die in the neonatal period, and up to 60% die prior to age 2. For those that survive, 25% to 30% have severe neurological impairment including CP, epilepsy, visual and hearing impairment, cognitive impairment, and social-behavioral disorders (Ristovska et al.) The pattern of brain injury in HIE depends on the severity and duration of the hypoxia and the degree of brain maturation.

The primary treatment for HIE is therapeutic hypothermia. Lowering the child's body temperature reduces the risk of neurological problems. Children who have experienced HIE are often diagnosed with learning and behavior problems, but complications vary between children depending on the severity of HIE. The most commonly seen problems include difficulties with learning and retention, attentional difficulties and hyperactive behaviors, seizures, and CP.

Periventricular Leukomalacia (PVL)

The human brain consists of both white matter and grey matter. White matter is where communication happens in the brain (e.g., it is responsible for transmitting information and impulses between the body and the brain). Grey matter is where the brain processes that information and where muscle control and sensory perceptions are located. PVL occurs when a lack of oxygen or blood flow to the brain softens the brain tissue and kills the brain's white matter. As a result, empty spaces in the brain develop in place of white matter and fill with fluid, causing motor spasticity and intellectual impediments. When the periventricular area (i.e., the space around the fluid-filled ventricles) is impacted, it affects the nerve fibers responsible for carrying information from the brain to the muscles to regulate movement. While PVL can impact any newborn, premature babies are at greatest risk. Periventricular white matter in the preterm infant is extremely sensitive to perfusion-related injury because the neurovascular structure of white matter in neonates is immature which results in poor ability to regulate blood flow (Huang et al., 2017). PVL is the most common form of white matter injury in preterm infants, and the most common cause of cerebral palsy (i.e., 60% to 100% of PVL survivors develop some form of CP).

Diagnosis is difficult as babies with PVL may have no visible signs of the disorder, but they are at risk for delays in cognitive development, motor movement disorders, difficulties with coordination, and/or vision and hearing impairments. Often there are no signs of PVL until at least eight weeks after birth (Huang et al., 2017). As time progresses, children may manifest a spectrum of symptoms including temporary pauses in breathing known as apnea, delayed motor development, issues with vision, low heart rates, seizures, and weakness or altered muscle tone primarily observed in the lower extremities. While a diagnosis of PVL is beneficial for the family and to guide intervention, there is not a specific treatment protocol. Long-term outcomes for individuals with PVL depend upon the severity of the brain damage as some may be mildly impacted while others may have greater physical or cognitive impairments.

Neonatal Brain Hemorrhage (NBH; AKA Intracranial or Intraventricular Hemorrhage [IVH])

NBH refers to any bleeding within the brain and surrounding meningeal spaces. NBH occurs approximately 3.5 times per 1000 live births and is the most common neurological disorder of newborns (Lekic et al., 2015). Risk factors for NBH include gestational age, vaginal delivery, low Apgar scores, seizure, RDS/HMD, hypoxia, infection, as well as issues with blood flow and clotting.

There are several types of NBH including epidural hemorrhage, subdural hemorrhage, subarachnoid hemorrhage, and intraparenchymal hemorrhage (Tenny & Thorell, 2023). Outcomes are rated and quantified into Grades I (least severe) to IV (most severe). Approximately 20% of infants born at 28 to 34 weeks experience an intraventricular hemorrhage, with the vast majority (> 60 percent) rated as Grade I or II. Whereas 60% of infants born between 24 to 28 weeks will have an intraventricular hemorrhage rated as Grade III or IV. The extent of bleeding is the factor that is ultimately most associated with increased morbidity and mortality. Grade I–II hemorrhage has been related to developmental disabilities; while grade III–IV hemorrhages are associated with increased risk of hydrocephalus, as well as long-term sequelae like intellectual deficits and CP. Post-hemorrhagic hydrocephalus often develops because of NBH with potential long-term neurological deficits as a result of expansion of the cerebroventricular system and compression of the brain tissues. Additionally, NBH results in observable white matter injury (damage to axons and reduced myelination) which contributes to long-term neuropsychological sequelae such as neuropsychiatric difficulties (e.g., increased rates of anxiety and depression) and behavioral struggles (e.g., poor social skill and attention deficit hyperactivity issues; Cheng & Ballabh, 2022). Ultimately, up to 85% of survivors of NBH will exhibit major cognitive dysfunction; the majority of which eventually require special educational intervention (Lekic et al., 2015; Tenny & Thorell).

Seizures are another significant neurological complication of preterm birth (see Chapter 13 discussing epilepsy). Additionally, preterm birth is often correlated to psychomotor impairments such as cerebral palsy (see Chapter 23).

Vision Impairments – Retinopathy of Prematurity (ROP)

Retinopathy of prematurity is an eye disease commonly seen in babies weighing less than 3 pounds at birth. ROP occurs when abnormal blood vessels grow in the retina (the light- sensitive tissue in the back of the eye). When diagnosing ROP, five stages are utilized based on level of impairment (Dammann et al., 2023; National Eye Institute, 2023). Stages 1 and 2 are considered mild, infants and children usually only require monitoring to ensure the ROP does not worsen. These children typically respond well to treatment, and many develop with healthy vision. Children with Stage 3 ROP usually need treatment to stop the abnormal blood vessels from damaging the retina and causing retinal detachment. In Stage 4 the retina is partially detached and in Stage 5 it is completely detached. Stage 4 and 5 are very serious, may result in vision loss or blindness, and need aggressive treatment. Babies with ROP often display shaking or wandering eye movements, lack of tracking with the eyes, white pupils, and difficulty recognizing faces. As the baby grows there may be long term impacts such as retinal detachment, nearsightedness, amblyopia (lazy eye), or crossed eyes. Children with severe ROP may evidence difficulty with visual-motor integration, visual attention, and motor coordination (Dammann et al.). Social communication impacts or challenges with writing and math skill development are often exhibited. Interventions utilizing visual supports, occupational therapy (OT), and physical therapy (PT) services, and learning skill interventions (e.g., alternative writing aids) may be needed (Msall, 2023).

Overview of Assessment and Interventions for Prematurity Associated Complications

Although prematurity is causative of several disorders diagnosed in childhood, it may be difficult to directly link prematurity to later neurodevelopmental difficulties. But it is important to consider preterm birth as a risk factor within the individual's developmental history to understand current challenges.

A primary principle for assessing the effect of prematurity on neurological outcome is to understand that the child's general developmental status and cognitive scores will tend to decrease with reductions in gestational age. An infant born at 24 weeks is at greater risk than an infant born at 26 or 28 weeks as brain development is less complete. This leads to a higher likelihood of adverse events (intracranial hemorrhage, mechanical ventilation) which in turn adversely impacts brain development. However, once a child moves out of the high-risk groups, the outcomes become more highly variable and difficult to connect. Assessment of developmental history becomes one of the most important tools for the clinician.

Assessment of cognitive status and learning will depend on what issues are being observed and the sequelae associated with the child's preterm presentation. Assessments are likely to involve multiple professionals and evaluations. For example, OT, PT, and adaptive physical education (APE) professionals evaluate motor challenges and issues related to exercise intolerance. The educational team should ask parents about prematurity and review any medical records provided. The team may need to consider a health support plan to assess issues involving exercise intolerance, asthma or breathing-related issues, or other medical problems which may require modifications to PE, recess, attendance, and absence policies. A school-based neuropsychological evaluation may be needed for children that have experienced complications such as NBH or PVL, or when their cognitive difficulties are more severe, diffuse, or vague. Special education classification and recommended interventions should focus on the unique presentation of symptoms. If educational need is present, the child may qualify under the eligibility of Other Health Impairment (OHI) dependent on the presentation of symptoms (i.e., ADHD, learning challenges, etc.). Given the variability of prematurity's impact, individualized assessment and treatment planning needs to be in place.

Conclusion

The overall survival rate of prematurely born infants has seen improvement in recent years, thanks to medical advancements. Research on long-term neurodevelopmental outcomes associated with prematurity is still emerging. Often, clinicians may not associate a middle school student's challenge in math reasoning or social communication with a potential long-term effect stemming from an early neurological insult due to prematurity. It is crucial for clinicians and families to comprehend the potential long-term effects of prematurity and offer necessary support, encompassing both physical and academic aspects.

Resources, Organizations, and Websites

Prematurity General Resources

- Birth Injury Center: https://birthinjurycenter.org/
- National Organization of Rare Diseases: https://rarediseases.org/
- March of Dimes: https://www.marchofdimes.org/

Complications Associated with Prematurity

- **Retinopathy of prematurity**

  a American Society of Retina Specialists: https://www.asrs.org/patients/retinal-diseases/17/retinopathy-of-prematurity

  b National Eye Institute: https://www.nei.nih.gov/

Bronchopulmonary dysplasia (BPD)

a BPD collaborative:

https://thebpdcollaborative.org/

b National Heart, Lung and Blood Institute:

https://www.nhlbi.nih.gov/

Necrotizing enterocolitis (NEC)

a NEC Society: https://necsociety.org/

Respiratory Distress Syndrome (RDS)/Hyaline Membrane Disease (HMD)

a The ARDS Center: https://ards.org/

Hypoxic ischemic-encephalopathy

a HIE Help Center: https://hiehelpcenter.org/
b Hope for HIE: https://www.hopeforhie.org/

- **Periventricular leukomalacia**

  a Child Neurology Foundation: https://www.childneurologyfoundation.org/disorder/periventricular-leukomalacia/

References

Canvasser, J., Patel, R. M., Pryor, E., Green, L., Hintz, S. R., Fagan, M., & Harrison, J. D. (2022). Long-term outcomes and life-impacts of necrotizing enterocolitis: A survey of survivors and parents. *Seminars in Perinatology*, 47(1), 151696. doi:10.1016/j.semperi. 2022.151696.

Cheng, B. & Ballabh, P. (2022). Recovery of the brain after intraventricular hemorrhage. *Seminars in Fetal and Neonatal Medicine*, 27(1), 101224. doi:10.1016/j.siny.2021.101224.

Cheong, J. L. Y., Burnett, A. C., Treyvaud, K., & Spittle, A. J. (2020). Early environments and long-term outcomes in preterm infants. *Journal of Neural Transmission*, 127(1), 1–8. DOI: https://doi.org/10.1007/s00702-019-02121-w.

Dammann, O., Hartnett, M. E., & Stahl, A. (2023). Retinopathy of prematurity. *Developmental Medicine & Child Neurology*, 65(5), 625–631. https://doi.org/10. 1111/dmcn.15468.

Davidson, L. M. & Berkelhamer, S. K. (2017). Bronchopulmonary Dysplasia: Chronic lung disease of infancy and long-term pulmonary outcomes. *Journal of Clinical Medicine*, 6(1), 4. doi:10.3390/jcm6010004.

De Asis-Cruz, J., Andescavage, N., & Limperopoulos, C. (2022). Adverse prenatal exposures and fetal brain development: Insights from advanced fetal MRI. *Biological Psychiatry: Cognitive Neuroscience and Neuroimaging*, 7(5), 480–490. https://doi.org/10.1016/j.bpsc.2021.11.009.

Gregory, K. E., DeForge, C. E., Natale, K. M., Phillips, M., & Van Marter, L. (2011). Necrotizing enterocolitis in the premature infant: Neonatal nursing assessment, disease pathogenesis, and clinical presentation. *Advanced Neonatal Care*, 11(3), 155–164. doi:10.1097/ANC.0b013e31821baaf4.

Huang, J., Zhang, L., Kang, B., Zhu, T., Li, Z., Zhao, F., Qu, Y., & Mu, D. (2017). Association between perinatal hypoxic-ischemia and periventricular leukomalacia in preterm infants: A system review and meta-analysis. *Plos one*, 12(9), e0184993. doi:10.1371/journal.pone.0184993.

Islam, J. Y., Keller, R. L., Aschner, J. L., Hartert, T. V., & Moore, P. E. (2015). Understanding the short- and long-term respiratory outcomes of prematurity and bronchopulmonary dysplasia. *American Journal of Respiratory and Critical Care Medicine*, 192(2), 134–156. https://doi.org/10.1164/rccm.201412-2142PP.

Lekic, T., Klebe, D., Poblete, R., Krafft, P. R., Rolland, W. B., Tang, J., & Zhang, J. H. (2015). Neonatal brain hemorrhage (NBH) of prematurity: Translational mechanisms of the vascular-neural network. *Current Medical Chemistry*, 22(10), 1214–1238.

Lanphear, B. P. (2015). The impact of toxins on the developing brain. *Annual Review of Public Health*, 36, 211–230. https://doi.org/10.1146/annurev-publhealth-031912-114413.

Manti, S., Galdo, F., Parisi, G. F., Napolitano, M., Decimo, F., Leonardi, S., & Maraglia Del Giudice, M. (2021). Long-term effects of bronchopulmonary dysplasia on lung function: A pilot study in preschool children's cohort. *Journal of Asthma*, 58(9), 1186–1193. https://doi.org/10.1080/02770903.2020.1779289.

Ment, L. R. & Vohr, B. R. (2008). Preterm birth and the developing brain. *Lancet Neurology*, 7(5), 378–379. doi:10.1016/S1474-4422(08)70073-5.

Msall, M. E. (2023). Improving neurodevelopmental trajectories after retinopathy of prematurity: challenges and opportunities. *Pediatric Research*, 94(5), 1598–1599.

National Eye Institute (2023). *Retinopathy of prematurity.* Retrieved January 14, 2024 from https://www.nei.nih.gov/learn-about-eye-health/eye-conditions-and-diseases/retinopathy-prematurity.

National Heart, Lung and Blood Institute (2018). *Prematurity and Respiratory Outcomes Program (PROP) Core Database Protocol.* National Heart, Lung, and Blood Institute. Retrieved January 14, 2024 from https://biolincc.nhlbi.nih.gov/studies/prop/.

National Research Council (2000). *From neurons to neighborhoods: The science of early childhood development.* National Academies Press. Retrieved January 15, 2024 from http://nap.nationalacademies.org/.

Quinn, J. A., Munoz, F. M., Gonik, B., Frau, L., Cutland, C., Mallett-Moore, T., Kissou A, Wittke, F., Das, M., Nunes, T., Pye, S., Watson, W., Ramos, A. A., Cordero, J. F., Huang, W-T., Kochhar, S., Buttery, J., & The Brighton Collaboration Preterm Birth Working Group (2016). Preterm birth: Case definition and guidelines for data collection, analysis, and presentation of immunization safety data. *Vaccine*, 34(49), 6047–6056. doi:10.1016/j.vaccine.2016.03.045.

Ristovska, S., Stomnaroska, O., & Danilovski, D. (2022). Hypoxic ischemic encephalopathy (HIE) in term and preterm infants. *Prilozi*, 43(1), 77–84.

Sasannejad, C., Ely, E. W., & Lahiri, S. (2019). Long-term cognitive impairment after acute respiratory distress syndrome: A review of clinical impact and pathophysiological mechanisms. *Critical Care*, 23(1), 352. doi:10.1186/s13054–13019–2626-z

Sewell, E., Roberts, J., & Mukhopadhyay, S. (2021). Association of infection in the neonate and long-term neurodevelopmental outcome. *Clinics in Perinatology*, 48(2), 251–261.

Tenny, S. & Thorell, W. (2023). *Intracranial Hemorrhage.* StatPearls. National Library of Medicine. National Center for Biotechnology Information. Retrieved January 4, 2024 from https://www.ncbi.nlm.nih.gov/books/NBK470242/.

Thompson, D. K., Matthews, L. G., Alexander, B., Lee, K. J., Kelly, C. E., Adamson, C. L., Hunt, R. W., Cheong, J. L. Y., Spencer-Smith, M., Neil, J. J., Seal, M. L., Inder, T. E., Doyle, L. W., & Anderson, P. J. (2020). Tracking regional brain growth up to age 13 in children born preterm and very preterm. *Nature Communications*, 11(1), 696. doi:10-10.38/s41467-020-14334-0-9.

Vasileiadis, G. T., Thompson, R. T., Han, V. K. M., & Gelman, N. (2009). Females follow a more “compact” early brain developmental model than males: A case-control study of preterm neonates. *Pediatric Research*, 66(5), 551–554. https://doi.org/10.1203/PDR.0b013e3181ba1ae7.

Walani, S. R. (2020). Global burden of preterm birth. *International Journal of Gynecology and Obstetrics, 150*, 31–33. doi:10.1002/ijgo:13195.

World Health Organization (2023). *Born too soon: Decade of action on preterm birth: A global report.* World Health Organization. Retrieved January 6, 2024 from http://who.int/publications/i/item/9789240073890.

Section II

Metabolic, Toxic, and Inflammatory Disorders

4 Inflammation of the Brain

Pediatric Encephalitis and Meningitis

Alison Wilkinson-Smith and Stephanie Nelson

Introduction

Encephalitis and meningitis are serious, potentially fatal inflammations of the central nervous system. Encephalitis is inflammation of the brain (Alam et al., 2023). Meningitis is inflammation of the meninges, the protective membranes that surround the brain and spinal cord (Al-Qahtani et al., 2022). While encephalitis and meningitis have both infectious or non-infectious triggers, both conditions are most often caused by infection (Alam et al; Al-Qahtani et al; Erickson et al., 2020). While our focus in this chapter is on children, encephalitis and meningitis may occur in people of all ages.

Understanding Encephalitis and Meningitis in Childhood

Young children are at greater risk of developing meningitis than older children or adults, and also at greater risk of dying from meningitis or viral encephalitis compared to individuals in other age groups (World Health Organization, 2021). Fortunately, young children represent our best opportunity to reduce encephalitis and meningitis, because childhood vaccines prevent some of the illnesses that can trigger these central nervous system inflammations. For example, reducing the number of children who contract measles through robust vaccination campaigns reduces the number of children who develop measles-related encephalitis (World Health Organization, 2023). Because children are uniquely vulnerable to encephalitis and meningitis, and because this age group presents a bright opportunity for mitigating future cases, the WHO has specifically targeted children in their strategic goals for addressing encephalitis (Why Encephalitis Matters virtual meeting; WHO, 2023) and meningitis (Defeating Meningitis by 2030: A Global Roadmap; WHO, 2021) worldwide.

Encephalitis and meningitis are serious conditions. Approximately 1 in 20 patients with encephalitis will die as a result of the disease (Britton et al., 2020). Worldwide, deaths from childhood meningitis have decreased in the past 30 years, but not as quickly as other vaccine-preventable causes of

DOI: 10.4324/9781032703923-6

death such as measles and tetanus (Wright et al., 2021). Pediatric viral meningitis is mostly benign and self-limiting, but it can be fatal. Mortality rates for children with bacterial meningitis are much higher and range from approximately 5% to 15% (Alamarat & Hasbun, 2020). Pediatric bacterial meningitis is nearly always fatal if not treated, and was always fatal prior to development of antibiotics (Castagno et al., 2023; Zainel et al., 2021). Accurately measuring the number of deaths from pediatric meningitis and encephalitis is challenging because of differences in quality of death registration data around the world, thus the mortality risk is likely underestimated (Wright et al.).

Most children with encephalitis or meningitis recover from the disease but often experience life-long complications. Children with histories of meningitis may have physical sequelae such as hearing loss and slower growth. These children are also at risk for neurocognitive problems including lower IQ and executive functioning impairment (Dezfouli & Khosravi, 2021). Outcomes of encephalitis in children are variable, but approximately 60% to 70% experience neurological or cognitive impairment (Brenner et al., 2024; Pöyhönen et al., 2021). Pediatric practitioners must be knowledgeable about the outcomes of these conditions so that we can guide families in understanding how encephalitis and meningitis affect children long term. This knowledge can also help advocate for these children's needs at home, at school, and in the community.

Note that patients may have inflammation of the brain and meninges concurrently. This condition is known as meningoencephalitis, and it combines features of both disorders. Meningoencephalitis can be difficult to distinguish from encephalitis based on clinical features, but having both tends to cause worse outcomes than meningitis alone. However, outcomes for these diseases vary depending on factors such as underlying cause, time to diagnosis and treatment, and demographic features of the patient (Ungureanu et al., 2021). Because of the overlap of symptoms and recovery of meningoencephalitis, meningitis, and encephalitis, we will not discuss meningoencephalitis as a separate condition.

Understanding Encephalitis

Definition and Causes

Encephalitis can be triggered by infectious or non-infectious factors. The most common cause of infectious encephalitis is a viral infection (Alam et al., 2023; Britton et al., 2020; Erickson et al., 2020), while the least common cause of infectious encephalitis is a bacterial infection. Non-infectious types of encephalitis include post-infectious paraneoplastic (cancer-related) and autoimmune encephalitis (Alam et al.). For both children and adults, infectious encephalitis is more common than non-infectious encephalitis. Viral encephalitis is relatively more common in younger children (infants and toddlers), while autoimmune encephalitis is more common in older children and adolescents (Britton et al.). See Table 4.1 for an overview of types of encephalitis and examples of each. Worldwide, the most common cause of pediatric viral encephalitis is West Nile virus, which is spread by mosquitos. Other viruses that can trigger viral encephalitis include those in the herpes simplex virus (HSV) family, Epstein-Barr, cytomegalovirus, and varicella zoster (the virus that causes chickenpox and shingles); enteroviruses; influenza; and other mosquito-borne viruses like Zika. While bacterial encephalitis is rare, the most common cause of pediatric bacterial encephalitis is *Bartonella henselae*, the bacterium that causes cat scratch disease (Erickson et al.).

Table 4.1 Causes of Encephalitis and Common Examples

Infectious	Viral	Insect-born: • West Nile • Zika Other viral: • HSV • Varicella Zoster
	Bacterial: • Bartonella henselae Other infections: • Fungal • Parasitic	
Non-infectious	Autoimmune	Post-infectious: • Streptococcus • COVID-19 Paraneoplastic: • ANMDARE associated with ovarian teratoma Other autoimmune: • Rasmussen • Hashimoto • Seronegative
	Other non-infectious: • Drug-induced • Unidentified	

The most common cause of non-infectious encephalitis in children and adults is autoimmune encephalitis. The most common type of autoimmune encephalitis is Anti-N-methyl-D-aspartate receptor encephalitis (ANMDARE), a condition that causes the body's immune system to attack the brain's NMDA receptors (Alam et al., 2023; De Bruijn et al., 2020). ANMDARE can occur without an identifiable trigger, but it can also develop following HSV encephalitis or as a paraneoplastic response to an ovarian teratoma (De Bruijn et al.). For one in five children with autoimmune encephalitis, a specific antibody trigger is never identified (Britton et al., 2020; De Bruijn et al.). Indeed, across all patients who develop encephalitis, even after extensive medical work-up, the exact cause of the encephalitis remains unknown in 30% to 40% of cases (Johns Hopkins Medicine, n.d.; Autoimmune Encephalitis Alliance Clinicians Network [AEACN], 2021).

Epidemiology in Children

Rates of encephalitis worldwide are difficult to determine precisely and likely underestimated (World Health Organization, 2023). Viral encephalitis incidence in children in the United States is seven per 100,000 per year, which translates to over 5000 children per year using 2024 population figures. Worldwide, the prevalence of viral encephalitis is estimated at 16 per 100,000 per year (Vova & Howarth, 2023). Autoimmune encephalitis in children worldwide is estimated between 1.16 and 1.54 per million children per year (Hardy, 2022; Vova & Howarth), which translates to about 3000 children per year using 2023 population estimates. Individuals assigned female at birth are at increased risk for autoimmune encephalitis, mostly because of the association between ovarian teratoma and ANMDARE (Hardy).

Clinical Presentation, Diagnosis, and Treatment

Pediatric encephalitis can be difficult to identify initially. Symptoms often appear rapidly, which can be frightening for children and families. The symptoms are often nonspecific at first, and may include headache, fever, nausea and vomiting, and loss of energy or appetite. Differential diagnosis, therefore, can be challenging. Infectious encephalitis often presents with fever, elevated C-reactive protein, and abnormal magnetic resonance imaging (MRI) of the brain (Pointon et al., 2022). Meanwhile, autoimmune encephalitis most commonly presents with seizures, psychiatric symptoms (changes in personality, behavior, or affect), sleep disturbance, and/or cognitive impairment (Adams et al., 2021; Cellucci et al., 2020; Pointon et al.).

Infectious encephalitis is typically diagnosed by testing cerebrospinal fluid (CSF) from lumbar puncture (LP). Autoimmune encephalitis can be diagnosed through analysis of blood or CSF if an antibody is detected. However, laboratory results can take days or weeks. Imaging (MRI) of the brain and spine are likely to be normal, which can help rule out other diagnostic considerations. However, a normal electroencephalogram (EEG) is unusual, especially a prolonged EEG. Multiple consensus criteria have been developed to identify autoimmune encephalitis early. Indeed, treatment may need to be started before a diagnosis is confirmed, due to the length of time needed to identify a specific antibody. Many patients will already be improving by the time diagnosis is confirmed (Hardy, 2022). Similarly, early detection in viral encephalitis is important because disease progression is rapid (Gundamraj & Hasbun, 2023).

In addition to anti-viral medications, viral encephalitis can be treated with corticosteroids and intravenous immunoglobulin (IVIG). Supportive care may be the only option for some viral etiologies. In some cases, supportive care is all that is needed as some patients will recover well from viral encephalitis on their own (Gundamraj & Hasbun). Children with autoimmune encephalitis are typically treated with immunotherapy, including corticosteroids, IVIG, and broad immunosuppressants like rituximab and cyclophosphamide (Hardy, 2022). For children with any etiology of encephalitis, symptom-specific interventions, such as inpatient rehabilitation, outpatient rehabilitation, anti-seizure medications, and behavioral health interventions, are often part of the treatment plan (Vova & Howarth, 2023).

Outcomes and Neuropsychological Impact

Outcomes for encephalitis in children and adolescents are mixed. The long-term neuropsychological impact of encephalitis varies by factors including etiology, type of treatment, age of onset, and access to medical care. Looking broadly across pediatric and adult outcomes, approximately two-thirds of patients show problems on detailed cognitive assessments two years after diagnosis with any kind of encephalitis (Brenner et al., 2024). Adults demonstrate impairment in autobiographical memory and report cognitive problems, depression, and fatigue that persists more than one year after encephalitis diagnosis (Harris et al., 2020). A small study of pediatric encephalitis outcomes found 71% of patients had minor neurological dysfunction, with IQ scores lower in this group of children (Pöyhönen et al., 2021). A sample of children with encephalitis of mixed etiologies showed lower quality of life compared to age- and sex-matched controls (Ramanuj et al., 2014).

For pediatric viral encephalitis, age plays a significant role in prognosis. More severe long-term impairments are associated with onset in infancy (Vova & Howarth, 2023). After the vulnerable infancy period, older age of onset becomes a significant risk factor for children with viral encephalitis. For example, in a large population-based study in Japan that excluded patients with onset in infancy, adolescent onset (onset between 12 and 18 years of age) was a risk factor for unfavorable outcomes (Hatachi et al., 2021). Seizures, lethargy, or reduced consciousness are also predictors for poor outcomes. Perhaps unsurprisingly, children with premorbid conditions and those who experience a delay in accessing treatment also tend to do worse long-term (Hatachi et al.; Vova & Howarth).

There are very few studies on neuropsychological impairments in pediatric patients with autoimmune encephalitis, and the few that are available have small sample sizes. Most studies focus almost exclusively on ANMDARE (Galioto et al., 2024). The most common areas of neuropsychological impairment for children with any type of autoimmune encephalitis are memory and executive functioning (Galioto et al.; Vova & Howarth, 2023). In children with ANMDARE specifically, memory and executive functioning are highly likely to be affected, and a majority of children show some degree of overall impairment on neuropsychological testing (Wilkinson-Smith et al., 2022). Children with a history of ANMDARE have lower quality of life overall. A small, mixed antibody sample of pediatric autoimmune encephalitis found significant morbidity when measured an average of two years later. More than 20% had moderate disability, and more than half had refractory seizures. Further, more than half had memory impairment, and more than 40% had cognitive impairment aside from memory (Sabanathan et al., 2022).

In summary, children with a history of encephalitis frequently experience cognitive and adaptive challenges post-recovery, and these challenges affect long-term development. Neuropsychological assessment of these children should include assessment of cognitive skills, memory, and executive functioning. Assessment of skills such as academic achievement, and adaptive functioning may help guide placement and intervention. Although data on psychological well-being and quality of life outcomes for children is limited, the available outcome data suggest increased risk for fatigue and emotional distress. As such, neuropsychologists should devote particular care to assessing and making appropriate recommendations to support emotional functioning and overall well-being for these children.

Case Study: ANMDARE

Julian (de-identified), a Latino male, was healthy until two and a half years of age, when he developed seizures. He was diagnosed with epilepsy and treated with levetiracetam. His condition deteriorated. He lost the ability to walk, talk, and swallow. He began displaying agitation, abnormal movements, and altered consciousness. Julian was hospitalized and eventually diagnosed with ANMDARE. He was treated with steroids and plasmapheresis. His abnormal movements and seizures improved; however, he continued to show developmental impairment and received outpatient therapies. He also continued to demonstrate abnormal EEG activity a year later and was treated with rituximab. Unfortunately, EEG remained abnormal. He continued to be prescribed levetiracetam.

At age 8, Julian was referred for neuropsychological assessment because his mother was concerned about communication. Julian had mixed language exposure; his family spoke Spanish at home during his early years, while his schooling had been in English. However, Julian's mother reported he barely understood or spoke Spanish. She therefore tried to talk to him in English, even though she had limited proficiency. Even in English, Julian spoke only a few words at a time. Language dominance testing with a bilingual neuropsychologist showed that he was more proficient in English than Spanish.

At the initial evaluation, Julian's mother described him as functioning at the level of a younger child. She noted that he needed more help than most children his age to complete adaptive living tasks. Testing of Julian's intellectual development revealed that his cognitive abilities were well below the average range (Standard Score=47), in the range consistent with intellectual disability. He performed better on tasks that were visual or hands-on in nature. He struggled most with tasks that were verbal, and his functional communication skills were profoundly impaired. Recommendations included special education support, speech therapy, and adaptive skill-building.

Julian was seen for a follow-up evaluation at age 10. In the interim, he had received two more treatments with rituximab. An EEG at age 9 had revealed continued abnormalities, but he was not having seizures. Also at age 9, serum and CSF were both negative for NMDA antibodies. He continued on levetiracetam. He received ongoing speech therapy and special education support. Although follow-up testing revealed that Julian's functioning was stable, he continued to demonstrate intellectual disability with severe language impairments.

At age 17, Julian's test scores remained stable, continuing to show intellectual disability and severe language impairments. Discussion with the family focused on increasing Julian's adaptive skills to allow him to become as independent as possible. Looking ahead to adulthood, Julian will need lifelong support, especially for complicated daily living tasks like managing money. He will also need help with job training and placement. A pivotal component of the assessment process included linking his family with services to ensure access to these supports.

Understanding Meningitis

Definition and Causes

The meninges are the three layers of protective membranes around the brain and spinal cord. Meningitis is an inflammation in these layers. Meningitis can be caused by infectious agents, such as viruses, bacteria, or fungi. It can also be caused by non-infectious factors, including systemic disease, drugs, and neoplasm. As with encephalitis, viruses are the most common cause of meningitis. Enteroviruses, especially coxsackieviruses, are the most common cause of viral meningitis (Faraj et al., 2021). Mumps was the most common cause prior to the availability of vaccines (Al-Qahtani et al., 2022). The most common causes of bacterial meningitis worldwide are *Streptococcus pneumoniae, Haemophilus influenzae* type b and *Neisseria meningitidis* (Alamarat & Hasbun, 2020; Faraj et al.). Fungal meningitis is most likely to be caused by *Coccidioides* (Faraj et al.), a genus of fungi commonly seen in the southwestern United States as well as Central and South America (Kirkland, 2016). Parasitic meningitis is relatively rare and can be caused by roundworms such as *Strongyloides stercoralis* and *Baylisascaris procyonis*, as well as the amoeba *Naegleria fowleri*. Drug-induced meningitis can be triggered by sulfa drugs and non-steroidal anti-inflammatory drugs (Faraj et al.). See Table 4.2 for an overview of types of meningitis and examples of each.

Epidemiology in Children

Similar to encephalitis, the incidence of meningitis is difficult to track. It is estimated to strike approximately 2.8 million people per year worldwide (Lee et al., 2022). Bacterial meningitis has an annual incidence of 1.33 cases per 100,000 people worldwide (Vasudeva, 2024).

Clinical Presentation, Diagnosis, and Treatment

Pediatric meningitis can be challenging to identify in its earliest stages, as it may present with nonspecific findings such as fever and CSF pleocytosis (increased cell count, such as white blood cells; Graff et al., 2021). The onset of symptoms is more noticeable when it is rapid, but symptom onset can be prolonged. Symptoms of meningitis are more severe in infants and children than in adults (Al-Qahtani et al., 2022) and bacterial meningitis in particular can be life-threatening.

Confirming a diagnosis of meningitis follows a similar process to diagnosing encephalitis. CSF analysis can be used to detect viral, bacterial, fungal, parasitic, and paraneoplastic etiologies. A high suspicion for bacterial meningitis will prompt administration of antibiotics prior to confirmation (Faraj et al., 2021), as delays, even as short as hours, can result

Table 4.2 Causes of Meningitis and Common Examples

Infectious	Viral: • Coxsackie • Mumps • Cytomegalovirus Bacterial: • Neisseria meningitidis • Group B Streptococcus • Haemophilus influenzae Fungal: • Coccidiodes Parasitic: • Naegleria fowleri
Non-infectious	Systemic diseases: • Systemic lupus erythematosus • Behcet's disease Drug-induced: • Non-steroidal anti-inflammatory drugs • Antibiotics Neoplastic: • Metastic • Leukemia/lymphoma

in significant increase in mortality. Treatments for viral meningitis include antiviral medications, IVIG, corticosteroids, and supportive care (Gundamraj & Hasbun, 2023). The use of steroids can decrease risk of hearing loss and other neurological sequelae (Alamarat & Hasbun, 2020).

Outcomes and Neuropsychological Impact

Long-term outcome studies beyond 5 years are rare in meningitis. Subtle persistent neuropsychological deficits are likely under-reported in the literature (Schiess et al., 2021). The studies that have been completed show a broad range of outcomes. Children with meningitis of any kind have increased risk for lower IQ, though mean differences are small. Executive functioning impairments have been noted up to 12 years later for survivors of childhood meningitis. Viral and bacterial meningitis increase the risk of hearing loss and language delays (Dezfouli & Khosravi, 2021).

Bacterial meningitis is associated with worse outcomes than viral encephalitis (Dezfouli & Khosravi, 2021). Hearing loss develops in about 10% of children with bacterial meningitis, and the risk of neurological complications in this population is approximately 50% (Zainel et al., 2021). Seizures and developmental delay are also common complications of bacterial meningitis (Alamarat & Hasbun, 2020). A long-term investigation of adults with a history of childhood bacterial meningitis showed increased risk for cognitive disabilities, seizures, and hearing loss (Mohanty et al., 2024). The risk for neurological complications in bacterial meningitis is higher when treatment is delayed. Additional predictors of poor outcome include neonatal onset, altered level of consciousness, and *S. pneumoniae* etiology (Teixeira et al., 2020; Zainel et al., 2021).

Children with histories of meningitis will benefit from neuropsychological follow-up. The literature suggests that we should emphasize assessment of language and executive functioning. As many complex academic, learning, social, and adaptive tasks depend on language and executive functioning skills, assessment of these areas will help identify any significant or subtle challenges. Assessment of IQ and adaptive skills may be especially salient for children with histories of bacterial meningitis, especially if complications were present.

Case Study: Neonatal Viral Meningitis

Mia (de-identified), a White female, was the product of an uncomplicated pregnancy and delivery. At 12 days of age, she developed a fever. She was taken to the hospital and immediately started on antibiotics due to suspicion of bacterial meningitis. A Meningitis/Encephalitis Pathogen PCR Panel following LP was positive for human parechovirus (PeV). Antibiotics were discontinued, and she was treated with intravenous fluids and acetaminophen. Mia improved and was discharged three days later.

Mia recovered and experienced a healthy infancy and toddlerhood. Her early motor development was normal, but her language development was delayed. Hearing and vision tested within normal. Mia received school-based speech and occupational therapies. At age 7, Mia developed headaches. An MRI revealed hyperintensity in the right frontal lobe intermediate white matter, likely gliosis (a fibrous proliferation of glial cells that occurs in injured areas of the CNS). Mia was subsequently referred for a neuropsychological evaluation.

At the time of testing, Mia had just started second grade. She received special education services but spent more than 80% of her time in the general education classroom. Mia's parents were concerned that she needed a long time to learn new information, that it was difficult for her to concentrate, and that she lacked confidence. Mia performed well below age expectations overall on language development tasks (Core Language Standard Score=66). On academic measures, she was unable to read and write beyond her first name and was inconsistent in identifying letters. She had difficulty on a computerized test of inattention and impulsivity. Her parents and teachers rated her as inattentive and hyperactive with challenges in executive functioning. Mia also showed many strengths. Her nonverbal reasoning skills were within or above age expectations (Visual Spatial Standard Score=122). She performed within the average range on math tests. There were no concerns about social skills, play skills, motor development, or overall adaptive functioning. While some anxiety was noted on parent and teacher rating scales, these concerns appeared secondary to her language, learning, and executive functioning challenges.

Mia was diagnosed with mixed receptive-expressive language disorder, dyslexia, and attention deficit/hyperactivity disorder (ADHD), combined presentation. Recommendations included speech/language therapy, a trial of stimulant medication, and dyslexia-specific interventions. Monitoring of her emotional functioning was also recommended. As children with neurocognitive sequalae of pediatric meningitis often present with subtle difficulties that can become more apparent when expectations increase, regular follow-up evaluations were also recommended.

Future Directions

Prevention

Childhood encephalitis and meningitis remain public health concerns worldwide. Both are significant causes of morbidity and mortality, and a variety of efforts are underway to reduce rates of encephalitis and meningitis in children. Vaccinations are the most effective prevention against many of the infections that can lead to CNS inflammation (Faraj et al., 2021; Zainel et al., 2021). The decrease in childhood meningitis since 2020 demonstrates that common strategies to decrease communicable diseases (e.g., hand hygiene, isolation of sick individuals) can be effective in decreasing encephalitis and meningitis (Lee et al., 2022). Neonatal meningitis caused by group B Streptococcus can be prevented with intrapartum screening and prophylactic antibiotics (Alamarat & Hasbun, 2020). Mosquito mitigation efforts can prevent encephalitis caused by viruses such as West Nile.

Challenges and Opportunities

Despite encouraging developments, meningitis and encephalitis are not preventable and the best treatments do not prevent all negative outcomes.

Pediatric practitioners will continue to play an ongoing role in supporting children with encephalitis and meningitis, such as helping to educate families about the long-term outcomes of these conditions and advocating for their needs. Additionally, more research about the neuropsychological sequalae of encephalitis and meningitis is needed. Given that impairments can be subtle and variable (Schiess et al., 2021), clinicians are in a unique position to contribute to future outcome research. Additionally, identifying clinical features of the acute phases of encephalitis and meningitis may lead to faster diagnosis and earlier treatment. This may be especially helpful in autoimmune encephalitis, as diagnostic confirmation can be a lengthy process and may not be possible at all. The commitment of pediatric practitioners to understanding and mitigating the long-term outcomes of pediatric encephalitis and meningitis will ensure better quality of life for affected children and their families.

References

Adams, A. V., Van Mater, H., Gallentine, W., & Mooneyham, G. C. (2021). Psychiatric phenotypes of pediatric patients with seropositive autoimmune encephalitis. *Hospital Pediatrics*, 11(7), 743–750. https://doi.org/10.1542/hpeds.2020-005298.

Alam, A. M., Easton, A., Nicholson, T. R., Irani, S. R., Davies, N. W., Solomon, T., & Michael, B. D. (2023). Encephalitis: Diagnosis, management and recent advances in the field of encephalitides. *Postgraduate Medical Journal*, 99(1174), 815–825. https://doi.org/10.1136/postgradmedj-2022-141812.

Alamarat, Z. & Hasbun, R. (2020). Management of acute bacterial meningitis in children. *Infection and Drug Resistance*, 13, 4077–4089. https://doi.org/10.2147/IDR.S240162.

Al-Qahtani, S. M., Shati, A. A., Alqahtani, Y. A., & Ali, A. S. (2022). Etiology, clinical phenotypes, epidemiological correlates, laboratory biomarkers and diagnostic challenges of pediatric viral meningitis: Descriptive review. *Frontiers in Pediatrics*, 10, 923125. https://doi.org/10.3389/fped.2022.923125.

Autoimmune Encephalitis Alliance Clinicians Network ([AECN] 2021). Autoimmune encephalitis: Proposed best practice recommendations for diagnosis and acute management. *Journal of Neurology, Neurosurgery and Psychiatry*. 92(7), 757–768. https://doi.org/10.1136/jnnp-2020-325300

Brenner, J., Olijslagers, S. H. C., Crijnen, Y. S., de Vries, J. M., Mandarakas, M. R., & Titulaer, M. J. (2024). Clinical outcome assessments in encephalitis: A systematic review. *Neurology Neuroimmunology & Neuroinflammation*, 11(1), e200168. https://doi.org/10.1212/NXI.0000000000200168.

Britton, P. N., Dale, R. C., Blyth, C. C., Clark, J. E., Crawford, N., Marshall, H., Elliott, E. J., Macartney, K., Booy, R., & Jones, C. A. (2020). Causes and clinical features of childhood encephalitis: A multicenter, prospective cohort study. *Clinical Infectious Diseases*, 70(12), 2517–2526. https://doi.org/10.1093/cid/ciz685.

Castagno, E., Aguzzi, S., Rossi, L., Gallo, R., Carpino, A., Ricceri, F., Urbino, A. F., & Bondone, C. (2023). Clinical predictors and biomarkers in children with sepsis and bacterial meningitis. *Pediatric Emergency Care*, 39(5), 311–317. https://doi.org/10.1097/PEC.0000000000002865.

Cellucci, T., Van Mater, H., Graus, F., Muscal, E., Gallentine, W., Klein-Gitelman, M. S., Benseler, S. M., Frankovich, J., Gorman, M. P., Van Haren, K., Dalmau, J., & Dale, R. C. (2020). Clinical approach to the diagnosis of autoimmune encephalitis in the pediatric patient. *Neurology Neuroimmunology & Neuroinflammation*, 7(2), e663. https://doi.org/10.1212/NXI.0000000000000663.

De Bruijn, M. A. A. M., Bruijstens, A. L., Bastiaansen, A. E. M., Van Sonderen, A., Schreurs, M. W. J., Sillevis Smitt, P. A. E., Hintzen, R. Q., Neuteboom, R. F., & Titulaer, M. J. (2020). Pediatric autoimmune encephalitis: Recognition and diagnosis. *Neurology Neuroimmunology & Neuroinflammation*, 7(3), e682. https://doi.org/10.1212/NXI.0000000000000682.

Dezfouli, S. M. M. & Khosravi, S. (2021). Impact of meningitis on cognitive skills and development in children. *Indian Journal of Forensic Medicine & Toxicology*, 15(1), 2674. https://doi.org/10.37506/ijfmt.v15i1.13802.

Erickson, T. A., Muscal, E., Munoz, F. M., Lotze, T., Hasbun, R., Brown, E., & Murray, K. O. (2020). Infectious and autoimmune causes of encephalitis in children. *Pediatrics*, 145(6), e20192543. https://doi.org/10.1542/peds.2019-2543.

Faraj, L. A., Alghamdi, K. M., Tayyib, E. M., Asiri, A. M., Al-Dhahry, S. A., Alzayer, E. K., Hubail, K. A., Ghazwani, M. H., Marhoon, J. A., Alsharif, M. F., Zaki, L., AlAanaz, M. I. H. (2021). An overview on pediatric meningitis diagnosis and management approach. *International Journal of Pharmaceutical Research And Allied Sciences*, 10(4), 84–88. https://doi.org/10.51847/8fnDhpmWUW.

Galioto, R., Grezmak, T., Swetlik, C., Abbatemarco, J. R., Titulaer, M. J., Finke, C., & Kunchok, A. (2024). Neuropsychological testing in autoimmune encephalitis: A Scoping review. *Neurology Neuroimmunology & Neuroinflammation*, 11(1), e200179. https://doi.org/10.1212/NXI.0000000000200179.

Graff, K., Dominguez, S. R., & Messacar, K. (2021). Metagenomic next-generation sequencing for diagnosis of pediatric meningitis and encephalitis: A review. *Journal of the Pediatric Infectious Diseases Society*, 10(Supplement_4), S78–S87. https://doi.org/10.1093/jpids/piab067.

Gundamraj, V. & Hasbun, R. (2023). Viral meningitis and encephalitis: An update. *Current Opinion in Infectious Diseases*, 36(3), 177–185. https://doi.org/10.1097/QCO.0000000000000922.

Hardy, D. (2022). Autoimmune encephalitis in children. *Pediatric Neurology*, 132, 56–66. https://doi.org/10.1016/j.pediatrneurol.2022.05.004.

Harris, L., Griem, J., Gummery, A., Marsh, L., Defres, S., Bhojak, M., Das, K., Easton, A., Solomon, T., & Kopelman, M. (2020). Neuropsychological and psychiatric outcomes in encephalitis: A multi-centre case-control study. *PLOS ONE*, 15(3), e0230436. https://doi.org/10.1371/journal.pone.0230436.

Hatachi, T., Michihata, N., Inata, Y., Takeuchi, M., Matsui, H., Fushimi, K., & Yasunaga, H. (2021). Prognostic factors among children with acute encephalitis/encephalopathy associated with viral and other pathogens. *Clinical Infectious Diseases*, 73(1), 76–82. https://doi.org/10.1093/cid/ciaa536.

Johns Hopkins Medicine (n.d.) *Encephalitis*. Retrieved 2023 from hopkinsmedicine.org/health/conditions-and-disease/encephalitis

Kirkland, T. N. (2016). The quest for a vaccine against coccidioidomycosis: A neglected disease of the Americas. *Journal of Fungi*, 2(4), 34. https://doi.org/10.3390/jof2040034.

Lee, J., Choi, A., Kim, K., Bin, J. H., Eom, T. H., Yoo, I. H., Yoon, D. H., Kim, S., & Kim, Y. H. (2022). Changes in the epidemiology and causative pathogens of meningitis in children after the outbreak of the coronavirus disease 2019: A multicenter database study. *Frontiers in Pediatrics*, 10, 810616. https://doi.org/10.3389/fped.2022.810616.

Mohanty, S., Johansson Kostenniemi, U., Silfverdal, S. A., Salomonsson, S., Iovino, F., Sarpong, E. M., Bencina, G., & Bruze, G. (2024). Increased risk of long-term disabilities following childhood bacterial meningitis in Sweden. *JAMA Network Open*, 7(1), e2352402. https://doi.org/10.1001/jamanetworkopen.2023.52402.

Pointon, T., Ward, R., Yeshokumar, A., Piquet, A., Schreiner, T., & Kammeyer, R. (2022). Evaluation of multiple consensus criteria for autoimmune encephalitis and temporal analysis of symptoms in a pediatric encephalitis cohort. *Frontiers in Neurology*, 13, 952317. https://doi.org/10.3389/fneur.2022.952317.

Pöyhönen, H., Setänen, S., Isaksson, N., Nyman, M., Nyman, A., Peltola, V., & Lähdesmäki, T. (2021). Neurological and cognitive performance after childhood encephalitis. *Frontiers in Pediatrics*, 9, 646684. https://doi.org/10.3389/fped.2021.646684.

Ramanuj, P. P., Granerød, J., Davies, N. W., Conti, S., Brown, D. W., & Crowcroft, N. S. (2014). Quality of life and associated socio-clinical factors after encephalitis in children and adults in England: A population-based, prospective cohort study. *PLoS ONE*, 9(7), e103496. https://doi.org/10.1371/journal.pone.0103496.

Sabanathan, S., Abdel-Mannan, O., Mankad, K., Siddiqui, A., Das, K., Carr, L., Eltze, C., Eyre, M., Gadian, J., Hemingway, C., Kaliakatsos, M., Kneen, R., Krishnakumar, D., Lynch, B., Parida, A., Rossor, T., Taylor, M., Wassmer, E., Wright, S., … Hacohen, Y. (2022). Clinical features, investigations, and outcomes of pediatric limbic encephalitis: A multicenter study. *Annals of Clinical and Translational Neurology*, 9(1), 67–78. https://doi.org/10.1002/acn3.51494.

Schiess, N., Groce, N. E., & Dua, T. (2021). The impact and burden of neurological sequelae following bacterial meningitis: A narrative review. *Microorganisms*, 9(5), 900. https://doi.org/10.3390/microorganisms9050900.

Teixeira, D. C., Diniz, L. M. O., Guimarães, N. S., Moreira, H. M. D. A. S., Teixeira, C. C., & Romanelli, R. M. D. C. (2020). Risk factors associated with the outcomes of pediatric bacterial meningitis: A systematic review. *Jornal de Pediatria*, 96(2), 159–167. https://doi.org/10.1016/j.jped.2019.07.003.

Ungureanu, A., van der Meer, J., Bicvic, A., Abbuehl, L., Chiffi, G., Jaques, L., Suter-Riniker, F., Leib, S. L., Bassetti, C. L. A., & Dietmann, A. (2021). Meningitis, meningoencephalitis and encephalitis in Bern: An observational study of 258 patients. *BMC Neurology*, 21(1), 474. https://doi.org/10.1186/s12883-021-02502-3.

Vasudeva, S. S. (2024, April 26). Meningitis: Practice essentials, background, pathophysiology. *Medscape*. https://emedicine.medscape.com/article/232915-overview#a5.

Vova, J. A. & Howarth, R. A. (2023). Evaluation, treatment, and outcomes of viral and autoimmune encephalitis in children. *Pediatric Clinics of North America*, 70 (3), 429–444. https://doi.org/10.1016/j.pcl.2023.01.007.

Wilkinson-Smith, A., Blackwell, L. S., & Howarth, R. A. (2022). Neuropsychological outcomes in children and adolescents following anti-NMDA receptor encephalitis. *Child Neuropsychology*, 28(2), 212–223. https://doi.org/10.1080/09297049.2021.1965110.

World Health Organization (2021). *Defeating meningitis by 2030: A global road map*.

World Health Organization (2023). *Why encephalitis matters: Report of the virtual meeting, 28–29 June 2022*. World Health Organization.

Wright, C., Blake, N., Glennie, L., Smith, V., Bender, R., Kyu, H., Wunrow, H. Y., Liu, L., Yeung, D., Knoll, M. D., Wahl, B., Stuart, J. M., & Trotter, C. (2021). The global burden of meningitis in children: Challenges with interpreting global health estimates. *Microorganisms*, 9(2), 377. https://doi.org/10.3390/microorganisms9020377.

Zainel, A., Mitchell, H., & Sadarangani, M. (2021). Bacterial meningitis in children: Neurological complications, associated risk factors, and prevention. *Microorganisms*, 9(3), 535. https://doi.org/10.3390/microorganisms9030535.

5 Neonatal Abstinence Syndrome

Denise E. Maricle and Amy Skinner

Introduction

Neonatal abstinence syndrome (NAS) is a spectrum of withdrawal symptoms that occurs in newborn babies shortly after birth as a result of exposure to addictive substances while in utero. Described by Dr. Laura Finnegan in the 1970s, NAS is most frequently associated with opioids (i.e., oxycodone or hydrocodone) but can also be caused by other drugs such as alcohol, nicotine, antidepressants, barbiturates or benzodiazepines (sleeping pills or anti-anxiety medications), the medications used to treat opioid addiction (such as methadone or buprenorphine), and illegal drugs such as heroin, cocaine, or methamphetamine. More recently, neonatal opioid withdrawal syndrome (NOWS) has been used to describe the constellation of withdrawal signs associated with in utero exposure to illicit or legally prescribed opioids. NAS/NOWS occurs because the baby becomes dependent on the substance during fetal development, hence the withdrawal symptoms after birth once the child is no longer exposed to the substance.

Drugs, legal or illegal, are easily passed through the placenta and umbilical cord as well as via breast milk from the mother to the fetus or infant. Most of these drugs easily pass through the blood–brain barrier. Drugs act on a fetal brain in the same way they act on an adult brain. The effect of drugs on the developing central nervous system (CNS) differs from the effect it has on a mature CNS. In utero it produces alterations in developmental trajectories of the developing brain, its communication systems and processing networks. Alterations to brain structures have been noted in some cases. The dosages ingested and the concentrations tolerated by adults quickly reach toxic levels in the developing brain. The immature or developing brain is flooded with large amounts of a drug that are too toxic to the infant's smaller and less developed CNS.

The statistics for drug use/abuse in the USA are staggering (National Center for Drug Abuse Statistics, n.d.). Eighty six percent of the population age 18+ have used alcohol with 56% using it within the past month. Over 138 million individuals self-reported regular alcohol use in 2020 and 57 million reported regular use of tobacco/nicotine. Fifty percent of people

DOI: 10.4324/9781032703923-7

age 12+ reported illicit drug use at least once, with 61 million (or 29.9%) reporting use within the last year. The most frequently used/abused drug is marijuana. The highest self-reported drug and alcohol use is seen from age 18 to 29 (73%). In 2017, the International Narcotics Control Board reported that 99.2% of global hydrocodone use occurred in the USA. Estimates suggest more than 10 million Americans age 12+ misuse opioids, with most abusing legally obtained prescription opioids. Approximately 16.5% of the population would meet the DSM 5 TR criteria for substance use disorder. Overdose is now the number one cause of accidental death in the USA with 109,000 fatal overdoses occurring between March 2021 and March 2022. Sixty percent of fatal overdoses are due to Fentanyl, which is now the leading cause of death in Americans age 18 to 41.

The 2020 National Survey on Drug Use and Health (Substance-Abuse and Mental Health Services Administration, 2020) indicates that 8% to 11% of pregnant women age 15 to 44 self-reported using illicit drugs, tobacco/nicotine, or alcohol in the past month. The National Institute on Drug Abuse (2021) Substance Use in Women Research Report estimates that 5% or more of pregnant women use one or more addictive substances throughout their pregnancies. Additionally, many women who are pregnant use prescription and OTC medications. The NIDA suggests that of the 6 million pregnancies each year, 9 out of 10 mothers will take medication at some time during their pregnancy, however fewer than 10% of legally prescribed or OTC medications have enough information to determine fetal risk. The Center for Disease Control and Prevention (CDC, 2019) cites a 2019 study noting that 7% of women report using prescription drugs during pregnancy with 1 in 5 self-reporting misuse.

The CDC notes that between 2010 and 2017 diagnoses of NAS/NOWS increased by 131%. Data from the 2020 Healthcare Cost and Utilization Project (Agency for Healthcare Research and Quality, 2020) reports six out of one thousand newborns are diagnosed with NAS/NOWS, or 59 newborns each day. Hirai and colleagues (2021) give the statistics as 7.3 per 1000 births diagnosed NAS/NOWS and 8.2 per 1000 women diagnosed with maternal opioid-related disorder (MOD). The USA has some of the highest rates of substance use during pregnancy. Winkelman and colleagues (2018) suggest that 94.3 per 1000 live births are at risk for developing NAS/NOWS due to intrauterine exposure. NAS/NOWS has been declared a national epidemic in the USA and is rapidly approaching a global public health crisis.

Despite the staggering numbers of infants born with NAS/NOWS, little is known about the long-term effects on child health, specifically the effects on neurodevelopment. Improved treatment has led to increased survival rates of infants with NAS/NOWS making the long-term impact of prenatal drug exposure of major international concern as these children are at increased risk of cognitive difficulties, mental health issues and physical problems. One major issue in understanding and working with children identified with NAS/NOWS is the likelihood of polysubstance exposure. Many children exposed in utero are not exposed to only one toxic substance but often to multiple substances. For example, 80% of children with a history of NAS/NOWS had polysubstance (i.e., two or more substances) exposure (including tobacco) (Wachman et al., 2018). Research summarized by the CDC (2023) has found that polysubstance use is common in pregnancy. Results indicate that pregnant women prescribed opioid pain medication were and more likely to smoke tobacco compared to those who did not use opioids; more than half of pregnant women who used opioids for nonmedical reasons reported drinking more than five drinks containing alcohol per day during a 1-month period of time. In addition, of those pregnant women who used marijuana before and during pregnancy, 74% also smoked cigarettes while pregnant. Individuals with prescription opioid use disorders report co-occurring substance use 50% of the time and those using heroin report co-occurring substance use 88.5% of the time.

Research shows that individual substances (i.e., tobacco, alcohol, cocaine, opioids, and benzodiazepines) have differing effects on infants with NAS/NOWS. However, little is known about the interaction effects of combinations of substances on newborns. There is currently no clear evidence for NAS/NOWS with drugs such as marijuana, nicotine, and amphetamines (i.e., Ritalin), although that does not mean these drugs have no impact on the developing fetus or lack long-term neuropsychological sequelae.

Characteristics and Symptoms of NAS/NOWS

NAS/NOWS is challenging to predict, diagnose and manage due to its highly variable expression (Yen et al., 2023). Signs of NAS/NOWS vary widely and reflect dysfunction in autonomic regulation, state control, and sensory-motor functioning. Immediate physical signs are classified or grouped into gastrointestinal, metabolic, vasomotor, respiratory, and CNS activity (Clark & Ronan, 2015). The symptoms of NAS/NOWS commonly begin 24 to 72 hours after birth, with the average time of onset dependent on the half-life of the substances ingested by the mother. For example, with short-acting opioids such as heroin, the onset of NAS/NOWS symptoms is 2 to 3 days whereas for long-acting drugs such as methadone or buprenorphine onset is about 4 days. Consequently, an infant with known exposure to drugs in utero requires at least 4 days (or 96 hours) in hospital to ensure capturing the symptoms of NAS/NOWS (Substance-Abuse and Mental Health Services Administration, 2018). Withdrawal in the newborn is a qualitatively distinct process from that of adults due to the complexity of immature neuronal circuitry.

Substance exposure is usually identified using toxicology screening of the newborn's urine and meconium. Urine testing generally reflects substance exposure within the past several days whereas meconium toxicology screening can reveal substance exposure for the past several months.

Umbilical cord tissue sampling is also used and can provide a longer history of prenatal drug use, but also reflects drugs used during labor and delivery.

Immediate neuropsychological sequelae include tremors, overactive reflexes and tight muscle tone, extreme fussiness or excessive crying characterized by a high-pitched tone, poor feeding due to an inability to suckle, abnormal breathing including tachypnea (rapid breathing), insomnia, and a higher rate of sudden infant death syndrome (SIDS) (Kocherlakota, 2014).

Metabolic and respiratory disturbance may include irregular body temperature (excessive sweating, fever), blotchy skin, excessive yawning, and difficulty breathing. Gastrointestinal dysfunction includes diarrhea, vomiting, dehydration, and slow weight gain. Jaundice is also common.

Long-term neuropsychological sequelae are not as well-known compared with the short-term effects, however, developmental delays particularly in motor, speech and language, behavior and learning are common. Long-term neuropsychological sequelae have been found to vary depending on the substance of abuse. Medically, these children have higher rates of ear infections (i.e., otitis media is associated with methadone) and visual concerns. Strabismus, nystagmus and refractive errors are more common, as is delayed visual motor development involving eye-hand movement/coordination and visual spatial organizational abilities. Fill and colleagues (2018) discussed common developmental trajectories in children identified with NAS/NOWS. They speculated that potential changes to brain matter and myelination due to prenatal exposure to drugs affects learning and language development in children with a history of NAS/NOWS.

The lingering effects of drug exposure on neuropsychological functions is most recognizable in areas such as attention, impulsivity, memory, perception and externalizing behaviors. Academic underachievement in reading, writing, and mathematics is common with executive functioning deficits influencing cognition and behavior (Fill et al., 2018). Children with drug exposure appear to have significantly more regulatory problems than their non-exposed peers especially in areas of attention, internalized anxiety and depression, and externalized aggression. These children exhibit less social responsiveness and poorer social engagement, and they are at risk for higher rates of mental health problems, delinquency or criminal behavior, and substance abuse (Shearer-Miller, 2019).

Table 5.1 Common Developmental Trajectories in Children with NAS

Percentage of NAS identified children	*Abnormal motor development*	*Abnormal behavioral development*	*Abnormal Cognitive development*
At 1 year of age	21%	8%	13%
At 5 years of age	5%	22%	22%
At 10 years of age	3%	18%	27%

Source Fill et al., 2018

Most Commonly Used Substances Related to NAS/NOWS

There is a plethora of research and literature addressing specific substance use and its impact on children exposed in utero. However, given the differing impact of various substances, a brief summary of the most common substances is provided.

Alcohol

Alcohol is the world's oldest drug and the teratogenic effects of prenatal alcohol exposure have been known for centuries. Fetal alcohol syndrome disorders (FASD) include fetal alcohol syndrome (FAS), fetal alcohol effect (FAE), alcohol related neurodevelopmental disorder (ARND), alcohol related birth defects (ARBD) and neurobehavioral disorder associated with prenatal alcohol exposure (ND-PAE). FASD is covered in Chapter 6.

Crack/Cocaine

Cocaine is the third most abused illicit drug with about 750,000 cocaine-exposed pregnancies each year (Substance-Abuse and Mental Health Services Administration, 2020). Cocaine is derived from the coca plant. In powdered form it is cocaine and in rock form it is crack. Cocaine/crack is a stimulant that easily crosses the placenta and the blood–brain barrier (BBB). It directly inhibits the reuptake of multiple monoamines at the presynaptic junction leading to increased concentrations of dopamine, serotonin, and norepinephrine within the synaptic cleft. The magnitude of the effect depends on dosage, gestational timing, duration of exposure, as well as postnatal care and subsequent environmental influences, such as parenting.

Cocaine metabolites can still be present in an infant's blood 5 to 7 days post-delivery (Substance-Abuse and Mental Health Services Administration, 2020). Cocaine/crack use during pregnancy is associated with polysubstance use, maternal migraines and seizures, premature membrane rupture, and separation of the placental lining prior to delivery. Infants exposed to prenatal cocaine/crack are often prematurely delivered, have low or very low birth weights, smaller head circumference, and shorter stature. Irritability, hyperactivity, tremors, a high pitched cry and excessive sucking may also be seen in an exposed newborn. Research suggests that exposure to cocaine/crack during fetal development may lead to subtle, yet significant deficits in children. These include behavior problems (i.e., difficulties with self-regulation, inhibitory control, and sustained attention) and deficits in cognition (i.e., language difficulties, information processing, and executive functioning deficits). Frequent use in utero is associated with severe behavior problems including aggression and delinquency, often beginning around age 9 (Cestonaro et al., 2022; Dodge et al., 2019).

Opiates

Opioids include morphine, codeine, heroin, hydrocodone, oxycodone, and fentanyl. Opiates originated from the opium poppy (i.e., morphine and codeine; with heroin then derived from morphine). More recently semi-synthetic (oxycodone; hydrocodone) and synthetic opiates (fentanyl) have been created. Opiates are G-protein coupled receptors which bind to the areas of the brain controlling pain and emotion, driving up dopamine and producing feelings of euphoria. As the brain habituates it takes more and more to produce the same effect. Prenatal opiate exposure disrupts maturation of the opiate receptor systems in the brain and induces tolerance for opiates, putting the child at risk for later addiction and subsequent misuse.

Mothers using opiates during pregnancy are at increased risk of preeclampsia, placental insufficiency, placental abruption, intrauterine growth retardation, birth defects, and stillbirth. Babies are often born premature exhibiting the classic signs of NAS/NOWS (i.e., excessive crying, stiff limbs, tremor, and diarrhea). Babies exposed to heroin in utero are treated with morphine, which is gradually titrated and replaced with a methadone maintenance program. Neuropsychological sequelae can vary with some children showing language delays, difficulty with inhibitory control, problems with selective attention (particularly visual attention), deficits in spatial learning, memory issues, and learning disabilities.

Methamphetamine/Amphetamine

Methamphetamines include speed, meth, chalk, and legal amphetamines such as Ritalin or Adderall. Methamphetamine abuse is versatile in that these drugs can be injected, smoked, snorted or taken orally or anally. Methamphetamine is a potent CNS stimulant that affects the reward centers of the brain by releasing massive amounts of dopamine, norepinephrine, and serotonin. It stimulates dopamine in the synaptic cleft while inhibiting the reuptake of both dopamine and norepinephrine. Methamphetamines have greater neurotoxic effects due to their ability to remain longer in the body mimicking the effects of neurotransmitters in the brain. Exposure to methamphetamine is known to alter brain structure. The caudate nucleus (a c-shaped subcortical structure deep in the brain near the thalamus) plays a critical role in various higher neurological functions such as learning, memory, and motor control, and has been found to be reduced in size and volume in methamphetamine-exposed children. Methamphetamines alter white matter tracts in the brain (Warton et al., 2018) and disrupt the normal development of the frontal cortex. Imaging studies have shown that a newborn exposed to methamphetamine has a brain that resembles asphyxiated infants.

Mothers using methamphetamines are at greater risk for preeclampsia, placental abruption, premature delivery, and LBW or VLBW babies. A newborn exposed to methamphetamine may appear acutely intoxicated (rapid heart rate, high BP, irritability, seizures, and stroke) or may be in withdrawal (classic signs of NAS/NOWS). Long-term impacts include emotional reactivity, higher risk for anxiety/depression, attentional difficulties and cognitive or learning delays. Long-term sequelae include deficits with inhibitory control, attention difficulties, challenges with visual-motor integration tasks, as well as impairments in verbal memory and long-term spatial memory tasks.

Amphetamines, such as Ritalin, Adderall, Dexedrine, or Focalin have not been proven to have a direct teratogenic effect, however since the cellular action is similar to methamphetamine, they are suspected to have similar negative outcomes when used prenatally. Use during pregnancy often results in preterm labor, LBW, and small size for gestational age. There also appears to be an increased prevalence of ADHD diagnoses, aggression, delinquency and learning deficits, particularly with attention, memory and motivation, in children exposed prenatally.

Inhalants

Inhalants include glue, paint, hairspray, deodorant, brake fluid, gasoline, or an aerosol propellant, refrigerant, or other solvent containing chlorofluorocarbons and related compounds (i.e., Freon). Neuropsychological impairments associated with use of inhalants during pregnancy have been well documented. Inhalant use during pregnancy significantly disrupts neural processing with structural deficits occurring in the basal ganglia, pons, and cerebellum as well as severe structural abnormalities in white matter. Inhalant use during pregnancy is linked with increased risk of premature birth, LBW, and physical effects. Prenatal exposure to highly concentrated inhalants may have impacts on the child's development, including delayed growth and problems with speech and motor skills.

Nicotine, Marijuana, and Caffeine

Nicotine

About 10% to 12% of pregnant women ingest nicotine. Nicotine interferes with oxygen supply to the fetus, and readily crosses the placenta with concentrations in fetal blood 15% higher than the mother. Nicotine is an agonist at the nicotine acetylcholine receptors of the brain and intrauterine exposure can disrupt the cholinergic system, a key modulator in brain development. Nicotine has been established as a neurotetragon that compromises the development of critical neural pathways in the developing brain (Wells & Lotfipour, 2023). It is associated with increased risk of ADHD, SLD, behavioral issues, and substance addiction (research strongly suggests that nicotine is a gateway drug—making the brain more sensitive to other drugs; Substance-Abuse and Mental Health Services Administration, 2020). Nicotine desensitizes neurotransmitter functions in prenatally exposed children thus reducing the levels of epinephrine, norepinephrine, and serotonin. It impairs limbic and cortical neuronal development, alters brain functions, and reduces brain size (Wells & Lotfipour). Infants exposed to nicotine have an increased risk of premature birth, miscarriage, and low birth weight. Children exposed to nicotine in utero often display decreased receptive language skills, deficits in memory processing, attention problems, and may be diagnosed more frequently with oppositional defiant disorder.

Marijuana

Marijuana is the most widely used illegal drug during pregnancy in the USA. Although it remains illegal at the federal level some states have legalized it for recreational and medicinal use. Additionally, a growing number of pregnant women view it as a safe, natural way to treat nausea and vomiting, or "morning sickness." But marijuana use during pregnancy is not safe and comes with serious, potentially deadly risks including stillbirth, preterm birth, and growth or development issues. Whether smoked, eaten in food (edibles), or vaped, marijuana is more potent than ever before, which makes use during pregnancy especially risky for a developing baby's health. Marijuana contains nearly 500 chemicals, including the mind-altering compound tetrahydrocannabinol (THC). These chemicals, particularly THC can cross the placenta quite easily and efficiently. Exposed newborns display sleep disturbance, altered responses to visual stimuli and an exaggerated startle response. Exposure has been linked to long-term sequelae including EF deficits, poor impulse control, and difficulty with visual–spatial perception.

CBD oil, a derivative of hemp from which marijuana is derived, has become increasingly popular for a variety of issues, from pain relief, suppressing nausea, and reducing anxiety. It's understandable that a pregnant person might consider taking it for pregnancy side effects. However, there is no comprehensive research studying the effects of CBD oil on the developing fetus, pregnant person, or breastfed baby. The FDA strongly advises against the use of CBD oil by pregnant and breastfeeding women since research on its safety among these populations is insufficient.

Caffeine

Epidemiological studies have revealed that caffeine consumption during pregnancy is associated with adverse gestational outcomes (Qian et al., 2020; Zhang et al., 2021). In the USA, approximately 70% of women continue to consume caffeine during pregnancy despite documentation that maternal caffeine consumption increases the risk of pregnancy failure or gestational complications. Caffeine blocks adenosine A_1 and A_{2A} receptors, increasing alertness and cognitive performance while regulating mood and disrupting sleep. During pregnancy, caffeine's metabolic rate in mothers is significantly decreased, especially after the first trimester, and the half-life of caffeine increases from 2.5–4.5 hours to approximately 15 hours towards the end of pregnancy. Caffeine is lipid soluble and freely transfers across all membranes, including the placental barrier, although neither fetus nor placenta has the enzymes for its metabolism. Thus, maternal caffeine intake during pregnancy likely leads to accumulation of caffeine in the fetal brain, which might affect early development and later childhood outcomes.

Caffeine consumption during pregnancy is associated with intrauterine growth retardation, low birth weight, and miscarriage. Daily intake of less than 300 mg caffeine (approximately three cups of coffee) during pregnancy has been deemed unlikely to harm gestational health. However, some studies (Qian et al., 2020; Zhang et al., 2021) have found that even daily intake as low as 100–200 mg during pregnancy is associated with an increased risk of miscarriage, fetal growth restriction and low birth weight. These studies raise concern that there may be no one absolute "safe" threshold of caffeine consumption during pregnancy. Long-term sequelae suggest greater likelihood of externalizing disorders, such as somatic concerns, oppositional defiant disorder, and conduct problems in older children prenatally exposed to caffeine.

Making Connections: Assessment and Intervention

Pediatric and school psychologists need to consider how prenatal, postnatal, and early developmental trajectories may be causal or correlational with the cognitive, learning, or behavioral manifestations being reported as concerns. Oftentimes, because the manifestation of the difficulties is so distant from its origination, contributing factors such as NAS/NOWS, prematurity, or anoxia at birth are often not considered.

The importance of a thorough and comprehensive developmental and medical history cannot be understated. Prenatal, birth, and postnatal data is critical to understanding possible cognitive, learning, or behavioral manifestations. In school practice, often a developmental history questionnaire is sent for the parents to complete, however by doing this, the clinician may be missing important information. Although medical and developmental milestone information is collected, the parent information obtained may not address areas of critical information needed. It is important to obtain more comprehensive and specific information regarding developmental attainments, language development, motor skills, social development, self-care and learning. It would be best practice to conduct history-taking as part of an in-person clinical interview, where it is possible to follow up with more specific questions if there is an indication of a problem or known information about intrauterine drug exposure. For example, if a child was in the NICU it is important to get more information about why (prematurity, VLBW, respiratory distress, etc.), the services, treatments or procedures (intubation, feeding tube, surgeries) conducted, and the child's response. If drug or alcohol use is indicated, the clinician should ask questions regarding each drug more specifically (i.e., frequency, duration, amount, gestational period of use).

Initially, children with NAS/NOWS are likely to receive diagnoses of developmental delay, or Speech-Language Impairment. Overall, older children with NAS/NOWS are more like to be diagnosed with learning disability, ADHD, or ODD (Fill et al., 2018). Children displaying difficulties stemming from intrauterine drug exposure may qualify for some disability categories under the IDEA (i.e., SLD, OHI, SLI, ED), whereas others may meet criteria under Section 504 of the Rehabilitation Act of 1973. Children exposed to alcohol and drugs in utero also tend to experience higher than average adverse childhood experiences (ACEs), which are known to impact an individual's cognitive, academic, and social-emotional-behavioral functioning. The effect of ACEs on neurological functioning and in relationship to other neurodevelopmental disorders is just now being explored. This can make differential diagnosis a challenge; what is caused by NAS/NOWS and what is due to other factors like genetics or ACEs is often impossible to determine.

Assessments Specific to NAS/NOWS

Several instruments may be used at birth to assess NAS/NOWS and these results may be seen in the child's medical record. The Finnegan Neonatal Abstinence Scoring System (FNASS) is a 31-item scale designed to quantify the severity of NAS and to guide treatment. It extensively catalogs signs and symptoms in three areas: CNS, metabolic/vascular/respiratory, and gastrointestinal (Grossman & Berkwitt, 2019). Other NAS/NOWS screening instruments include The Neonatal Withdrawal Inventory, the Neonatal Narcotic Withdrawal Index and the Lipsitz Neonatal Drug Withdrawal Scoring System.

Assessment in childhood will vary significantly depending upon each child's individual circumstance and presenting problems (Kocherlakota, 2014). But in general, the following aspects should be considered:

1 Neurodevelopmental assessments to identify motor deficits and cognitive delays, particularly in the areas of visual-spatial motor issues, visual and spatial memory deficits, attention and executive function difficulties, as well as receptive language challenges.
2 Psycho-behavioral assessments to identify hyperactivity, impulsivity, attention-deficit, and other behavioral problems.

3 Ophthalmologic assessment to identify nystagmus, strabismus, refractive errors, and other potential visual defects.
4 Growth and nutritional assessment to identify failure to thrive and short stature.
5 Family support assessments to rule out continuous maternal substance abuse and child abuse.

Interventions Specific to NAS/NOWS

Ultimately, recommendations and interventions will depend on the individual child and the unique presentation of NAS/NOWS at home and in the classroom, but in general, psychologists/educators need to consider several critical areas including attention, memory, visual-spatial problems, and social emotional difficulties.

Postnatal and Infancy

Infants identified with NAS/NOWS can be treated pharmacologically and non-pharmacologically. Pharmacological treatment is typically instituted when 3 consecutive Finnegan scores are >8 or when the average of 2 scores is >12. Approximately 50% to 75% of infants exposed to opioids in utero will require pharmacological treatment for opioid withdrawal. Morphine is the first line treatment, but phenobarbital may be added or used in conjunction if polysubstance exposure is suspected. Non-pharmacological interventions include swaddling, rocking, maintenance of temperature stability, and minimizing sensory or environmental stimulation (dimness, reduction of sound and visual stimulation, weighted blankets). If excessive sucking is an issue, consider alternating the bottle and pacifier. Breastfeeding when appropriate can help reduce the need for pharmacological treatment but is contraindicated if the mother continues to have drugs in her system.

Preschool and Childhood

Attentional interventions or accommodations might include teaching the child self-monitoring techniques, access to quiet or secluded study spaces, frequent checks for understanding, or access to fidget gadgets. Interventions for memory difficulties might include teaching external executive function skills, such as organizational charts or electronic calendars, as well as teaching strategies that utilize repetition and scaffolding. Visual spatial difficulties might be addressed by using grid paper or covering unneeded material on a worksheet. Social-emotional interventions might include individual or group therapy with a cognitive behavioral focus, check in–check out monitoring, or other appropriate behavioral interventions. Due to the higher rates of these children following a more criminogenic path, it will be pertinent to monitor their behaviors and provide prosocial activities. Assigning a mentor both in the community and in school might be beneficial for the child.

Conclusion

A staggering number of children have been exposed to drugs in utero, altering both brain structure and function permanently. Many will develop neurodevelopmental disorders and exhibit neuropsychological deficits as a result of this early exposure. We know very little about the long-term outcomes for babies born drug exposed. Future research should focus on understanding the role of drug exposure in fetal development, newborn withdrawal, and long-term outcomes.

Resources

SAMHSA (2018). Clinical Guidance for Treating Pregnant and Parenting Women with Opioid Use Disorder and Their Infants. Publication ID # SMA18–5054. Available from samhsa.gov

University of Maryland Medical Center Video (https://vimeo.com/101299947). Describes NAS.

National Center on Birth Defects and Developmental Disabilities (cdc.gov/ncbddd)

National Center on Substance Abuse and Child Welfare (ncsacw.acf.hhs.gov)

References

Agency for Healthcare Research and Quality (2020). *Healthcare cost and utilization project*. Retrieved August 15, 2024 from https://hcup-us.ahrq.gov.

Center for Disease Control and Prevention. (2023, March 23). *What we do*. https://www.cdc.gov/ncbddd/aboutus/what-we-do.html.

Center for Disease Control and Prevention (2019). *About opioid use during pregnancy*. https://www.cdc.gov/pregnancy/opioids/basics.html.

Cestonaro, C., Menozzi L., & Terranova, C. (2022). Infants of mothers with cocaine use: Review of clinical and medico-legal aspects. *Children*, 9(1), 67. doi:10.3390/children9010067.

Clark, L. & Ronan, A. (2015). Identifying and assessing the substance-exposed infant. *The American Journal of Maternal/Child Nursing*, 40(2), 87–95. doi:10.109/NMC.0000000000000117.

Dodge, N. C., Jacobson, J. L., & Jacobson, S. W. (2019). Effects of fetal substance exposure on offspring substance use. *Pediatric Clinics*, 66(6), 1149–1161. doi:10.1016/j.pcl.2019.08.010.

Fill, M. A., Miller, A. M., Wilkinson, R. H., Warren, M. D., Dunn, J. R., Schaffner, W., & Jones, T. F. (2018). Educational disabilities among children born with neonatal abstinence syndrome. *Pediatrics*, 142(3), e20180562. doi:10.1542/peds.2018-0562.

Grossman, M. & Berkwitt, A. (2019). Neonatal abstinence syndrome. In *Seminars in Perinatology*, 43(3), 173–186. https://doi.org/10.1053/j.semperi.2019.01.007.

Hirai, A. H., Ko, J. Y., Owens, P. L., Stocks, C., & Patrick, S. W. (2021). NAS and maternal opioid related disorders in the USA, 2010–2017. *JAMA* 325(2), 146–155. doi:10.1001/j1m1.2020.24991.

Kocherlakota, P. (2014). Neonatal abstinence syndrome. *Pediatrics*, 134(2), e547–e561. doi:10.1542/peds.2013-3524.

National Center for Drug Abuse Statistics (n.d.). *Drug abuse statistics.* Retrieved August 17, 2024 from https://drugabusestatistics.org.

National Institute on Drug Abuse (2021). *Substance use in women research report: Summary.* NIDA. Retrieved August 15, 2024 from https://nida.nih.gov/publications/research-reports/substance-use-in-women/summary.

Qian, J., Chen, Q., Ward, S. M., Duan, E., & Zhang, Y. (2020). Impacts of caffeine during pregnancy. *Trends in Endocrinology and Metabolism*, 31(3), 218–227. doi:10.1016/j.tem.2019.11.004.

Substance-Abuse and Mental Health Services Administration (2020). *2020 national survey on drug use and health.* Retrieved August 17, 2024 from https://www.samhsa.gov.

Substance-Abuse and Mental Health Services Administration (2018). *Clinical guide for treating pregnant and parenting women with opioid use disorder and their infants.* Retrieved August 18, 2024 from https://store.samhsa.gov/sites/default/files/d7/priv/sma18-5054.pdf.

Shearer-Miller, J. S. (2019). *The long-term effects of neonatal abstinence syndrome on neurodevelopmental health outcomes.* Unpublished Dissertation. University of Tennessee-Knoxville.

Wachman, E., Schiff, D., & Silverstein, M. (2018). Neonatal abstinence syndrome: Advances in diagnosis and treatment. *JAMA* 319(13), 1362–1374. doi:1001/jama.2018.2640.

Warton, F. L., Taylor, P. A., Warton, C. M. R., Molteno, C. D., Wintermark, P., Lindinger, N. M., Zöllei. L., van der Kouwe, A., Jacobson, J. L., Jacobson, S. W., & Meintjes, E. M. (2018). Prenatal methamphetamine exposure is associated with corticostriatal white matter changes in neonates. *Metabolic Brain Disease* 33(2), 507–522. doi:10.1007/s11011-017-0135-9.

Wells, A. C., & Lotfipour, S. (2023). Prenatal nicotine exposure during pregnancy results in adverse neurodevelopmental alterations and neurobehavioral deficits. *Advances in Drugs and Alcohol Research*, 3. doi:10.3389/adar.2023.1.1638.

Winkelman, T. N. A., Villapiano, N., Kozhimannil, K.B., Davis, M. M., & Patrick, S. W. (2018). Incidence and costs of neonatal abstinence syndrome among infants with Medicaid: 2004–2014. *Pediatrics, 14(14)*: e2017–3520. doi:10.1542/peds.2017-3020.

Yen, E., Gaddis, N., Jantaie, L., & Davis, J. (2023). A review of the genomics of neonatal abstinence syndrome. *Frontier in Genetics*, 14, 1140400. doi:10.3389/fgen.2023.1140400.ecollection2023.

Zhang, R., Manza, P., & Volkow, N. D. (2021). Prenatal caffeine exposure: Association with neurodevelopmental outcomes in 9-to-11-year-old children. *Journal of Child Psychology and Psychiatry*, 63(5), 563–578. https://doi.org/10.1111/jcpp.13495.

6 Fetal Alcohol Spectrum Disorders (FASDs)

Ann Marie Leonard-Zabel

Introduction

Prenatal exposure to alcohol is never planned, but a result of an unknowing or alcohol-addicted mother who may not realize that alcohol is considered teratogenic and may produce disabilities in a developing fetus (Levinthal, 2023). Raising a child with FASDs can be both challenging and rewarding. With appropriate understanding and assistance a mother's guilt may evolve to love, care, and support despite the challenges encountered. This chapter will promote a deeper understanding of FASDs from a neurodevelopment standpoint to empower families and professionals to engage and inspire these children toward a future of hope.

Identification and Categorization of Fetal Alcohol Spectrum Disorders (FASDs)

According to Popova et al. (2016), FASDs involve three major alcohol-related diagnostic categories: (1) Fetal alcohol syndrome (FAS), (2) Partial fetal alcohol syndrome (pFAS), and (3) Alcohol-related neurodevelopment disorder (ARND). Each presents differently from the other by symptomatology and with a range of neurodevelopmental patterns of strengths and weaknesses. Recently, the DSM-5-TR (American Psychiatric Association, 2022) noted within Section II of the Emerging Measure and Models heading, that FASDs should be included in the future under the category of Neurobehavioral Disorders Associated with Prenatal Alcohol Exposure (ND-PAE) (Levinthal, 2023). According to the DSM-5-TR, the proposed criteria are not intended yet for clinical use until further sufficient evidence is obtained to warrant full inclusion in a future DSM edition. FASDs, along with FAS, are known as non-heritable routes of intrauterine impact from alcohol exposure (Denny et al., 2017).

The differences between FASDs and FAS are due to a broad continuum of effects. FASDs involve children who do not meet the full criteria of FAS. They are more challenging to identify since they may have no significant FAS physical features or may only exhibit a few of these features.

DOI: 10.4324/9781032703923-8

This can make affected children more at risk for school failure due to not being seen as having a visible disability. Their behaviors may be the only issue alerting parents and professionals to a disability needing to be explored further. FASDs are often referred to as the invisible disability (Bell et al., 2016). On the other hand, FAS is a medical diagnosis that involves both physical and cognitive symptoms due to confirmed prenatal exposure to alcohol during pregnancy. It has specific criteria involving three key features: (1) small stature/size involving head circumference/decreased cranial size, weight, and height, (2) difference with central nervous system issues involving learning, activity level, sensory concerns, and (3) specific facial features such as smaller eye openings, upper thin lip, flattened philtrum and flat midface, and smaller jaw for age. Structural brain abnormalities may include microcephaly, agenesis of the corpus callosum, and cerebellar hypoplasia. Neurological hard or soft signs may include fine motor skill impairments, hearing loss, difficulty with tandem gait, and poor eye-hand coordination (Malbin, 2017).

Two other alcohol-related FASDs are known as partial fetal alcohol syndrome (pFAS), and alcohol-related neurodevelopment disorder (ARND). A diagnosis of pFAS combines confirmation of maternal prenatal alcohol exposure and matches some, but not all, of the characteristics of FAS. Evidence of pFAS components blends characteristics of a facial anomaly with cognitive and/or behavioral patterns inconsistent with peer developmental level. It cannot be explained by familial background or environment only, such as learning issues, poor school performance, difficulty with impulse control problems involving social perception, higher-order language skills, or poor metacognition (Malbin, 2017). According to Levinthal (2023), "If only some of these characteristics are observed, the condition is referred to as partial fetal alcohol syndrome (pFAS). FAS and pFAS cases are included in a range of diagnoses in which congenital disabilities have been related to maternal alcohol consumption, collectively referred to as FASD" (p. 222). On the other hand, children diagnosed with ARND may have intellectual disabilities and problems with behavior and learning. They can struggle with math, memory, attention, judgment, and poor impulse control (Centers for Disease Control and Prevention, CDC, n.d.; Reid et al., 2022). Additional terms noted within the medical community include neurobehavioral disorder associated with prenatal alcohol exposure (ND-PAE) and alcohol-related birth defects (ARBD). Children diagnosed with ND-PAE exhibit problems in three main areas: thinking and memory; behavior problems involving irritability, moodiness, and difficulty shifting attention; and day-to-day living coupled with adaptive behavior skills. For a child to be diagnosed with ND-PAE, the mother must have consumed more than 13 alcoholic drinks per month within any 30 days of pregnancy. In addition, children with ARBD are at risk for problems with the heart, kidneys, bones, and hearing (Flannigan et al., 2022; Hagen et al., 2016).

Genetics and FASDs

It is commonly understood amongst professionals in the substance use disorders profession that excessive alcohol consumption can lead to a variety of issues, involving biological impact especially when pregnant. According to Kaminen-Ahola (2020), "Genetics and environmental factors contribute to the broad phenotype: chromosomal rearrangements, risk, and protective alleles, environmental-induced epigenetic alternations, as well as gene-environment interactions are all involved" (p.1). FASDs etiology is further complicated by deficits involving overall growth, congenital disabilities, and neurodevelopmental impairments, which continue to be studied to determine which biomarkers contribute to these concerns to assist with early diagnosis and intervention.

Epidemiology

According to May et al., (2018) and Denny et al., (2020), research studies involving trends in alcohol use among pregnant women in the United States of America from 2011 to 2018 validated alcohol as the leading preventable cause of intellectual developmental disability (IDD) and the leading cause of FASDs. The results of the study pointed to alcohol use increasing among reproductive-aged women. The incidence of these conditions is observed to be between 1.1% and 5.0% in first-grade students, particularly in four regions of the United States: the Rocky Mountains, Midwest, Southeast, and Pacific Southwest. This increase can be attributed to changing gender roles and economic development, targeted alcohol marketing, reduced social stigma, and shifts in women's workplace and educational roles. As such, there has been a notable rise in alcohol consumption among women of childbearing age.

In the United States, the rate of FAS is estimated to be about 0.2 to 1.5 per 1000 births. However, the rates can fluctuate. For instance, within the Native American population, FASDs are estimated to be three times higher than FAS (CDC, n.d.). The estimated prevalence of FASDs has challenges, but various methods have been employed to gauge their occurrence in the population. FASDs encompass a range of diagnoses stemming from prenatal alcohol exposure, with FAS representing the most severe manifestation characterized by multiple physical and developmental impairments. The CDC (n.d.) studies conducted in specific United States locales have identified approximately one infant with FAS per 1000 live births, as revealed by medical analyses. Within recent assessments of children aged 7 to 9 years, the CDC identified FAS in 0.3 out of 1000 cases. Conversely, studies that employ direct evaluations of school-aged children across various United States communities have yielded higher prevalence estimates, ranging from 6 to 9 cases per 1000 children. Comprehensive estimations covering the entire spectrum of FASDs remain scarce, but community studies funded by the National Institutes of Health suggest that the prevalence of FASDs in the United States and certain Western European countries could range from 1 to 5 cases per 100 school age children (May et al., 2018).

Diagnosis of FASDs

FASDs are a group of conditions that can be prevented and are caused by maternal alcohol use during pregnancy. These disorders are characterized by a range of physical, behavioral, and cognitive challenges. While healthcare and research professionals recognize FASDs as a distinct clinical condition, there is still no consensus on a diagnostic standard that is accepted worldwide (Brown et al., 2019). Furthermore, Wozniak, Riley, and Charness (2019) conducted an in-depth review of FASDs, addressing the diagnostic criteria, the disorders' prevalence, assessment methods, pathophysiological basis, and management options. They reported neuroimaging results showing irregularities in brain structure, disrupted cortical development, and compromised white matter tracts and their functional connections. The authors emphasize the significant public health implications of FASDs due to prenatal alcohol exposure, which leads to enduring neurodevelopmental and physical difficulties. They call attention to the urgent need for a universally standardized diagnostic approach for FASDs, a goal that remains unfulfilled despite its importance in clinical practice.

The prenatal brain may be affected by alcohol exposure in many ways at different stages of development. The variability in FASDs' manifestation among children can be attributed to factors such as the timing of alcohol exposure during pregnancy, the quantity of alcohol consumed, genetic influences, maternal stress, the mother's age, and nutritional status, along with the mother's mental health. For example, according to the DSM-5-TR (American Psychiatric Association, 2022), diagnostic features of ND-PAE encompass impairments in neurocognitive, behavioral, and adaptive functioning associated with prenatal alcohol exposure. ND-PAE may be diagnosed with or without physical effects. ND-PAE is complicated by neurocognitive, behavioral, and adaptive functioning, with the present needs varying from one child to another. In addition, the DSM-5-TR reports that the central nervous system (CNS) dysfunction seen in individuals with ND-PAE can often lead to multiple organ system issues, including but not limited to heart, kidney, gastrointestinal abnormalities, higher levels of school disruptive experiences, poor employment records, involvement with law enforcement, legal or psychiatric confinement, dependent living, and suicidal thoughts and behaviors with impaired affect regulation, especially in adolescents.

When looking at neuropsychological implications, what is important is the timing of exposure to brain development that individuals with FASDs experience. Alcohol's relentless toxic impact may hijack various parts or entire portions of the fetal brain. Therefore, memory, attention, sensory responses, executive functioning, planning, foresight ability, visual and auditory processing speed, and psychosocial developmental growth may be affected. Slower processing speed involving thinking and hearing, retrieving information just learned, difficulties forming links and associations to material learned, and generalization difficulties can impact learning and psychosocial developmental progress. (Geddes, 2021).

According to Malbin (2017), there are primary, secondary, and tertiary behavioral characteristics associated with FASDs. Primary characteristics are reflective of brain structure and function and vary in degree. Some noted behaviors include appearing or acting younger than their stated chronological age, impulsivity, distractibility, and over-or-under sensitivity to stimuli with personal strengths in some areas such as music, art, interpersonal skills, and basic computer use. Secondary characteristics are behaviors developed over time but have a poor fit between the child and the environment. Behaviors may include frustration and fatigue, anxiousness, fear, being rigid, argumentativeness, becoming overwhelmed, having poor self-esteem, and getting picked on or bullied. These children often experience school problems leading to detention or expulsion, victimization (sexual or emotional abuse) coupled with depression and exhibit self-destructive or self-harm behaviors coinciding with suicidal ideation. Tertiary characteristics involve delinquent and criminal involvement, trouble at home, school, and in the community, involvement of social services, drug use, or addiction. Children and adolescents may be given the diagnoses of oppositional defiant disorder or intermittent explosive rage reaction, among others. Parents, school officials, and the mental health community need to work together to be proactive so that no child with FASDs will enter the secondary or tertiary behavioral characteristics, which can impact the trajectory of the individual's life.

Characteristics, Symptoms, and Neuropsychological Implications of FAS and FASDs

The research on FASD is rich with information involving neurological implications. In a recent study by Boateng and colleagues (2023), they investigated how brain structures differ between individuals with fetal alcohol spectrum disorders (FASDs) and typically developing controls. Their research aimed to quantify differences and explore various FASD subtypes. Specifically, they hypothesized that the FASD group would show smaller brain volume, reduced cortical thickness, and decreased surface area compared to controls. However, the partial fetal alcohol syndrome (pFAS) and fetal alcohol syndrome (FAS) subtypes exhibited the most significant effects, while the PAE/alcohol-related neurodevelopmental disorder (ARND) subtype demonstrated intermediate effects. Despite these findings, the research reports there is no safe level of alcohol intake at any time during pregnancy and total abstinence is recommended.

When reviewing the neuropsychological implications from Glass et al. (2014) general intellectual functioning is reported to range from a standard score of 40 (severe intellectual disability) to 112 (above average intellectual functioning), with the average standard score frequently reported as 70 (low in comparison to same-age peers but average for the FAS child). Verbal and nonverbal abilities are both affected but remain stable over the child's life span. In addition, a study by Kully-Martens and colleagues (2022), delved further into the cognitive profile of individuals with fetal alcohol spectrum disorders (FASDs). While trying to pinpoint specific strengths proved challenging, they noticed trends indicating that nonverbal reasoning, learning, and memory abilities tended to be stronger than verbal abilities. Acknowledging these relative strengths can guide more effective intervention approaches.

In addition, Lange et al. (2019) identified several subtests that effectively detect the neuropsychological characteristics of FASDs. The study retained ten observed indicator variables, eight of which were obtained from three neurodevelopmental test batteries such as the Wechsler Abbreviated Scales of Intelligence, Second Edition (WAIS-II; Wechsler, 2011) involving Block Design, Similarities, and Vocabulary; the Wechsler Intelligence Scale for Children Fourth Edition (WISC-IV; Wechsler, 2003) using the Coding and Symbol Search subtests, and the Developmental Neuropsychological Assessment Second Edition (NEPSY-II; Korkman et al., 2007) using the Response Set, Arrows, and Word Generation (letters) subtests. The remaining two variables were derived from the Child Behavior Checklist (CBCL; Achenbach, 2010), specifically involving two syndrome scales known as attention problems and rule-breaking behaviors. Australia's National Voice on Fetal Alcohol Spectrum Disorders (FASD United, 2024) suggests the following formulation of assessments depending on the child's need and stamina: (1) motor skills including fine and gross motor, graphomotor skills, and visuospatial integration; (2) cognitive skills involving verbal and nonverbal reasoning, visual and verbal processing speed, and working memory; (3) language skills including expressive and receptive language, (4) academic achievement encompassing literacy areas such as reading, writing, spelling, and written or oral expression; (5) memory involving both verbal and visual domains; (6) attention including selective, divided, and alternating attention, particularly skills involving switching focus or sustaining attention; (7) executive functioning specifically reviewing for higher-level skills such as organization, efficiency, and controlling one's thoughts and behaviors; (8) affect regulation assessing mood and anxiety; (9) adaptive behaviors involving life skills and adaptability to everyday tasks; and (10) if appropriate, ruling in or out significant social-emotional concerns.

According to Malbin (2017, p.21), neurological impacts from FASDs include the following:

- Slow visual and auditory processing speeds involving metacognitive thinking and reasoning.
- Slow processing speed impacting retrieval of information.
- Gaps with associations of information leading to difficulty linking coherent thought processes.
- Gaps with forming links and associations when learning.
- Difficulty with abstract thoughts.
- Having a challenging time seeing outcomes.
- Difficulty following through with saying one thing but doing something else.
- Difficulty grasping concepts holistically, only able to understand in a piecemeal fashion.

Keeping the above neurological impacts in mind, these children would benefit from a comprehensive school neuropsychological assessment and intervention plan to include cognitive, achievement, visual and auditory processing, higher-order reasoning skills, and memory involving immediate and delayed recall, executive functioning, verbal and nonverbal language, fine and gross motor, attention, and emotional regulation.

Treatment and Intervention Strategies for FAS/FASDs

Children with FAS and FASDs exhibit a range of neurocognitive challenges that affect their learning, memory, focus, and executive functions. The severity of these challenges can vary widely. The (CDC, n.d.) notes that while there is no definitive cure for FAS or FASDs, early intervention services can be beneficial. These services include medical care, behavioral therapies, and family support systems. A multidisciplinary team of health professionals may be involved in the care of these children, which could include a pediatrician, geneticist, immunologist, ear, nose, and throat specialist, audiologist, speech therapist, physical and occupational therapists, neurologist, ophthalmologist, gastroenterologist, nutritionist, and various psychologists specializing in clinical, school, and neuropsychological domains, and include parents and/or caregivers. To manage symptoms such as hyperactivity, concentration issues, impulsiveness, mood swings, sleep disturbances, irritability, antisocial actions, aggression, anxiety, and other neurobehavioral concerns, a combination of medical treatments may be prescribed, including stimulants, mood stabilizers, antipsychotics, and anxiolytics, tailored to the individual needs of the child. Additionally, alternative therapies such as biofeedback, auditory integration training, pet therapy, relaxation techniques, yoga, and physical exercise may also be considered as part of the treatment plan.

Treatment intervention strategies designed to support children and their families might include participation in the Good Buddies program (O'Connor, 2023), which focuses on imparting suitable social skills across a span of 12 weeks. Additionally, the Families Moving Forward (FMF) program (Seattle Children's Hospital, 2024a), spanning a year with 16 biweekly sessions, offers guidance on constructive behavioral support strategies for parents or caregivers. Furthermore, the neurocognitive initiative called Parents and Children Together (PACT) (Wells et al., 2012) aims to bolster self-regard and executive function abilities through a series of 12-week sessions, as reported by the CDC (n.d.).

Implications for School Services and Educational Progress

One of the advantages of the United States educational system is the federal and state laws that surround special education and disability. Two laws in particular that may apply to children with FAS or FASDs are the Individuals with Disabilities Education Act (IDEA) and Section 504 of the Rehabilitation Act of 1973. A child may qualify for either, or both, or none depending on an assortment of variables. IDEA focuses on specialized instruction and related services via an Individualized Education Plan (IEP) whereas a 504 plan is developed to provide accommodation that will ensure academic success in the learning environment. The difference between these two laws involves the services offered or required.

However, not all children who have a disability will meet the legal requirements for specialized instruction. Having a diagnosis of FAS or FASDs does not automatically qualify a child for an IEP and/or a 504 plan. Although FAS and FASDs are not listed as one of the 13 categories for special education under United States federal laws, if a child with FAS or FASDs meets specific legal parameters specified in these laws, he, she, or they, may receive modifications and/or accommodations. One major area under IDEA law that a child with FAS or FASDs might qualify for is under the category of Other Health Impairment depending upon additional involved health factors.

According to Popova et al. (2016) and Streissguth et al. (2004), children affected by prenatal alcohol exposure are at risk of developing what are called secondary disabilities, which involve school failure and dropout, mental health problems, risk of substance use and/or abuse, unemployment, homelessness, and being lured into criminal activity, resulting in reduced quality of life and significant societal and economic costs. Due to their neurocognitive and learning risks, most children do require special education, especially with the comorbid impact of attention, executive functioning, processing speeds, language, and memory, all of which impact the ability to learn.

Enhancing Support for Students with FAS or FASDs: A Guide for Educators and Parents

The pivotal role of educators and parents lies in thoughtfully selecting and implementing a range of strategies and support mechanisms specifically designed for children with fetal alcohol syndrome (FAS) or fetal alcohol spectrum disorders (FASDs). Initially endorsed by Williams et al. (2015), ongoing research has been instrumental in shaping evidence-based FASD education for professionals, parents, and the broader public. Through screening, assessment, intervention, and comprehensive management of educational and medical needs, educators and healthcare providers can significantly contribute to fostering academic achievement and social skills in children, both at home and within educational institutions.

Children with FAS or FASDs may encounter significant obstacles in mastering academics especially mathematical concepts. The Math Interactive Learning Experience (MILE; Seattle Children's Hospital, 2024b) responds to this need by providing exhaustive resources for both parents and educators, aimed at improving mathematical literacy and motor coordination. Furthermore, Do2Learn (2024) offers a collection of materials tailored to aid children with FASDs. The Alert Program (William & Shellenberger, 2024), initially conceived for occupational therapy, has been adapted effectively for those with FASDs, enhancing executive functions, emotional stability, self-regulation, and social engagement.

Another contributor of interventions is FASD United (2024) which provides a comprehensive suite of educational content and tools. This includes the K-12 FASD Education and Prevention Curriculum, the enlightening video "8 Magic Keys: Strategies for Students with FAS or FASD," the brochure "Ain't Misbehaving: Understanding Behaviors in Students with FASD," and personalized educational profiles "Meet Your Student (Teen)" and "Meet Your Student (Youth)." FASD United's portal is a reservoir of information for parents and educators seeking further guidance. Additionally, the work of Petrenko and Alto, (2017) offers a plethora of strategies and methods to support children with FAS or FASDs, including the Visual Performance Attention Training (VPAT), Rehearsal Training for working memory enhancement, Cognitive Control Therapy (CCT), GoFar for metacognitive strategy development, the Alert Program for Self-Regulation, Literacy and Language Training (LLT), Project Step-Up, the Coaching Families Program (CF), and the Families Moving Forward Program (FMF). These interventions represent a beacon of hope, potentially transforming the lives of children with FAS or FASDs and paving the way for a fulfilling life they richly deserve.

Summary

This chapter has explored the complex neurodevelopmental effects of fetal alcohol spectrum disorders (FASDs) on children. Prenatal alcohol exposure can lead to a range of neurocognitive, behavioral, and physical impairments, underscoring the critical need for early diagnosis and intervention. These measures can significantly improve the developmental outcomes for affected children. The literature emphasizes the importance of timely identification and tailored interventions to address the unique needs of each child, thereby enhancing their potential for success in various aspects of life.

Resources

Websites

Fetal Alcohol Exposure National Institute on Alcohol and Alcoholism (NIAAA): www.nih.gov

Organizations

National Association on Fetal Alcohol Spectrum Disorders: www.nofas.org FASD United (formerly NOFAS): https://fasdunited.org

Fetal Alcohol Spectrum Consultation, Education and Training Services (FASCETS): https://fascets.org

The National Voice on Fetal Alcohol Spectrum Disorders (FASD United): www.fasunited.org

Books

Catterick, M. & Curran, L. (2014). *Understanding fetal alcohol spectrum disorder: A guide to FASD for parents, carers, and professionals.* Jessica Kingsley Publishers.

Do2Learn. (2024). Title of the website. Retrieved August 2, 2024 from Do2Learn.

FASD_National_Directory_2022–2.pdf (www.uw.edu) Fetal Alcohol Spectrum Disorders (FASD) National Resource Directory: National & State Organization and Resources Addressing FASD

Malbin, D. (2017). *Fetal alcohol spectrum disorders: Trying differently rather than harder.* Fetal Alcohol Syndrome Consultation. Education and Training Services.

References

Achenbach, T. M. (2010). *Child behavior checklist (CBCL).* Achenbach System of Empirically Based Assessment.

American Psychiatric Association (2022). *Diagnostic and statistical manual of mental disorders* (5th ed., text rev.). American Psychiatric Association. https://doi.org/10.1176/appi.books.9780890425787.

Bell, E., Andrew, G., Di Pietro, N., Chudley, A. E., Reynolds, J., & Racine, E. (2016). It is a shame! Stigma against fetal alcohol spectrum disorder: Examining the ethical implications for public health practices and policies. *Public Health Ethics*, 9(1), 65–77. https://doi.org/10.1093/phe/phv012.

Boateng, T., Beauchamp, K., Torres, F., Ruffaner-Hanson, C. D., Pinner, J. F. L., Vakamudi, K., Cerros, C., Hill, D. E., & Stephen, J. M. (2023). Brain structural differences in children with fetal alcohol spectrum disorder and its subtypes. *Frontiers in neuroscience*, 17, 1152038. https://doi.org/10.3389/fnins.2023.1152038.

Brown, J. M., Bland, R., Jonson, E., & Greenshaw, A. J. (2019). The standardization of diagnostic criteria for fetal alcohol spectrum disorder (FASDS): Implications for research, clinical practice, and population health. *The Canadian Journal of Psychiatry. Revue Canadienne De Psychiatrie*, 64(3), 169–176. https://doi.org/10.1177/0706743718777398.

Centers for Disease Control and Prevention (n.d.). *Fetal alcohol spectrum disorders: Data and statistics on FASDs.* Retrieved May 27, 2024, from https://www.cdc.gov/fasd/data/index.html.

Denny, C. H., Acero, C. S., Terplan, M., & Kim, S. Y. (2020). Trends in alcohol use among pregnant women in the U.S., 2011–2018. *American Journal of Preventive Medicine*, 59(5), 768–769. https://doi.org/10.1016/j.amepre.2020.05.017.

Denny, L., Coles, S., & Blitz, R. (2017). Fetal alcohol syndrome and fetal alcohol spectrum disorders. *American Family Physician*, 96(8), 515–522A. https://doi.org/10.1080/09362835.2015.1064415.

Do2Learn (2024). *Do2Learn: Educational resource for special needs.* Retrieved July 16, 2024 from https://do2learn.com.

FASD United (2024). *The national voice on fetal alcohol spectrum disorders.* Retrieved July 24, 2024 from www.fasdunited.org.

Flannigan, K. R., Coons-Harding, K. D., Turner, O., Symes, B. A., Morrison, K., & Burns, C. (2022). A survey of measures used to assess brain function at FASD clinics in Canada. *Canadian Psychology / Psychologie canadienne*, 63(1), 106–119. https://doi.org/10.1037/cap0000245.

Geddes, A. (2021). *A Complicated Beautiful Brain.* Self-Published.

Glass, L., Ware, A. L., & Mattson, S. N. (2014). Neurobehavioral, neurologic, and neuroimaging characteristics of fetal alcohol spectrum disorders. *Handbook of Clinical Neurology*, 125, 435–462. https://doi.org/10.1016/B978-0-444-62619-6.00025-2.

Hagan, J. F., Jr, Balachova, T., Bertrand, J., Chasnoff, I., Dang, E., Fernandez-Baca, D., Kable, J., Kosofsky, B., Senturias, Y. N., Singh, N., Sloane, M., Weitzman, C., Zubler, J., Neurobehavioral Disorder Associated with Prenatal Alcohol Exposure Workgroup, & American Academy of Pediatrics (2016). Neurobehavioral disorder associated with prenatal alcohol exposure. *Pediatrics*, 138(4), e20151553. https://doi.org/10.1542/peds.2015-1553.

Kaminen-Ahola, N. (2020). Fetal alcohol spectrum disorders: Genetic and epigenetic mechanisms. *Obstetrics & Gynecology Prenatal Diagnosis, 40*(9), 1185–1192. https://doi.org/10.1002/pd.573.

Korkman, M., Kirk, U., & Kemp, S. (2007). *NEPSY-II: A developmental neuropsychological approach*. The Psychological Corporation.

Kully-Martens, K., McNeil, A., Pei, J., & Rasmussen, C. (2022). Toward a strengths-based cognitive profile of children with fetal alcohol spectrum disorders: Implications for intervention. *Current Developmental Disorders Reports*, 9, 53–62. https://doi.org/10.1007/s40474-022-00245-5.

Lange, S., Shield, K., Rehm, J., Anagnostou, E., & Popova, S. (2019). Fetal alcohol spectrum disorder: Neurodevelopmentally and behaviorally indistinguishable from other neurodevelopmental disorders. *BMC Psychiatry*, 19, 1–10. https://doi.org/10.1186/s12888-019-2289-y.

Levinthal, C. F. (2023). *Drugs, behavior, and modern society* (9th ed.). Pearson.

Malbin, D. (2017). *Trying differently rather than harder: Fetal alcohol spectrum disorders*. FASCETS, Inc.

May, P. A., Chambers, C. D., Kalberg, W. O., Zellner, J., Feldman, H., Buckley, D., Kopald, D., Hasken, J. M., Xu, R., Honerkamp-Smith, G., Taras, H., Manning, M. A., Robinson, L. K., Adam, M. P., Abdul-Rahman, O., Vaux, K., Jewett, T., Elliott, A. J., Kable, J. A., … Hoyme, H. E. (2018). Prevalence of fetal alcohol spectrum disorders in 4 US communities. *JAMA*, 319(5), 474–482. https://doi.org/10.1001/jama.2017.21896.

O'Connor, M. J. (2023). *Good Buddies program for children with fetal alcohol spectrum disorders (FASD)*. University of California, Los Angeles.

Petrenko, C. L. & Alto, M. E. (2017). Fetal alcohol spectrum disorder: Neurodevelopmentally and behaviorally indistinguishable from other neurodevelopmental disorders. *European Journal of Medical Genetics*, 60(1), 79–91. https://doi.org/10.1016/j.ejmg.2016.10.005.

Popova, S., Lange, S., Burd, L., & Rehm, J. (2016). Special education of children with fetal alcohol spectrum disorder. *Exceptionality*, 42(3), 165–175. https://doi.org/10.1080/09362835.2015.1064415.

Reid, N., Shanley, D. C., Logan, J., White, C., Liu, W., & Hawkins, E. (2022). International survey of specialist fetal alcohol spectrum disorder diagnostic clinics: Comparison of diagnostic approach and considerations regarding the potential for unification. *International Journal of Environmental Research and Public Health*, 19(23), 15663. https://doi.org/10.3390/ijerph192315663.

Seattle Children's Hospital (2024a). *Families moving forward program*. Seattle Children's Hospital FMF Program. Retrieved July 15, 2024 from familiesmovingforward@seattlechildrens.org.

Seattle Children's Hospital (2024b). *Math interactive learning experience (MILE)*. Retrieved from Seattle Children's Hospital FMF Program. Retrieved July 15, 2024 from Math Interactive Learning Experience Mile (cebc4cw.org).

Streissguth, A. P., Bookstein, F. L., Barr, H. M., Sampson, P. D., O'Malley, K., & Young, J. K. (2004). Risk factors for adverse life outcomes in fetal alcohol syndrome and fetal alcohol effects. *Journal of Developmental and Behavioral Pediatrics*, 25(4), 228–238.

Wechsler, D. (2003). *Wechsler Intelligence Scale for Children–Fourth Edition (WISC-IV)*. Pearson.

Wechsler, D. (2011). *Wechsler Abbreviated Scale of Intelligence–Second Edition (WASI-II)* [Database record]. APA PsycTESTS.

Wells, A. M., Chasnoff, I. J., Schmidt, C. A., Telford, E., & Schwartz, L. D. (2012). Neurocognitive habilitation therapy for children with fetal alcohol spectrum disorders: An adaptation of the Alert Program ®. *American Journal of Occupational Therapy*, 66(1), 24–34. https://doi.org/10.5014/ajot.2012.002691.

William, M. S. & Shellenberger, S. (2024). *The alert program: Self-regulation made easy.* TherapyWorks, Inc.

Williams, J. F., Smith, V. C., & Committee on Substance Abuse (2015). Behavioral interventions in fetal alcohol spectrum disorders. *Pediatrics*, 136(5), e20153113. https://doi.org/10.1542/peds.2015-3113.

Wozniak, J. R., Riley, E. P., & Charness, M. E. (2019). Diagnosis, epidemiology, assessment, pathophysiology, and management of fetal alcohol spectrum disorders. *The Lancet Neurology*, 18(8), 760–770. https://doi.org/10.1016/S1474-4422(19)30150–30154.

7 Neurotoxins and Pediatric Poisoning

Nadia Webb, Brandy Machado and Tessah Joseph

Introduction

People are exposed to many different toxins or poisons during their lives. Self-exposure occurs to drugs, alcohol, or tobacco. Other toxic substances are present in our environment, often without our knowledge. Heavy metals, petroleum products, radioactive substances, asbestos, and lead-related products are some common, hidden, environmental toxins. Other toxins include mold and infectious lifeforms, such as tick-borne and mosquito-borne illnesses. These compounds are categorized as neurotoxins since they are considered toxic, or potentially toxic, to the nervous system. Neurotoxins show neuropsychological patterns analogous to fingerprints that may identify which toxin is the culprit and help identify practical consequences and service needs.

The brain is acutely vulnerable to toxicity due to its metabolic demands and biochemical sensitivity and particularly in children who have faster metabolisms than adults. Younger children are even more likely to experience accidental poisoning since they have greater contact with contaminated surfaces while crawling, exploring, and oral ingestion. The data reflects this vulnerability as most calls to Poison Control concern children under six years old, particularly toddlers. According to the data, most poisonings happen at home when children find pills on the floor (27%), in a purse or wallet (20%), or left out on a counter or nightstand (20%). Families that require a high number of medications are at particular risk, such as those with medically fragile children who are often prescribed multiple medications—some of which are colorful and sweet-tasting—and households with elderly members who may require non-childproof containers.[1]

While poisonings are more frequent in young children, they are typically less severe. Serious poisonings occur about six times more often among adolescents and are frequently the result of intent to self-harm.[2] Data from the National Poison Data System show a rise in suicide attempts by self-poisoning among children aged 10–18 (Spiller et al., 2020). Boys account for most poison exposures until age 13, after which there is a significant increase among young women. Those suicide attempts are correlated with

DOI: 10.4324/9781032703923-9

high stress levels, with school stressors posing a unique risk. Individuals with ADHD, a condition that can cause added stress in school settings, have higher suicide rates regardless of gender or age (Balazs & Kereszteny, 2017). Suicide attempts among children and teens increase during school months between Monday through Thursday (Matsubayashi, Ueda, & Yoshikawa, 2016). This pattern fades after age 18, further suggesting the unique risks of school stressors.

Direct and Indirect Effects

Poisons have both direct and indirect effects on the brain. Toxins can directly or indirectly harm the brain by disrupting the brain's oxygen supply (e.g., metabolic acidosis); triggering chronic inflammation in brain tissue or altering the brain's immune response; reducing cerebral blood flow and creating oxidative stress (an imbalance in the free radicals); disrupting neurotransmitters and the complex chemical balance of the brain; or directly damaging and killing brain cells causing neuronal necrosis. Indirect effects are often the result of a cascade of events that negatively impact the individual's physical, cognitive, or neuropsychological functions following the direct damage sustained. The toxins introduced below were chosen because they are common and relevant to school psychologists and also introduce the direct and indirect effects in a practical way.

Carbon Monoxide

Carbon monoxide (CO) is a colorless, odorless gas released by incomplete combustion, typically from faulty heating systems or poor ventilation. CO poisoning can lead to brain damage, impairing vision, movement, auditory processing, attention, executive functioning, learning, and memory. CO poisoning can also lead to cardiac compromise. Brains exposed to CO poisoning appear to age more rapidly, eventually leading to cognitive collapse. When exposure occurs at a young age, it not only contributes to rapid cognitive decline but also impedes brain development because the brain develops in an injured state (Hedges et al., 2019). CO poisoning has a threshold—if an individual is symptomatic, there is a 50/50 chance of developing long-term impairments. Some individuals are more vulnerable than others, and while it's difficult to pinpoint exactly why, genetics and preexisting health conditions play a role.

CO poisoning often impairs vision, including eye movement, visual field cuts, and damage to primary vision regions in the occipital cortex (Bi et al., 2020). A normal routine eye examination does not rule these out. It's prudent to assess visual field cuts, judgment of line orientation, color perception, visual tracking, movement perception, visual motor integration, object recognition, etc. Visual symptoms can show delayed onset in children and may be the primary symptom. Auditory processing deficits may co-occur with visual processing impairments. Difficulties may be seen with expressive and receptive language, phonological processing, reading fluency, reading comprehension, and written language.

Hyperbaric oxygen therapy (HBOT) is the best-researched treatment for cognitive impairment or delayed neurological sequelae (DNS) (see Lead section below). Double-blind studies indicate that HBOT may reverse some of the effects of CO poisoning, as well as other brain injuries, in children. While this is an emerging literature, the results appear promising (Hadanny et al., 2022; Karaman et al., 2016; Siewiera et al., 2019).

Lead

The CDC states there is no safe level of lead exposure, equating any lead exposure to lead poisoning. Even at lower levels, such as 5 mcg/dL, the consequences are measurable. For each 1 mcg/dL increase in blood lead concentration, there is a 0.7-point decrement in arithmetic scores, an approximately 1-point decrement in reading scores, a 0.1-point decrement in scores on measures of nonverbal reasoning, and a 0.5-point decrement in scores on short-term memory (Lanphear et al., 2000). Duration and dose of exposure correlate with the severity of the outcome. Lead poisoning is usually caused by lead-based paint or contaminated soil. Lead's sweet taste increases the risk for children who are young or have pica in settings with peeling lead paint.

Lead poisoning lowers intelligence (Bellinger, 2016; Surkan et al., 2007). It can also damage hearing and auditory processing through the loss of outer hair cells in the ear, degeneration of spiral ganglion neurons in the cochlea, and damage to central auditory processing networks. Performance on central auditory processing disorder (CAPD) tasks declines as blood lead levels increase (Schneider, 2023).

Moderate to severe lead poisoning also causes anemia by interfering with the normal use of iron in forming heme in red blood cells. Lead poisoning includes a wide range of cellular and intracellular damage mechanisms (e.g., apoptosis, excitotoxicity, disruption of second messenger systems, mitochondrial function, neurotransmitter synthesis and release, abnormal myelin formation, and dendritic branching patterns (Schneider)).

Lead may cause delayed neurological sequelae (DNS), meaning symptoms develop well after the poisoning. DNS, however, is not unique to lead, and the proposed causal factors include:

- Disrupting critical periods.
- Triggering neuroinflammatory responses in the brain.
- Impairing synaptic function, reducing the efficiency of neurotransmission.
- Promoting apoptosis (programmed cell death).
- Interfering with myelination and disrupting neural communication.
- Compromising the blood–brain barrier.

- Contributing to global atrophy, particularly frontal gray matter, such as the anterior cingulate cortex (ACC). Atrophy can be noted in other regions (e.g., poor fine motor skills correlated with the loss of cerebellar volume).

Lead Mitigation

Once lead has entered the body, especially the bones, it is difficult to remove. Dietary zinc and iron can mitigate lead absorption through competitive inhibition. When there is an adequate intake of zinc and iron, they can outcompete lead for binding to transport proteins and receptor sites in the intestinal cells. Chelation therapy, a medical procedure that uses a chemical solution to remove heavy metals and minerals from the body, may decrease circulating blood lead concentrations by binding to metals and facilitating excretion. The common agents are Dimercaptosuccinic Acid (DMSA), Edetate Calcium Disodium (CaNa2EDTA), and British anti-Lewisite (BAL, Dimercaprol). However, chelating agents can strip away necessary minerals, destabilize cardiac function, and increase seizure risk if managed improperly.[3]

An enriched environment that includes elements such as complex toys, social interactions, and varied physical spaces mitigates lead's impact on behavior and cognition (Schneider et al., 2001). Environmental enrichment can reverse long-term deficits in spatial learning caused by lead exposure, although the biological mechanisms remain unclear. Studies have considered deficits in N-methyl-D-aspartate (NMDA) receptors, brain-derived neurotrophic factor (BDNF), and alterations in mRNA signaling pathways as underlying factors (Guilarte et al., 2003). Longitudinal studies suggest cognitive enrichment programs can improve IQ scores and are most effective when paired with reduced lead exposure. One such study found that comprehensive interventions largely closed the gap with age- and demographically matched peers if the lead-poisoned children received lead remediation, nutritional assessment, medical evaluation, developmental surveillance, and public assistance referrals (Billings & Schnepel, 2018). Head Start and other early interventions improve cognitive and developmental outcomes in children with lead poisoning. Home-based interventions that provide cognitive stimulation and support to parents also improve children's cognitive development (Moodie et al., 2013).

Iron

Although iron is essential for brain functions, such as neuronal development, myelination, synthesis of neurotransmitters, electronic transport, and respiration, the same features that make iron useful and indispensable for life can make it toxic and dangerous when too much or too little iron is present. Children's or gummy vitamins containing iron look like candy, and children may eat them, accordingly, causing acute iron poisoning. This presents as stomach pain, vomiting, and diarrhea, typically prompting parents to seek medical care. If treatment is delayed or the poisoning is severe, it can lead to liver failure, permanent gastrointestinal (GI) damage, cognitive impairment from blood loss, or seizures (Tarango & Liu, 2016). Like many poisons, iron produces a cascade of indirect effects that can damage the brain.

In high doses, iron ions react with gastric acids to form corrosive compounds like ferrous sulfate, which damages the GI lining. This can cause GI bleeding, which reduces hemoglobin levels and diminishes the blood's oxygen-carrying capacity in the brain (Huo et al., 2022). GI scarring can then impede the absorption of nutrients, such as vitamin B12. Insufficient B12 can cause tingling and numbness in the extremities, muscle weakness, and difficulties with coordination. If untreated, it can cause permanent damage, affecting gait, balance, and cognitive functions (Hunt, Harrington, & Robinson, 2014).

Pesticide Poisoning

Pesticides, such as organophosphates or carbamates, can lead to CNS toxicity. Poisoned individuals may experience DNS, including neuropathy, muscle weakness, and cognitive impairments. Poisoning while in utero typically produces the most global, nonspecific impact. For example, prenatal exposure to chlorpyrifos, a common pesticide, was associated with a decrease in communication scores, both at 12 months and 18 months of age ($P < 0.01$). Higher concentrations of an organophosphate pesticide predicted lower gross motor abilities in 12- and 18-month-old children ($P < 0.01$) per research by Wei and colleagues (2023).

Many pesticides are organophosphates—essentially, low-level nerve agents that bind irreversibly to acetylcholinesterase (AChE) receptors. Because of the irreversible binding, the effects can remain over 2–3 weeks until new AChE receptors form. Long-term effects may include neurodevelopmental delays, learning disabilities, and behavioral issues. A study of neuropsychological assessment results in healthy school-aged children who had been hospitalized in infancy after exposure to organophosphate pesticides found the exposed children seemed to have overcome the acute one-time exposure incident by global measures (e.g., all attended regular schools). However, compared to peers, there were deficits on testing, such as inhibitory motor control (Kofman et al., 2006).

Poisonings: Drugs and Medications

Unintentional poisoning is the leading cause of injury death in the United States, comprising nearly 42% of the fatalities in 2020. About 75% of these deaths involved an opioid, and drug overdose deaths have quadrupled since 1999, largely because of Fentanyl.[4] Fentanyl is now appearing in street drugs, such as marijuana—exposing individuals who would otherwise not knowingly take an opiate and have no opiate tolerance.

Most non-fatal poisonings are from over-the-counter remedies. The two most frequent were ibuprofen (8%) and vitamins (8%), followed by acetaminophen, diphenhydramine, and dextromethorphan. Among prescription drugs, most overdoses involve benzodiazepines, atypical antipsychotics, methylphenidate, clonidine, antihypertensives (excluding diuretics), and beta blockers. Exposures in teens and adults were more serious, with 21% of teens and 19% of adults having a moderate, major, or fatal effect compared to 1% of children younger than 6 years old.[5] Timeliness of medical intervention was often crucial (e.g., liver failure from acetaminophen overdose presents after a delay and can be prevented with prompt intervention). Some pharmaceutical poisonings with lasting CNS effects include:

- **Benzodiazepines**: Ingestion of benzodiazepines, such as diazepam (Valium) or alprazolam (Xanax), cause CNS depression, leading to respiratory distress. Severe poisoning can cause cognitive deficits and memory problems.
- **Tricyclic Antidepressants (TCAs):** TCAs can lead to CNS toxicity causing seizures, cardiac arrhythmias, and neurological damage.
- **Atypical antipsychotics:** Certain antipsychotic medications, such as haloperidol or risperidone, can cause CNS depression and extrapyramidal symptoms in children. In severe cases, they may cause long-term motor and cognitive issues.
- **Antiepileptics**: Poisoning with antiepileptics, such as phenytoin or carbamazepine, can produce seizures and altered mental status. Lasting neurological deficits can occur in severe cases.
- **Clonidine:** Clonidine is used to treat high blood pressure as well as attention deficit hyperactivity disorder (ADHD). Overdose can cause CNS depression as well as a drop in blood pressure. The latter can produce fainting episodes and falls, as well as decreased perfusion of the brain.
- **Opioids:** Opioid poisoning causes CNS and respiratory depression, with decreased perfusion of the brain, oxygen deprivation (hypoxia), and brain damage. In toxic doses, opioids can cause potentially lethal acute leukoencephalopathy, which has a predilection for the cerebellum in young children (Reisner et al., 2015).

Ethylene Glycol and Methanol

Methanol and ethylene glycol are used as antifreeze additives in windshield wiper and radiator fluids. Ethylene glycol tastes sweet and is often packaged with bright colors or a fruity scent, making it appealing to children. Denatonium benzoate is frequently added because it tastes bitter, but young children typically consume 1–2 teaspoons before the bitter taste stops them (Nelson et al., 2019). Even after the acute phase, individuals may experience DNS, such as visual disturbances, seizures, and movement disorders. In severe cases, it can cause CNS damage, including optic nerve damage and blindness.[6] Prompt treatment minimizes these neurotoxic effects.

Treatment in School Settings

Children with neurological injuries are usually treated in parallel by the medical and educational systems, requiring effort to reduce gaps and inefficiencies. An Individualized Education Program (IEP) often includes information a physician needs to plan and coordinate care. Similarly, injuries noted in medical records, such as subcortical injuries or visual field cuts, have curriculum implications. The skills of school neuropsychologists are particularly helpful in this context since they are often best able to efficiently gather information from community neuropsychologists and medical providers and to make the links between a specific toxin, the known neuropathology of the brain associated with it, and the practical consequences that present on testing and in the classroom. Clinical neuropsychologists provide a wealth of information on neuropathology and are encouraged to work closely with schools to assist in the transition of that information to recommendations for academic success. Coordinating the timing of medical and school evaluations streamlines the IEP process and reduces plan revisions while improving medical care. In both settings, families often need guidance to manage emotional and practical challenges, particularly since the entire family may have been poisoned, causing health problems and cognitive impairment in caregivers (Piantadosi, 2002).

Collaborative treatment should be considered for children with neurodevelopmental disorders as they are more likely to have comorbid medical conditions and a higher rate of medication use, combined with heightened sensitivity to changes in environment or internal sensations. These children have a lower reserve capacity to rebound from poisoning or subsequent neurological insults. In addition, some interventions occur in the context of a developmental disorder, including managing heightened tactile sensitivity. This can make simple tasks, like pill swallowing, a challenge.

Schools are increasingly serving as informal rehabilitation services, especially in underserved communities facing numerous challenges, in remote areas, or for children who cannot travel. They also serve as interventionists and one of the few avenues for systematic prevention. Schools address the cognitive consequences of toxic exposure through enrichment and services and may serve a role in mitigating poisonings. For example, meal programs can reduce lead absorption in children by ensuring they have enough zinc and iron.

Chelation Therapy and Its Misuse

Autism is at the center of chelation therapy misuse and vaccine avoidance. This section reviews factual information to address some of the common arguments related to autism and chelation therapy (Offit, 2007). The conflict is sometimes framed as a battle between Western and alternative medicine, ignoring that many alternative therapies that started on the fringe, such as acupuncture, have become conventional as the research supported its efficacy (Gill & Bell, 2004; Vickers & Zollman, 1999). However, some alternative therapies have harmful elements, such as lead in Ayurvedic remedies (Saper et al., 2008).

Half a million patients with autism spectrum disorder (ASD) undergo chelation therapy in the US annually, mostly for non-accepted indications (Brent, 2013). Chelation was introduced as a treatment for autism in 2001 when Bernard et al. published a review comparing symptoms of mercury poisoning to those of autism (Bernard et al., 2001). Chelating agents bind to metals and form complexes excreted through urine or feces (Vilensky & Redman, 2003). Most home chelators use oral dimercaptosuccinic acid (DMSA) and a "lead mobilization model," which measures metal excretion in response to chelation in urine. DMSA chelates free, circulating lead from the kidneys and circulating blood but does not remove lead bound in bones and tissues. Thus, "lead mobilization" is ineffective in predicting lead burden (Lowry, 2010).

Mercury and Thimerosal

Although mercury poisoning has been raised as a potential source of rising ASD diagnoses, the history of mercury use (and biochemistry) doesn't support this. If mercury exposure caused autism, the diagnosis frequency would rise and fall in tandem with exposure rates. If so, autism prevalence should have peaked in the early 20th century when mercury compounds, such as Calomel, were widely used for teething pain, rashes, and constipation in babies and children. Mercury was banned from most household products, including paint, by 1990 (Nelson et al., 2019). Today, mercury exposure happens in agriculture, industry, and crafts like stained glass or taxidermy—settings with few children. The rising ASD diagnoses occurred after most mercury was moved, and even safer forms of it, such as thimerosal, have been restricted.

Thimerosal has been at the center of anxious speculations about autism, as well as vaccinations in general, so school psychologists would be aware of the biochemistry. Thimerosal is a mercury-based preservative used in contact lens solutions, antiseptics, and some vaccines. However, it has a very different chemical structure and risk level compared with its poisonous relative. Mercury, particularly methyl mercury, accumulates in the body over time and is highly toxic. Thimerosal contains ethyl mercury, which breaks down quickly, is excreted from the body, and is more benign. Thimerosal was removed from most vaccines as a precaution, although there was no evidence of harm. Andrew Wakefield, the British physician who proposed the link between thimerosal and autism, failed to disclose that he had a financial stake in an alternate vaccination method, so the attempts to link thimerosal were built not only on a shaky premise but also a conflict of interest. Dr. Wakefield was charged with malpractice and lost his license but has since moved to the United States and opened a consulting business for parents.[7]

Risks of Home Chelation Therapy

The fear of mercury contributes to vaccine avoidance and the risk of neurological damage associated with preventable illnesses; it also drives the home use of chemical compounds, chelators, that can strip away metals necessary for life. Again, conflict of interest and financial gain are factors. The FDA issued warning letters to companies marketing chelation products and home test kits that claimed to diagnose metal and environmental toxicities, faulting them for misleading claims and an inherent conflict since their poorly regulated tests provided a rationale for buying their chelators. Home chelation therapy can pose significant health risks and complications, including:

- Stripping essential minerals like calcium, magnesium, and zinc, leading to muscle cramps, cardiac arrhythmias, and neurological symptoms (Chappell et al., 2006).
- Impairing renal function or kidney injury (Risher & Amler, 2005).
- Nausea, vomiting, diarrhea, abdominal pain, dehydration, and electrolyte imbalances (Bradberry & Vale, 2009).
- Allergic reactions, including rashes, swelling, and anaphylaxis (Kosnett, 2010).
- Cardiac arrhythmias, low blood pressure, and cardiac arrest (Risher & Amler, 2005).
- Neurological symptoms such as confusion, tremors, seizures, and peripheral neuropathy (Chappell et al.).
- Depleting iron, causing anemia (Bradberry & Vale).
- Decreasing bone density and increasing fracture risk (Risher & Amler).
- The Cochrane Institute found no evidence of behavioral improvement in children with ASD after chelation therapy, including in a placebo-controlled study using glutathione lotion and DMSA (James et al., 2015). Given the risks, including hypocalcemia, renal failure, and death, they did not support further research on chelating agents in autistic children without better safety measures (Adams et al., 2009).

Conclusion

School neuropsychologists are in a unique position to identify and consider poisoning as part of the diagnostic and intervention planning for individual students since the direct and indirect effects can have lasting consequences and predictable future needs. This chapter includes terms and core concepts that are probably unfamiliar, but they were included to introduce language that may appear in medical records, conversations with physicians, and scientific articles. It is simply a set of information that can be mastered, like learning the tests or curriculum development. These ideas and terms will be relevant to toxins this chapter did not address and should provide a starting point, particularly if the next step is overviews designed for medical or nursing students.

Each direct and indirect effect of a toxin could be a dissertation or a professional specialization, but this is true for many of the medical conditions school psychologists work with. Rather than being intimidated, consider this the opportunity to better serve a community of students who have been missed by encouraging simple prevention methods (such as meal programs); appreciating the value of social, developmental, and academic enrichment on the final neurological outcome; and serving as a steadying presence as parents navigate medical decision-making after a suspected poisoning, or which therapies to prioritize when a child has developmental delays or neurological injury. Or by supporting a community trying to weigh the risks of exposure to one compound, such as fluoride in water or vaccinations. Medical decisions involve risk. Treatment decisions have costs. They may be direct, like money, or indirect, like giving up one therapy for another. It's about the risks, alternatives, and benefits of each therapy, as well as the impact on quality of life. These are the conversations that happen in an eligibility or IEP meeting or within a medical treatment team. Medical decision-making, like educational planning, is a collaborative process with all stakeholders involved. The more mutual understanding there is, the better quality of care and service a student will receive. Conversations about the risks, alternatives, and benefits are simply discussions about the best route for achieving this, ideally in all the significant domains of a child's life.

Notes

1 https://www.poison.org/-/media/files/pdf-for-article-dowloads-and-refs/safekids-medicine-safety-2015.pdf.

2 https://www.poison.org/-/media/files/pdf-for-article-dowloads-and-refs/safekids-medicine-safety-2015.pdf.

3 ATSDR (2007). *Toxicological Profile for Lead.* Retrieved from https://www.atsdr.cdc.gov/toxprofiles/tp13.pdf.

Healthline (2023). *How to Reduce Lead Exposure.* Retrieved from https://www.healthline.com/health/how-to-reduce-lead-exposure.

Mayo Clinic (2023). *Lead Poisoning*. Retrieved from https://www.mayoclinic.org/diseases-conditions/lead-poisoning/diagnosis-treatment/drc-20354723.

4 American Board of Family Medicine. (n.d.). Abuse of Prescription and Over-the-Counter Medications. Retrieved from https://www.jabfm.org

Oregon Health & Science University (OHSU). (n.d.). Medicine-Related Poisonings. Retrieved from https://www.ohsu.edu

American Academy of Family Physicians (AAFP). (n.d.). Recognition and Management of Acute Medication poisoning. Retrieved from https://www.aafp.org

5 American Board of Family Medicine (n.d.). Abuse of Prescription and Over-the-Counter Medications. Retrieved from https://www.jabfm.org.

Oregon Health & Science University (OHSU) (n.d.). Medicine-Related Poisonings. Retrieved from https://www.ohsu.edu.

American Academy of Family Physicians (AAFP). (n.d.). Recognition and Management of Acute Medication poisoning. Retrieved from https://www.aafp.org.

6 American Academy of Family Physicians (AAFP). (n.d.). Recognition and Management of Acute Medication Poisoning. Retrieved from https://www.aafp.org.

7 https://time.com/5175704/andrew-wakefield-vaccine-autism/.

References

Adams, J. B., Baral, M., Geis, E., Mitchell, J., Ingram, J., Hensley, A., Zappia, I., Newmark, S., Geh, E., Rubin, R. A., Mitchell, K., & El-Dahr, J. (2009). Safety and efficacy of oral DMSA therapy for children with autism spectrum disorders: Part A—medical results. *BMC Clinical Pharmacology*, 9(1), 1–22. https://doi.org/10.1186/1472-6904-9-16.

Balazs, J. & Kereszteny, A. (2017). Attention-deficit/hyperactivity disorder and suicide: A systematic review. *World Journal of Psychiatry*, 7(1), 44–59. doi:10.5498/wjp.v7.i1.44.

Bellinger, D. C. (2016). Lead contamination in Flint—an abject failure to protect public health. *New England Journal of Medicine*, 374(12), 1101–1103. doi:10.1056/NEJMp1601013.

Bernard, S., Enayati, A., Redwood, L., Roger, H., & Binstock, T. (2001). Autism: A novel form of mercury poisoning. *Medical Hypotheses*, 56(4), 462–471. https://doi.org/10.1054/mehy.2000.1281.

Bi, W-K., Wang, J-L., Zhou, X-D., Li, Z-K., Jiang, W-W., Zhang, S-B., Zou, Y., Bi, M-J., & Li, Q. (2020). Clinical characteristics of visual dysfunction in carbon monoxide poisoning patients. *Journal of Ophthalmology 2020* (1), 9537360. https://doi.org/10.1155/2020/9537360.

Billings, S. B. & Schnepel, K. T. (2018). Life after lead: Effects of early interventions for children exposed to lead. *American Economic Journal: Applied Economics*, 10 (3), 315–344. doi:10.1257/app.20160056.

Bradberry, S. M. & Vale, J. A. (2009). A comparison of arsenic, cadmium, mercury, and lead pharmacokinetics and toxicity. *Journal of Toxicology: Clinical Toxicology*, 47(5), 383–396.

Brent, J. (2013). Commentary on the abuse of metal chelation therapy in patients with autism spectrum disorders. *Journal of Medical Toxicology*, 9, 370–372. https://doi.org/10.1007/s13181-013-0345-4.

Chappell, W. R., Abernathy, C. O., & Calderon, R. L. (2006). *Health effects of arsenic and its chemical interactions with other environmental contamination*. Taylor & Francis.

Gill, A. L. & Bell, C. N. A. (2004). Hyperbaric oxygen: Its uses, mechanisms of action and outcomes. *QJM*, 97(7), 385–395. https://doi.org/10.1093/qjmed/hch074.

Guilarte, T. R., Toscano, C. D., McGlothan, J. L., & Weaver, S. A. (2003). Environmental enrichment reverses cognitive and molecular deficits induced by developmental lead exposure. *Annals of Neurology: Official Journal of the American Neurological Association and the Child Neurology Society*, 53(1), 50–56. https://doi.org/10.1002/ana.10399.

Hadanny, A., Catalogna, M., Yaniv, S., Stolar, O., Rothstein, L., Shabi, A., Suzin, G., Lang, E., Finci, S., Polak, N., Fishlev, G., Harpaz, R. T., Adler, M., Goldman, R-L., Zemel, Y., Bechor, Y., & Efrati, S. (2022). Hyperbaric oxygen therapy in children with post-concussion syndrome improves cognitive and behavioral function: A randomized controlled trial. *Scientific Reports*, 12(1), 15233. https://doi.org/10.1038/s41598-022-19395-y.

Hedges, D., Farrer, T. J., Bigler, E. D., & Hopkins, R. O. (2019) Carbon monoxide poisoning and cognitive impairment. *The brain at risk: Associations between disease and cognition*. 225–244. https://doi.org/10.1007/978-3-030-14260-5_16.

Hunt, A., Harrington, D., & Robinson, S. (2014). Vitamin B12 deficiency. *BMJ*, 349. https://doi.org/10.1136/bmj.g5226.

Huo, C., Li, G., Hu, Y., & Sun, H. (2022). The impacts of iron overload and ferroptosis on intestinal mucosal homeostasis and inflammation. *International Journal of Molecular Sciences*, 23(22), 14195. https://doi.org/10.3390/ijms232214195.

James, S., Stevenson, S. W., Silove, N., & Williams, K. (2015). Chelation for autism spectrum disorder (ASD). *Cochrane Database of Systematic Reviews*, (5). https://doi.org/10.1002/14651858.CD010766.pub2.

Karaman, D., Metin, S., Kara, K., Ozdemir, A., Yildiz, S., Durukan, I., Almbaidheen, M., Uzun, G., & Turkbay, T. (2016). Neuropsychological evaluation of children and adolescents with acute carbon monoxide poisoning. *Pediatric Emergency Care*, 32(5), 303–306. doi:10.1097/PEC.0000000000000441.

Kofman, O., Berger, A., Massarwa, A., Friedman, A., & Jaffar, A. A. (2006). Motor inhibition and learning impairments in school-aged children following exposure to organophosphate pesticides in infancy. *Pediatric Research*, 60(1), 88–92. https://doi.org/10.1203/01.pdr.0000219467.47013.35.

Kosnett, M. J. (2010). Chelation for heavy metals (arsenic, lead, and mercury): Protective or perilous? *Clinical Pharmacology & Therapeutics*, 88(3), 412–415. https://doi.org/10.1038/clpt.2010.132.

Lanphear, B. P., Dietrich, K., Auinger, P., & Cox, C. (2000). Cognitive deficits associated with blood lead concentrations <10 microg/dL in US children and adolescents. *Public Health Reports*, 115(6), 521–529. doi:10.1093/phr/115.6.521.

Lowry, J. A. (2010). Oral chelation therapy for patients with lead poisoning. *American Academy of Pediatrics*, 116, 1036–1046.

Matsubayashi, T., Ueda, M., & Yoshikawa, K. (2016). School and seasonality in youth suicide: Evidence from Japan. *Journal of Epidemiology and Community Health*, 70(11), 1122–1127. https://doi.org/10.1136/jech-2016-207583.

Moodie, S., Ialongo, N., López, P., Rosado, J., García-Vargas, G., Ronquillo, D., & Kordas, K. (2013). The conjoint influence of home enriched environment and lead exposure on children's cognition and behaviour in a Mexican lead smelter community. *Neurotoxicology*, 34, 33–41. https://doi.org/10.1016/j.neuro.2012.10.004.

Nelson. L. S., Howland, M. A., Lewin, N. A., Smith, S. W., Goldfrank, L. R., & Hoffman, R. S. (2019). *Goldfrank's Toxicologic Emergencies, Eleventh Edition.* McGraw Hill.

Offit, P. A. (2007). *Vaccinated: One man's quest to defeat the world's deadliest diseases.* Smithsonian Books.

Piantadosi, C. A. (2002). Carbon monoxide poisoning. *New England Journal of Medicine*, 347(14), 1054–1055. doi:10.1056/NEJMp020104.

Reisner, A., Hayes, L. L., Holland, C. M., Wrubel, D. M., Kebriaei, M. A., Geller, R. J., Baum, G. R., & Chern, J. J. (2015). Opioid overdose in a child: Case report and discussion with emphasis on neurosurgical implications. *Journal of Neurosurgery: Pediatrics*, 16(6), 752–757. https://doi.org/10.3171/2015.4.PEDS14667.

Risher, J. F. & Amler, S. N. (2005). Mercury exposure: Evaluation and intervention—the inappropriate use of chelating agents in the diagnosis and treatment of putative mercury poisoning. *Neurotoxicology*, 26(4), 691–699. https://doi.org/10.1016/j.neuro.2005.05.004.

Saper, R. B., Phillips, R. S., Sehgal, A., Khoury, R., Davis, R. B., & Paquin, J. (2008). Lead, mercury, and arsenic in US- and Indian-manufactured Ayurvedic medicines sold via the Internet. *JAMA*, 300(8), 915–923. doi:10.1001/jama.300.8.915.

Schneider, J. S. (2023). Neurotoxicity and outcomes from developmental lead exposure: Persistent or permanent? *Environmental Health Perspectives*, 131(8), 085002. https://doi.org/10.1289/EHP123.

Schneider, J. S., Lee, M. H., Anderson, D. W., Zuck, L., & Lidsky, T. I. (2001). Enriched environment during development is protective against lead-induced neurotoxicity. *Brain Research*, 896(1–2),48–55. https://doi.org/10.1016/S0006-8993(00)3249–3242.

Siewiera, J., Mews, J., Królikowska, K., Kalicki, B., & Jobs, K. (2019) Hyperbaric oxygenation in pediatrics: Indications in the light of evidence-based medicine. *Developmental Period Medicine*, 23(2), 142–148. doi:10.34763/devperiodmed.20192302.142148.

Spiller, H. A., Ackerman, J. P., Smith, G. A., Kistamgari, S., Funk, A. R., McDermott, M. R., & Casavant, M. J. (2020). Suicide attempts by self-poisoning in the United States among 10–25-year-olds from 2000 to 2018: Substances used, temporal changes and demographics. *Clinical Toxicology*, 58(7), 676–687. https://doi.org/10.1080/15563650.2019.1665182.

Surkan, P. J., Zhang, A., Trachtenberg, F., Daniel, D. B., McKinlay, S., & Bellinger, D. C. (2007). Neuropsychological function in children with blood lead levels <10 μg/dL. *Neurotoxicology*, 28(6), 1170–1177. https://doi.org/10.1016/j.neuro.2007.07.007.

Tarango, S. M. & Liu, D. R. (2016). Pediatric ingestions: Emergency department management. *EB Medicine*, 13(4), 1–24.

Vickers, A. & Zollman, C. (1999). ABC of complementary medicine: Acupuncture. *BMJ: British Medical Journal*, 319(7215), 973–976. doi:10.1136/bmj.319.7215.973.

Vilensky, J. A. & Redman, K. (2003). British anti-Lewisite (Dimercaprol): An amazing history. *Annals of Emergency Medicine*, 41(3), 378–383. https://doi.org/10.1067/mem.2003.72.

Wei, H., Zhang, X., Yang, X., Yu, Q., Deng, S., Guan, Q., Chen, D., Zhang, M., Gao, B., Xu, S., & Xia, Y. (2023). Prenatal exposure to pesticides and domain-specific neurodevelopment at age 12 and 18 months in Nanjing, China. *Environment International*, 173, 107814. https://doi.org/10.1016/j.envint.2023.107814.

8 Viral Infections

Denise E. Maricle

Introduction

It is estimated that approximately 1.6 million viruses are circulating world-wide at any given time, with about half thought to be capable of infecting humans (Baker et al., 2022; Schulze-Markuch, 2020). Infections caused by viruses are universal during childhood and adolescence. Medical professionals regularly care for youth who present with infections caused by a variety of viral pathogens. These infections have varied presentations. Many infections have clinical presentations that are specific to the infecting virus but also present differently based on the age and immunocompetence of the individual. Some children are directly impacted early in their lives when maternal disease causes in-utero infection (e.g., cytomegalovirus, rubella, Zika virus, parvovirus B19). Other viruses may infect children in a predictable pattern as they grow older (e.g., rhinovirus, respiratory syncytial virus, influenza). Many viral infections encountered in the past (e.g., mumps, measles, polio) are no longer extant due to widespread immunization efforts. However, anti-vaccine movements in the United States and around the world have caused a resurgence of these once almost eradicated viruses. Moreover, an increasing number of sexually transmitted viral infections (e.g., herpes simplex virus, varicella zoster virus, cytomegalovirus) are being seen in children and adolescents. Additionally, linkages between viral infections and autoimmune conditions are being increasingly identified. Many viruses are known to trigger autoimmune responses, including fibromyalgia, myalgic encephalomyelitis/chronic fatigue, multiple sclerosis, and type 1 diabetes (See chapters 10, 20, and 24, for more information on these disorders). There are many disorders that this chapter could focus upon but publishing constraints have resulted in a sampling of viral infections to represent those most likely to be encountered in psychological practice.

DOI: 10.4324/9781032703923-10

Common Viral Diseases Impacting Children and Adolescents

SARS-CoV-2 (COVID-19)

Beginning in 2020, the world became acutely aware of viruses when the SARS-CoV-2 pandemic began. SARS-CoV-2 and long COVID in children will not be addressed here but is covered in detail in Chapter 9.

Influenza and Respiratory Syncytial Virus (RSV)

Influenza

Influenza is a well-known respiratory and potential neurotropic virus in children and adolescents (Jantarabenjakul et al., 2023; Robinson & Le Saux, 2020). It is a contagious virus that causes upper and lower respiratory tract infections. Each year 3% to 11% of children and adults develop asymptomatic influenza, while 5% to 20% experience symptoms that range from mild to lethal. Typical clinical presentations in children include high fever and gastrointestinal issues, and almost all symptomatic cases manifest with upper or lower respiratory tract infections. However, children are more likely than adults to exhibit non-respiratory symptoms, including neurologic manifestations. Neurological complications are seen in 10% to 30% of pediatric cases, the most common being seizures and encephalopathy. Influenza has a well-recognized etiology of encephalopathy and encephalitis in children. Other neurological complications include meningitis, stroke, acute disseminated encephalomyelitis, and Guillain–Barré syndrome.

The primary treatment for influenza is over-the-counter medications and antivirals. An annual flu vaccine is recommended for prevention for 6 months of age or older. Various studies report that the mortality rate for pediatric influenza varies from 7% to 30%. Although most children experience no sequelae, up to 10% of hospitalized children with influenza have neurological abnormalities at discharge and up to 40% of these cases have severe complications (Jantarabenjakul et al., 2023; Robinson & Le Saux, 2020). The clinical manifestations of influenza-associated neurological complications vary from mild symptoms (e.g., headache, numbness, and drowsiness) to moderate and severe symptoms (e.g., seizure and acute encephalopathy). It is unclear whether neurological complications are due to direct viral infection, immunological, or inflammatory responses. No research is currently available on long-term neuropsychological outcomes related to influenza in youth.

Respiratory Syncytial Virus (RSV)

RSV is a common respiratory virus that usually causes mild, cold-like symptoms. Most people recover in a week or two, but RSV can be serious and dangerous for infants and young children. Each year in the United States, an estimated 58,000–80,000 children younger than 5 years are hospitalized due to RSV. Children at greatest risk for severe illness from RSV include:

- Premature infants
- Infants up to 12 months, especially those 6 months and younger
- Children younger than 2 years with chronic lung disease or congenital heart disease
- Children with weakened immune systems
- Children who have neuromuscular disorders, including those with difficulty swallowing or clearing mucus secretions

Virtually all children contract RSV by age two. Typically, RSV will be mild, but it can also cause severe illness such as bronchiolitis (inflammation in the small airways in the lung) and pneumonia. Two to three of every 100 infants with RSV need hospitalization. Those who are hospitalized may require oxygen, IV fluids (if they aren't eating and drinking), and mechanical ventilation to aid breathing. Most children with RSV will improve with supportive care and are discharged in a few days.

In terms of treatment, the CDC recommends the RSV vaccine be given to women during pregnancy and the RSV immunization vaccination to infants and older babies if mother was not vaccinated during pregnancy. These vaccines provide protection against severe RSV for up to 6 months after birth. However, the protection wanes over time. Thus, RSV antibody immunization is recommended for all infants who are younger than 8 months, born during or entering their first RSV season. RSV antibodies can help protect babies and young children from severe disease. Most infants whose mothers received an RSV vaccine do not need the RSV antibody. A preventive antibody is not a treatment for those who already have RSV infection but can provide an extra layer of defense that helps fight RSV infections. Finally, a dose of RSV antibody is also recommended for children between the ages of 8–19 months and entering their second RSV season who are in at least one of these groups: children with chronic lung disease due to premature birth and requiring medical therapy for their lung disease; children who are severely immunocompromised; children with cystic fibrosis who have severe disease; and American Indian and Alaska Native children. No research is available delineating the long-term consequences of RSV and its treatments on the developing brain and later neurological functioning.

Zika Virus (ZIKV) and Congenital ZIKV Syndrome

ZIKV is a mosquito-borne flavivirus. The *Flaviviridae* are a family of positive, single-stranded, enveloped RNA viruses found primarily in ticks and mosquitoes, but which can infect humans. ZIKV originated in Africa but spread to the Americas in 2015 and is now emerging as a worldwide, mosquito-transmitted illness (Masmejan et al., 2020). The primary mode of transmission is by mosquito; however, other forms of transmission have been identified. Vertical transmission from mother to infant in utero results in congenital ZIKV syndrome. ZIKV can also be transmitted sexually, and potentially via blood transfusion and solid organ transplantation. The World Health Organization has declared ZIKV infection a Public Health Emergency of International Concern because of its association with severe central nervous system anomalies in fetuses and neonates exposed to ZIKV in utero. Research is just beginning to evaluate the biological pathways and outcomes of congenital ZIKV and is very limited. Long-term neurodevelopmental surveillance of infants born with ZIKV exposure is recommended.

Symptoms of infection include fever, headache, lethargy, myalgia, arthralgia, retro-orbital pain, conjunctivitis, and rash. ZIKV-infected hallmarks of neurological problems (e.g., fatigue, memory loss/confusion, difficulty concentrating/reduced speed of thought, and sensory problems) have been self-reported by both children and their parents. Prenatal exposure, particularly in the first trimester to ZIKV presents a significant threat to the developing neonate. Severe malformation (craniofacial, musculoskeletal, pulmonary, ocular or optic nerve abnormalities) structural brain abnormalities (microcephaly, corpus collosum abnormalities, abnormal cortical gyri patterns, cortical atrophy) and fetal death are associated with in utero exposure. These infants present with microcephaly, optic neuropathy, congenital glaucoma, global neuropsychological delay, epilepsy, and deafness. Not all exposed fetuses exhibit congenital ZIKV syndrome. Many newborns exposed in the 2nd or 3rd trimester do not exhibit the full manifestation of ZIKV. They are more likely to have mild neurodevelopmental delays, impaired neuromotor development, subependymal and choroid plexus cysts, and lenticulostriate vasculopathy (i.e., mineralization deposits on thalami and basal ganglia; Mulkey et al., 2020).

Children with congenital ZIKV syndrome are likely to be seriously impaired and meet criteria for special education services with classifications under intellectual delay/cognitive impairment, multiple disabilities, and developmental delay. Those with mild neurodevelopmental delays may not meet the criteria for an Individuals with Disabilities Education Act (IDEA) classification but might meet criteria under Section 504 of the Rehabilitation Act of 1973. Children with congenital ZIKV syndrome are likely to need the most restrictive special education placements, institutionalization, specialized classrooms, one-to-one instruction/monitoring, and altered programming. The services for children with mild neurodevelopmental sequelae will be dependent on the child's presenting issues or concerns. There is no treatment for ZIKV infection, no antiviral drug, and no preventative vaccine.

Lyme Disease

Lyme disease is caused by the bacterium Borrelia burgdorfei or Borrelia mayonii. It is transmitted via black-legged ticks (deer ticks). Lyme disease is more common in the upper Midwest, Northeast, and Mid-Atlantic regions of the United States but is also in European and Baltic regions as well. Symptoms occur differently in each child, but they usually appear within 3 to 30 days after a tick bite. Lyme disease has early- and late-stage symptoms. Early-stage Lyme disease is more easily cured with antibiotics than the late-stage. Most cases of late-stage disease occur when early-stage disease is not treated. Several days or weeks after a bite from an infected tick, the child may exhibit flu-like symptoms, including:

- Headache
- Stiff neck
- Aches and pains in muscles and joints
- Low fever and chills
- Tiredness
- Loss of appetite
- Swollen glands
- A skin rash known as erythema migrans occurs in 70% to 80% of people. It takes the shape of a bull's eye rash and is often seen about 7 days post-bite. It usually occurs at the site of the bite but can appear anywhere on the body

If untreated in the weeks or months following the bite, symptoms can worsen to include:

- Nervous system symptoms, including inflammation of the nervous system (meningitis) and weakness/paralysis of the facial muscles (Bell's palsy)
- Heart problems, including inflammation of the heart (myopericarditis) and problems with heart rate
- Inflammation of the eyes
- Skin disorders
- Severe tiredness
- Weakness

Months to a few years after an untreated bite, symptoms advance to include:

- Joint inflammation (arthritis)
- Nervous system symptoms such as numbness in the arms and legs, tingling and pain, and trouble with speech, memory, and concentration

Treatment at all stages is with antibiotics. Intravenous antibiotics are used with more severe cases and late-stage cases. Some children develop post-Lyme disease syndrome (PLDS; also called post treatment Lyme disease—PTLD) or chronic Lyme disease. This means that some symptoms last longer than 6 months. Symptoms include:

- Ongoing muscle and nerve pain
- Tiredness
- Problems with memory

PLDS does not respond to antibiotics, because there isn't an active infection anymore. Treatment is aimed at helping to control symptoms. PLDS/PTLD remains poorly understood, and more research is needed to better understand these prolonged symptoms and identify treatment targets. Children with PLDS/PTLD would meet criteria for other health impairment under IDEA or for Section 504 accommodations. Children and adolescents with chronic Lyme disease present similarly to children and adolescents with chronic fatigue, fibromyalgia, or juvenile arthritis. See chapters 10, 11 and 20 for more information about these conditions.

Subacute Sclerosing Panencephalitis (SSPE)

Subacute sclerosing panencephalitis (SSPE) is a progressive neurological disorder of children and young adults that affects the central nervous system (CNS). It is a slow and persistent viral infection related to measles. Most children with SSPE have a history of measles infection at an early age, usually younger than age 2, followed by a latent period of six to eight years before neurological symptoms begin. Despite the long interval between the measles infection and onset of SSPE, researchers think that the infection of the brain occurs soon after the primary bout with measles and progresses slowly. Why it persists and progresses isn't clear.

The initial symptoms of SSPE include:

- Mild cognitive decline (e.g., memory loss)
- Changes in behavior (e.g., irritability)
- Disturbances in motor function, including uncontrollable jerking movements of the head, trunk, or limbs (myoclonic jerks)
- Seizures
- Blindness in some instances

In advanced cases, individuals may lose the ability to walk as their muscles stiffen or spasm. There is progressive deterioration to a comatose state, and then to a persistent vegetative state. Death is usually the result of fever, heart failure, or the brain's inability to continue controlling the autonomic nervous system. Currently, there is no cure for SSPE. Prevention in the form of the measles vaccination is the only real "cure" for SSPE. It is important to understand that viral infections such as measles and mumps are not necessarily benign diseases with no adverse outcomes.

HIV/AIDS

Human immunodeficiency virus (HIV) and acquired immunodeficiency syndrome (AIDS) result from a viral infection that progressively destroys certain white blood cells and creates vulnerability to other infections and some cancers (Cachay, 2023). The HIV causes AIDS. HIV can be transmitted during sexual intercourse, pregnancy, childbirth, breastfeeding, and other forms of exposure to bodily fluids that carry the virus. When the virus enters the body, it injects itself into vital immune cells called CD4 cells. In the absence of treatment, HIV continues to replicate itself within the body, eventually leading to severe immunodeficiency, chronic illness, and death. More than 90% of HIV infections in children result from mother-to-child-transmission, where the virus is passed from a mother with HIV to her baby. The risk of transmission increases in direct relation to the severity of the mother's HIV infection.

Data provided by UNAIDS (UNAIDS.org) estimates 39 million people worldwide were living with HIV/AIDS in 2022, of which approximately 1.7 million are children under 15 years of age. There were about 1.3 million new infections in 2022 with 500 children newly infected with HIV every day. In 2022, 630,000 people died of AIDS-related illnesses worldwide, with about 100,000 of these being children or adolescents. However, HIV infections among children have been declining, and only about 1% of the people infected with HIV in the United States were diagnosed as children. This decline is due to greater testing and treatment for pregnant women with HIV. Treatment with antiretroviral medications before and during birth can help prevent transmission from mother to child. Although the number of infants and children with HIV living in the United States continues to decrease, the number of adolescents and young adults with HIV is increasing (Weinberg, 2023). This number is increasing because children who were infected as infants are surviving longer, and new cases are developing in adolescents and young adults, particularly in young men who have sex with men.

There are two human immunodeficiency viruses, HIV-1 and HIV-2. Infection with HIV-1 is more common. Both progressively destroy certain types of white blood cells (lymphocytes), which are an important part of the body's immune defense system. When these lymphocytes are destroyed, the body becomes susceptible to attack by other infectious organisms. Many of the symptoms and complications of HIV, including death, are the result of these other infections and not the HIV infection itself. HIV can lead to infections with organisms that do not ordinarily infect healthy people, and such opportunistic infections may result from viruses, parasites, fungi, or bacteria. Because children's immune systems are not fully developed, children living with HIV are more vulnerable and frequently become more severely ill than adults. They may experience the same common pediatric infections as HIV-negative children but cannot fight them as effectively. Common infections in HIV-positive children include ear and sinus infections, sepsis, pneumonia, tuberculosis, urinary tract infections, intestinal illness, skin disease, and meningitis. In developing countries in particular, tuberculosis, diarrhea, and respiratory illnesses are common in HIV-positive children.

There is no cure for HIV. Early diagnosis is critical. When antiretroviral therapy (ART) is administered as early as possible, it helps children living with HIV lead longer, healthier lives. Taken every day, these medicines drastically reduce the concentration of HIV in the bloodstream and increase levels of CD4 cells, slowing the progression of the disease. Sadly, most children worldwide do not have access to ART. Without diagnosis and treatment, one-third of infected infants will die before the age of one, and almost one-half before their second birthday. In western European countries access to combination antiretroviral therapy (cART) has resulted in HIV being considered a chronic disease rather than a terminal illness.

The exact pathophysiological mechanism of how HIV affects the developing brain, compounded by long-term effects of cART, is unclear and remains under study, but the cognitive dysfunction associated with HIV infection has long been recognized as an important and disabling aspect of the disease. Although cART clearly improves neurodevelopmental outcomes, increased rates of developmental, cognitive, and behavioral problems continue to be seen in children living with HIV. The term HIV-associated neurocognitive disorder (HAND) describes the spectrum of neurocognitive dysfunction associated with HIV that includes asymptomatic neurocognitive impairment (ANI), mild neurocognitive disorder (MND), and HIV-associated dementia (HAD). Despite entering the era of cART, HAND remains prevalent; however, less severe forms of HAND now predominate, and the most severe form, HIV-associated dementia, is rare. Typically, HAND presents with executive dysfunction and memory impairment with disruption of attention, multitasking, impulse control, judgment, and memory encoding and retrieval. HAND is also associated with motor dysfunction, including bradykinesia, loss of coordination, and gait imbalance. Most common symptoms seen in HIV-positive children are deficits in learning, memory, and executive function, and these neuropsychological deficits persist despite adequate viral suppression (Van Opstal et al., 2021). It is unclear if these HIV-related difficulties are connected to the residual effect of HIV, medications, or psychosocial-environmental factors. Recent research suggests that ongoing neuroinflammation, vascular dysfunction, and hypercoagulability impact the developing brain, resulting in significant damage to neuronal structures, white and grey matter volume, and the integrity of white matter (Van Opstal et al.), which may account for the high co-morbidity of executive function deficits.

Given the prevalence of HIV among youth, it is important for school/pediatric psychologists to understand how HIV impacts academic and social–emotional functioning, as well as the legal and ethical implications of HIV. Because of effective treatment options, youth with HIV can enjoy good health and are increasingly present in school settings. Nonetheless, students with HIV are at risk for academic deficits associated with the neuropsychological effects of untreated or poorly treated HIV, such as short-term memory difficulties, attention deficits, expressive and receptive language disorders, and visual–spatial problems. Further, students living with HIV may experience high rates of absenteeism due to illness from opportunistic infections, side effects of medication, and/or clinic visits. Peer relationships can also be impacted and create difficulties for children with HIV/AIDS. Children may fear disclosure of their HIV status but feel uncomfortable living with the secret. They may be teased or bullied and develop symptoms of depression or anxiety. These effects on learning and academic functioning often result in the need for accommodations and special education services. It is important to recognize that academic deficits may also be affected by social, economic, and environmental factors associated with HIV, including poverty, stigma, discrimination, and homophobia.

In the United States, the Office of Civil Rights (OCR) has indicated that youth with HIV/AIDS meet criteria for "disability" under IDEA as OHI or via Section 504. In fact, Section 504 protects individuals with HIV/AIDS of any current, previous, or perceived effect of HIV infection that substantially limits major life activities. Similar laws are present in other countries. Since HIV/AIDS damages many of the body's systems, such as the hemic (blood), lymphatic, reproductive, and other systems, persons with HIV/AIDS are often substantially limited in major life activities due to physical impairment. Children or adolescents with HIV/AIDS may also be substantially limited by the reaction of others to their perceived contagiousness. OCR has ruled that discrimination based solely on the fear of contagion is discrimination based on handicap. School professionals are further reminded that HIV infection status alone should not factor into decisions about eligibility, placement, services, or participation. A child living with HIV/AIDS poses no risk to others, requires no additional insurance, and typically requires no specific or additional resources.

Assessment

Linking a child's viral infection to the symptoms they are exhibiting is often difficult, primarily as symptom development and infection may not be time adjacent. Additionally, parents may be hesitant to share information, such as HIV status, for fear of stigma and possible negative reactions or discrimination. For many psychologists, obtaining a child's medical history is a cursory request. Parents are asked if their child has had certain medical conditions, but little to no follow through occurs on what they report. Obtaining a more thorough and comprehensive medical history should be considered for every referral. At a minimum, when information regarding viral infections is reported, asking for more information can elicit information that should be considered for diagnosis, educational classification, or treatment/intervention. Following up with more detailed information-seeking if a child does exhibit known symptoms associated with a particular viral disorder is also recommended. Asking specifically about children's exposure to common viral infections should become a routine part of clinical history-taking.

The structure of an assessment battery will be dependent upon presenting concerns and referral questions. It is suggested that for disorders with known neuropsychological patterns and sequelae, specific assessments be chosen to measure possible strengths and weaknesses in those areas. For example, in HIV/AIDS, visual spatial ability is often implicated, so it should be specifically measured and monitored. Professionals, such as school psychologists, should be cognizant of the neuropsychological characteristics of various viral infections commonly seen in children and adolescents and familiar with assessment tools to measure them.

Intervention

As with other nebulous disorders where the exhibited difficulties may include a wide variety of issues, intervention needs to be focused on the individual child's needs. A few areas deserve mentioning. A major issue is the need for educating ourselves and school professionals on basic skills such as universal precautions for blood-borne pathogens or using personal protective equipment to minimize viral transmission. Expectations for overall wellness and health should be part of every school's daily routine (e.g., basic human hygiene, surface cleaning, consideration for others when feeling unwell).

Communication, consultation, and collaboration are important intervention tools in the case of viral infections. It is not unusual for children and adolescents impacted by viral infection complications to be dismissed by other professionals as having psychosomatic problems. As a result, no comprehensive assessment is conducted to evaluate reported difficulties. Dismissal of symptoms and illness may cause psychological damage. Our greatest tool might be acknowledging their lived experience and responding to their concerns. Psychologists are not physicians and as such are not expected to be familiar with all aspects of medical conditions, but when a medical condition has known neurological, cognitive, or behavioral effects that impact learning and performance in schools, it is an obligation of school professionals to assist in assessing and intervening.

Flexibility in expectations and program planning is a necessary component in our response to children who are living with immediate or long-term consequences of a viral infection. It may be necessary to adjust entrance requirements; for example, children with HIV/AIDS cannot be inoculated with live viruses (e.g., measles, polio) so mandatory requirements for vaccination may need to be waived for them (Van Opstal et al., 2021). Alterations to attendance and participation requirements may be necessary, such as the number of absences permitted, homebound schooling, or waiving participation in physical education.

Some children will need an Education Health Care Plan (EHCP), Individualized Healthcare Plan (IHP), or an Emergency Procedures Plan (EPP) attached to their Individualized Education Program (IEP) or Section 504 plan. Some children may need to be able to use/take medications during school hours that might normally be prohibited, or may need specified rest periods and altered schedules, which can be addressed with these forms. Privacy and confidentiality may also become issues. For instance, parents are not required to divulge their child's HIV status, but when they do, invariably there may be discrimination or stigma. Although some school personnel may need to be aware of the child's health status, it should be kept to the minimum on a "need-to-know" basis.

Finally, education and support that is not commonly available in schools may need to be offered to the child or adolescent. For example, children with chronic illness may require counseling to navigate learning about their illness, taking responsibility for their health and well-being, adhering to medication or treatment regimes, and learning to advocate for themselves. Children may need counseling to assist in dealing with peer relationships, bullying or peer pressure, depression, or anxiety, and working through issues as they arise (i.e., adolescents who are HIV-positive may benefit from education about methods to prevent transmission if they are sexually active or have injury with bleeding complications).

Conclusion

There are many viral disorders not covered in this chapter, like acute disseminated encephalomyelitis, acute transverse myelitis, congenital cytomegalovirus, Epstein Barr virus, Ebola, Dengue and yellow fever, hepatitis, etc. School personnel are in a unique position to coordinate interdisciplinary services for children living with chronic viral infection and complications. Through facilitating suitable assessment and intervention, school personnel can substantially improve long-term outcomes for these students.

Why some viral infections are associated with neurological conditions is complex and still being researched. Addressing issues related to viral infections is challenging since the evidence base is limited. Despite recent advances in the understanding of long-term complications after acute infectious diseases, the pathogenesis of late effects remains unknown. Also, while non-specific conditions like chronic fatigue syndrome/myalgic encephalomyelitis have been historically linked with viral infections, causative mechanisms have never been demonstrated. Currently it is only speculation that infections in genetically predisposed patients can lead to immune dysregulation, chronic inflammatory processes, or neuro-inflammation. Viral persistence may also play a role in triggering such mechanisms. It is important to highlight that research is advancing quickly within the field, and as new knowledge is gained, further treatments and support should become available.

Resources

AIDS Alliance for Children, Youth & Families: aids-alliance.org

Children's HIV Association (CHIVA): royal.uk/chiva

Elizabeth Glaser Pediatric AIDS Foundation: pedaids.org

International Maternal Pediatric Adolescent AIDS Clinic Trials (IMPAACT): impaactnetwork.org

National Institute of Allergy and Infectious Diseases (NIAID): niaid.gov

References

Baker, R. E., Mahmud, A. S., Miller, I. F., Rajeev, M., Rasambainarivo, F., Rice, B. L., Tatem, A. J., Wagner, C. E., Wang, L-F., Wesolowski, A., & Metcalf, C. J. E. (2022). Infectious disease in an era of global change. *Nature Reviews Microbiology*, 20(4), 193–205.

Cachay, E. (2023). HIV infection. *Merck Manual*. Retrieved December 15, 2023 from https://www.merckmanuals.com.

Jantarabenjakul, W., Paprad, T., Paprad, T., Anugulruengkitt, S., Pancharoen, C., Puthanakit, & Chomtho, K. (2023). Neurological complication associated with influenza in hospitalized children. *Influence and Other Respiratory Viruses*, 17 (1), e13075. doi:10.1111/irv.13075.

Masmejan, S., Musso, D., & Vouga, M. (2020). Zika Virus. *Pathogens*, 9(11), 898. https://doi.org/10.3390/pathogens9110898.

Mulkey, S. B., Arroyave-Wessel, M., Peyton, C., Bulas, D. I., Fourzali, Y., Jiang, J., Russo, S., McCarter, R., Msall, M. E., du Plessis, A. J., DeBiasi, R. L., & Cure, C. (2020). Neurodevelopmental abnormalities in children within utero Zika virus exposure without congenital Zika syndrome. *JAMA Pediatrics*, 174(3), 269–276. doi:10.1001/jamapediatrics.2019.5204.

Robinson, J. L. & Le Saux, N. L. (2020). Neurologic manifestations of influenza in children. *Journal of the Association of Medical Microbiological Infectious Disease*, 5(1), 1–3. https://doi.org/10.3138/jammi.2020-01-07.

Schulze-Markuch, D. (2020). There are more viruses on earth than there are stars in the Universe. *Smithsonian Magazine*. Retrieved December 15, 2023 from Sm ithsonianmag.org.

Van Opstal, S., Dogterom, E., Wagener, M., et al. (2021). Neuropsychological and psychosocial functioning in children with perinatal HIV-infections in The Netherlands. *Viruses*, 13(10), 1947. DOI.org/10.3390/v13101947.

Weinberg, G. A. (2023) HIV infection in children and ddolescents. *Merck Manual*. Retrieved December 20, 2023 from https://www.merckmanuals.com.

9 COVID-19 and Long COVID in Children

Christine Koterba, Kristen Hoskinson, Gray Vargas and Rowena Ng

Introduction

Since the beginning of the pandemic, over 15 million youth have tested positive for COVID-19. This number is likely higher, with seroprevalence rates suggesting that over 90% of children have contracted COVID-19 (Centers for Disease Control and Prevention; CDC, 2024). As documented, youth with COVID-19 infections fare better than adults, with a mild acute course and few to no symptoms. However, they are not immune from the consequences of COVID-19. Indeed, although rare, a minority are at risk for severe COVID-19 infection and a small number may develop multisystemic inflammatory syndrome in children (MIS-C). Similar to adults, research suggests that a subgroup of youth may also experience persistent symptoms consistent with long COVID (Koterba, Hoskinson et al., 2024).

Severe COVID-19 and MIS-C

Children comprise around 20% of reported cases of COVID-19 and most make a full recovery. While very young children and those with pre-existing medical conditions (e.g., obesity, asthma, diabetes) are at higher risk for severe illness, fewer than 2% of children require hospitalization (Centers for Disease Control and Prevention, 2021). The mortality rate in children is fortunately much lower than in adults, with an estimated 0.5% of hospitalized children dying from COVID-19 (Castagnoli et al., 2020; Lu et al., 2020). Nevertheless, research suggests that children with severe acute illness may be at risk for developing additional medical issues following illness recovery (Francoeur et al., 2024).

A very small group of children have also experienced a rare but serious condition called multisystemic inflammatory syndrome in children (MIS-C). MIS-C involves fever and multiorgan symptoms (e.g., swollen lymph nodes, lung/heart inflammation, rash/swelling, toxic shock, abdominal pain, redness of the eyes) following COVID-19 infection/exposure (Patel, 2022). MIS-C typically occurs 2–6 weeks after infection and often leads to an ICU

DOI: 10.4324/9781032703923-11

admission and treatment (Feldstein et al., 2021). Unlike severe COVID-19 alone, MIS-C tends to occur more in healthy children than those with preexisting conditions (Zachariah, 2022).

While limited, studies of the neurological impact of acute COVID-19 infection are evolving (Fink et al., 2022; Francoeur et al., 2024). Evidence suggests that 5% to nearly 20% of children may present with neurological involvement/non-specific neurological symptoms, which could impact the developing nervous system (Panda et al., 2021; Stafstrom, 2022). Neurological symptoms are defined broadly and include fatigue, cognitive difficulties, mood concerns, physical symptoms, headache, muscle weakness, and in rare cases, stroke, encephalopathy, and seizures (Valderas et al., 2022). Overall, research suggests that children with underlying medical conditions, younger in age, and those who develop MIS-C are at greatest risk for neurological impact. Mechanisms are unknown and could include microvascular infarcts, multisystem failure, increased risk of hypoxia and hypotension, invasion of the cerebral cortex via the olfactory neurons, depletion of enzymes which lead to impaired blood flow, and immune dysregulation leading to hyperinflammation (Davis et al., 2023). For children with clear neurological injuries, psychological or neuropsychological consultation is similar to non-COVID-related neurological injuries and will not be discussed in this chapter.

Long COVID

Long COVID likely represents a unique condition (separate from severe COVID-19/MIS-C) and is not clearly associated with disease factors. Long COVID symptoms can emerge immediately following COVID-19 illness, shortly after resolution, or after several weeks. Symptoms can wax and wane and follow an unpredictable course that varies by the individual. A few definitions of long COVID are available (e.g., CDC, WHO), with the most recent definition being released in June 2024 by the National Academies of Science, Engineering, and Medicine. Their definition is intentionally broad and includes the following: symptoms can include over 200 different issues, must be attributed to a known or suspected infection, be present for at least 3 months, and lead to functional impairment.

Several mechanisms of long COVID have been proposed in adults, including primary (e.g., neurobiological causes), secondary (non-neurological medical conditions that lead to dysfunction), tertiary (psychological and stress-induced symptoms), and quaternary pathways (environmental/social factors) (Ballering et al., 2022; Koterba, Considine et al., 2024; Liu et al., 2022; Mainali & Darsie, 2021; Nalbandian et al., 2021; Reiss et al., 2023). Identifying a single cause of long COVID appears overly simplistic. In reality long COVID is a heterogeneous condition, and multiple causes may interact in the same individual leading to symptoms and functional impairment.

Research examining the mechanisms of long COVID in children is limited, and in many cases, we must extrapolate from adult literature. While frank neurological injuries are rare, COVID-19 can result in neuroinflammation, which can impact neuronal regulation and myelin production/repair potentially resulting in symptoms (e.g., brain fog, fatigue, headache, and impaired memory and attention) (Monje & Iwasaki, 2022). Alternatively, COVID-19 can impact vascular function resulting in disruption of the blood–brain barrier and oxygen saturation of circulating blood, leading to hypoxia and metabolic disturbance (Monje & Iwasaki).

Neuroimaging studies of long COVID are emerging, mostly in adults. We recommend interpreting these findings cautiously, as they remain isolated and inconsistent. For example, one study found that a quarter to over half of adults with long COVID had non-specific neurological symptoms; however, only 4 of the 41 participants who also underwent brain MRI had notable "non-specific" findings (Taruffi et al., 2023). This suggests that an identifiable structural abnormality is uncommon outside of cases with frank CNS involvement. In contrast, Besteher and colleagues (2022) studied brain structural changes in relation to neuropsychiatric symptoms in 30 adults with long COVID and 20 healthy controls and documented enlarged gray matter volume in fronto-temporal areas extending into subcortical structures. Further, Serrano Del Pueblo and colleagues (2024) studied 83 adults with long COVID relative to 22 adults with a history of SARS-CoV-2 infection without persistent symptoms and found reduced cortical thickness in one region of the posterior superior temporal gyrus. Additional white matter findings, specifically reduced fractional anisotropy and increased radial diffusivity, are potentially more compelling as they align with the white matter hypothesis noted above. That said, further research is needed in this area.

Long COVID and Neuropsychiatric Symptoms

Most relevant to neuropsychologists are the neuropsychiatric symptoms which can be associated with long COVID, including emotional/behavioral, cognitive, and psychiatric issues. Cognitive difficulties, including concentration problems, brain fog, memory problems, and slowed processing speed, are among the most frequently reported (Berg et al., 2022; Radtke et al., 2021). When compared to controls, reviews and meta-analyses suggest that there is a small but increased prevalence of cognitive difficulties in children post COVID-19 (Lopez-Leon et al., 2022). Relatively small differences between children with long COVID and controls suggest that the pandemic has increased rates of self-reported cognitive difficulties in youth, irrespective of long COVID status.

In one of the most robust studies of long COVID cognitive symptoms in children, Luedke and colleagues (2024) found that around 30% to 35% of children with long COVID struggled with performance-based measures of attention, and to a lesser extent, processing speed. Caregivers also reported executive dysfunction, as well as poor study skills. However, this could be an exacerbation of pre-illness weaknesses as many patients had pre-existing attention difficulties. Many also presented with anxiety and depression and/or reported pre-illness mood concerns.

The link between mental health and cognitive functioning has been well-established. Indeed, in adults, attention and cognitive test performance is susceptible to the effects of mood, fatigue, pain, and other physical symptoms (Badenoch et al., 2022; Premraj et al., 2022; Whiteside et al., 2022). When attention is impacted, other domains such as memory and processing speed may also be impacted. In the adult literature, those with pre-existing mental health conditions are more vulnerable to developing persisting symptoms after COVID-19 (Bobak et al., 2024). The pandemic has exacerbated mental health conditions for youth, including anxiety and depression, regardless of COVID-19 status (Deng et al., 2023; Gotlib et al., 2023; Powell et al., 2024). Taken together, results suggest that children with long COVID are likely at a slightly higher risk for both self-reported cognitive difficulties, and potentially objective cognitive difficulties, and that mental health concerns also contribute to these difficulties. Fortunately, emerging adult research indicates that symptoms improve over time and symptom reduction is possible.

Assessment Considerations

Long COVID remains a relatively new condition with symptom variability, leading to potential underdiagnosis (Thaweethai et al., 2023). In addition, fewer than 20 dedicated pediatric long COVID clinics exist in the United States, making it difficult for many children to get accurately assessed and diagnosed. Psychologists affiliated with or near one of the few specialty clinics may receive referrals to assess the cognitive and psychosocial impact of long COVID. However, for many, long COVID may not be identified, or providers may not be familiar with how to assess and treat concerns. In cases where a diagnosis is not clearly documented, psychologists are encouraged to evaluate the patient's presentation, determine whether symptoms and duration meet diagnostic criteria, consider other contributing factors, and advocate for the medical team to consider a diagnosis of and treatment for long COVID.

Diagnostic Interview

In addition to standard practice, psychologists are encouraged to gather information regarding pre and post illness functioning to understand the symptom course and exacerbating factors. In general, the following can be gathered when assessing a child with long COVID symptoms:

- COVID-19 diagnosis or exposure(s)
- COVID-19 vaccination(s)
- Post-COVID-19/long COVID symptoms—including subacute (4–12 weeks post-infection) and chronic (>12 weeks) neuropsychiatric symptoms, treatments, and new diagnoses (e.g., postural orthostatic tachycardia syndrome (POTS)), including whether these were new or exacerbated symptoms and how they changed over time
- COVID-19 hospitalization/treatment
- COVID-19 complications
- Detailed psychosocial, developmental, and behavioral history (including attention and mood problems and treatments) pre-COVID-19 and currently
- Family history of long COVID
- Academic history including pandemic-related effects, changes to performance, and symptom impact (e.g., absences, homebound instruction, online learning)
- School's response to symptoms and accommodations
- Assessment of psychosocial stressors (e.g., pandemic-related disruptions and stress)

Assessment

Not all children with long COVID need neuropsychological assessments. Sometimes children may be referred with mild cognitive complaints, but other symptoms may be more predominant. In these cases, after gathering a thorough history, psychologists may help the family determine when and if cognitive testing is needed. If testing is not needed, the provider may gather background information and provide recommendations (see below). When testing is warranted, batteries can be short and targeted as the effects on areas such as overall intelligence/IQ or reasoning would not be expected. In addition, as testing is brief, it can be completed via telehealth, which has been shown to be equivalent to in-person assessments in a small long COVID sample (Luedke et al., 2024). Telehealth testing can be ideal for children with long COVID as they may experience fatigue or have trouble traveling to in-person visits. See below for assessment domains:

- Attention (including sustained attention)
- Working memory
- Memory—immediate and delayed recall
- Processing speed
- Verbal fluency
- Executive functioning (e.g., shifting attention, cognitive flexibility)
- Caregiver, self, and teacher report of emotional/behavioral functioning, attention, and executive functions

Conceptualization and Recommendations

As most children have had COVID-19, and as rates of mental health issues are higher for everyone since the pandemic, it can be hard to determine whether symptomology is related to long COVID or the pandemic itself. However, rather than tease apart the underlying cause, psychologists are encouraged to identify and address a child's needs. Indeed, whether a child is reporting subjective cognitive complaints or has objective impairments, research indicates that those with long COVID experience distress and functional difficulties. (Luedke et al., 2024). Based on the federal definition, long COVID could qualify a student for school services under the IDEA or Section 504 of the Rehabilitation Act of 1973 (even without objective documentation of deficits). As long COVID is new, clear guidance is limited, and we encourage professionals to focus on an individual's symptoms and level of impairment in developing educational plans.

In general, recommendations are tailored to each patient based on objective impairments relative to testing and reported dysfunction. In working with children with long COVID, psychologists are encouraged to validate their symptom experience, provide information about what might be contributing to their difficulties and strategies to improve functioning, and express a shared belief that gradual symptom improvement is possible. Additional recommendations are included below:

- Strategies to address attention, executive functions, memory, and processing speed consistent with standard of care.
- Return to school: children with long COVID often do not have a medical reason to stay home from school or transition to online learning, so we recommend returning to school as soon as possible. The focus should be on regular attendance with consideration of a gradual return and/or a modified schedule to help get children back to school. Help the child, family, and school personnel understand there will be "good days and bad days." Focus on attendance rather than academic success. Provide extra time, help with writing, schedules, and copies of notes if the child has trouble keeping up. Allow preferential scheduling when the child is most alert or alternate between challenging classes and electives. Consider 1–2 study halls or opportunities to work with an intervention specialist, especially if a child has frequent absences.
- Physical symptoms: focus on small successes to build confidence and avoid repeated symptom assessment. Express understanding and support along with a shared belief that the child will feel better. If needed, consider physical therapy and medication, as well as healthy lifestyle changes (e.g., hydration, healthy eating, improving sleep).
- Pacing: this is key to reducing fatigue and avoiding post-exertional crashes experienced by many patients. Modify schedules, activities, and workload to avoid overdoing it or underdoing it. Consider

reducing workload and gradually work up to a regular volume. If a child has missed out on physical activities for an extended period, gradually ease back with a modified schedule. For example, return to athletic practice for 10 minutes at first and work up to a full practice as shorter periods are tolerated. Physical therapists can also help with pacing.
- Sleep: provide basic recommendations for sleep hygiene, as sleep can be disrupted after COVID-19 (e.g., aim for 8 hours of sleep per night, have a consistent time to wake up and go to bed, avoid naps/caffeine, get regular exercise, make the bedroom conducive to sleep).
- Emotional health: focus on functioning and gradually returning to activities, encourage behavioral activation principles, along with a regular schedule for activities. Acknowledge and address worries and encourage reframing of biased thoughts (e.g., instead of "I'm never going to get better," say "This won't last forever" or "I have strategies that can help"). Consider behavioral health services through school or outpatient clinics.
- Referrals to medical specialties: psychologists may sometimes advocate for referrals to medical specialists depending on symptoms. For instance, the following physical symptoms may warrant specific referrals: symptoms of postural orthostatic tachycardia syndrome (POTS; see Chapter 12 for information on this disorder), headaches (neurology), respiratory issues or chest pain (pulmonology), sleep disruption (sleep medicine/neurology). Medication monitoring and follow-up with a primary care physician or psychiatrist may also be considered depending on the patient's presentation (e.g., review of poly-medication for potential weaning of those that may have cognitive side effects, trial of stimulants for brain fog) (Fine et al., 2022).

Schools can be instrumental in improving a child's functioning. If a child's educational setting has changed due to long COVID (e.g., previously attended in-person school and transitioned to online learning), efforts can be made to return to their pre-illness setting. This will help to reinforce a sense of normalcy and will also help the child get back into a regular routine. The recommendations above can be shared with schools and can be implemented informally or through a Section 504 Plan. It is unlikely that most children with long COVID would need an Individualized Education Plan (IEP), although this could be considered depending on their functional impairment. A child could qualify for a Section 504 Plan or an IEP based on a medical diagnosis of long COVID (e.g., for an IEP, this could likely fall under Other Health Impairment). Over time, as symptoms hopefully improve academic accommodations could be reduced.

In addition to the recommendations listed above, some manualized therapy programs have been adapted for use with long COVID. For example, the Comfort Ability Program (CAP), which was developed for chronic pain, has been applied in symptom management for children with long COVID given the overlapping clinical presentation. The basis of CAP is a focus on improving functioning by learning strategies to manage discomfort. CAP is available in several locations throughout North America and may also be available via telehealth (https://www.thecomfortability.com). If providers are interested in referring patients, they can first ask if the particular location is able to serve children with long COVID.

Some adult research and to-be-published pediatric research also suggest that group therapy using a biopsychosocial approach may be effective (Vaes et al., 2021). Group-based treatment could be considered as findings from pilot trials yielded accounts that highlight the supportive nature of groups, validation from meeting others who understand symptoms of long COVID and functional effects, and the benefit of hearing and learning from shared experiences (Koterba et al., 2023). Finally, Project ECHO offers a virtual community healthcare approach (www.kennedykrieger.org/training/programs/project-echo/current-echo-series/pediatric-long-covid-echoref). Project ECHO provides training and mentorship to allied health professionals on best practices for care of children with long COVID. The goal of the program is to disseminate evidence-based assessment/intervention approaches to community providers and school health professionals and enable those in areas without specialty long COVID clinics to obtain equitable care. Hopefully, other options are or will become available over time as we learn more about how to address and treat long COVID. We recommend that psychologists guide families to the most empirically supported treatments (even those that have been validated in similar populations like chronic pain or chronic symptoms after concussion) and avoid treatments that are cost prohibitive and/or may be associated with medical risks.

Conclusion

Although children tend to experience less severe COVID-19 illnesses, they are far from being spared from the broader adverse impacts of the pandemic. Indeed, certain children are at risk for severe acute illnesses and MIS-C and some emerging evidence suggests that rates of neurological symptoms may be higher than expected. In addition, while rates are lower than in adults, youth are still at risk of experiencing long COVID. Finally, children have been disproportionately impacted by pandemic-related factors, including lockdowns, virtual learning, and reduced socialization. Taken together, COVID-19 has impacted children both directly and indirectly and may have long-term developmental impacts that are yet to be realized. As research continues to emerge, we will learn more about how COVID-19 has influenced children, and hopefully future research will focus on interventions to support the unique needs of youth impacted by the pandemic.

References

Badenoch, J. B., Rengasamy, E. R., Watson, C., Jansen, K., Chakraborty, S., Sundaram, R. D., Hafeez, D., Burchill, E., Saini, A., Thomas, L., Cross, B., Hunt, C. K., Conti, I., Ralovska, S., Hussain, Z., Butler, M., Pollak, T. A., Koychev, I., Michael, B. D., Holling, H., … & Rooney, A. G. (2022). Persistent neuropsychiatric symptoms after COVID-19: A systematic review and meta-analysis. *Brain Communication*, 4(1), 297. doi:10.1093/braincomms/fcab297.

Ballering, A. V., van Zon, S. K. R., olde Hartman, T. C., & Rosmalen, J. G. M. for the Lifelines Corona Research Initiative (2022). Persistence of somatic symptoms after COVID-19 in the Netherlands: An observational cohort study. *The Lancet*, 400(10350), 452–461. doi:10.1016/S0140-6736(22)01214-4.

Berg, S. K., Nielsen, S. D., Nygaard, U., Bundgaard, H., Palm, P., Rotvig, C., & Christensen, A. V. (2022). Long COVID symptoms in SARS-CoV-2-positive adolescents and matched controls: A national, cross-sectional study. *The Lancet Child & Adolescent Health*, 6(4), 240–248. doi:10.1016/S2352-4642(22)00004-9.

Besteher, B., Machnik, M., Troll, M., Toepffer, A., Zerekidze, A., Rocktäschel, T., Heller, C., Kikinis, Z., Brodoehl, S., Finke, K., Reuken, P. A., Opel, N., Stallmach, A., Gaser, C., & Walter, M. (2022). Larger gray matter volumes in neuropsychiatric long-COVID syndrome. *Psychiatry Research*, 317, 114836. DOI.org/10.1016/j.psychres.2022.114836.

Bobak, L., Dorney, I., Kovacevich, A., Barnett, B., & Kaelber, D. C. (2024). Pre-existing psychiatric conditions as risk factors for diagnosed long COVID-19 syndrome within aggregated electronic health record data. *Psychosomatic Medicine*, 86(3), 132–136.

Castagnoli, R., Votto, M., Licari, A., Brambilla, I., Bruno, R., Perlini, S., Rovida, F., Baldanti, F., & Marseglia, G. L. (2020). Severe acute respiratory syndrome coronavirus 2 (SARS-CoV-2) infection in children and adolescents: A systematic review. *JAMA Pediatrics*, 174(9), 882–889. doi:10.1001/jamapediatrics.2020.1467.

Centers for Disease Control and Prevention (2021). Hospitalizations associated with COVID-19 among children and adolescents – COVID-NET, 14 States, March 1, 2020-August 14, 2021. *CDC Morbidity and Mortality Weekly Report*, 70(36), 1255–1260. https://www.cdc.gov/mmwr/volumes/70/wr/mm7036e2.htm.

Centers for Disease Control and Prevention (2024) *2022–2023 Nationwide COVID-19 infection- and vaccination-induced antibody seroprevalence (blood donations)*. Department of Health and Human Services, CDC. Retrieved May 24, 2024, from https://covid.cdc.gov/covid-data-tracker/#nationwide-blood-donor-seroprevalence-2022.

Davis, H. E., McCorkell, L., Vogel, J. M., & Topol, E. J. (2023). Long COVID: Major findings, mechanisms, and recommendations. *Nature Reviews Microbiology*, 21(3), 133–146.

Deng, J., Zhou, F., Hou, W., Heybati, K., Lohit, S., Abbas, U., Silver, Z., Wong, C. Y., Chang, O., Huang, E., Zuo, Q. K., Moskalyk, M., Ramaraju, H. B., Heybati, S., & Heybati, S. (2023). Prevalence of mental health symptoms in children and adolescents during the COVID-19 pandemic: A meta-analysis. *Annals of the New York Academy of Sciences*, 1520(1), 53–73. https://doi.org/10.1111/nyas.14947.

Feldstein, L. R., Tenforde, M. W., Friedman, K. G., Newhams, M., Rose, E. B., Dapul, H., Soma, V. L., Maddux, A. B., Mourani, P. M., Bowens, C., Maamari, M., Hall, M. W., Riggs, B. J., Giuliano, J. S., Singh, A. R., Li, S., Kong, M., …

& Overcoming COVID-19 Investigators. (2021). Characteristics and outcomes of US children and adolescents with multisystem inflammatory syndrome in children (MIS-C) compared with severe acute COVID-19. *Jama*, 325(11), 1074–1087. doi:10.1001/jama.2021.2091.

Fine, J. S., Ambrose, A. F., Nyaz, D., Fleming, T. K., Glashan, L., Longo, M., Merlino, A.Ng, R., Nora, G. J., Rolin, S., Silver, J., Terzic, C. M., Verduzco-Gutierrez, M., & Sampsel, S. (2022). Multi-disciplinary collaborative consensus guidance statement on the assessment and treatment of cognitive symptoms in patients with post-acute sequelae of SARS-CoV-2 infection (PASC). *PM & R: Journal of Injury, Function & Rehabilitation*, 14(1). doi:10.1002/pmrj.12745.

Fink, E. L., Robertson, C. L., Wainwright, M. S., Roa, J. D., Lovett, M. E., Stulce, C., Yacoub, M., Potera, R. M., Zivick, E., Holloway, A., Nagpal, A., Wellniz, K., Czech, T., Even, K. M., Brunow de Carvalho, W., Rodriguez, I. S., Schwartz, S. P., Walker, T. C., … & Schober, M. E. (2022). Prevalence and risk factors of neurologic manifestations in hospitalized children diagnosed with acute SARS-CoV-2 or MIS-C. *Pediatric Neurology, 128, 33–44*. https://doi.org/10.1016/j.pediatrneurol.2021.12.010.

Francoeur, C., Alcamo, A. M., Robertson, C. L., Wainwright, M. S., Roa, J. D., Lovett, M. E., Stulce, C., Yacoub, M., Potera, R. M., Zivivk, E., Holloway, A., Nagpal, A., Wellnitz, K., Even, K. M., Brunow de Carvalho, W., Rodriguez, I. S., Schwartz, S. P., Walker, T. C., Campos-Mino, S., Dervan, L. A., … & Fink, E. L. (2024). Severe pediatric neurological manifestations with SARS-CoV-2 or MIS-C hospitalization and new morbidity. *JAMA Network Open*, 7(6), e2414122-e2414122. doi:10.1001/jamanetworkopen.2024.14122.

Gotlib, I. H., Miller, J. G., Borchers, L. R., Coury, S. M., Costello, L. A., Garcia, J. M., & Ho, T. C. (2023). Effects of the COVID-19 pandemic on mental health and brain maturation in adolescents: Implications for analyzing longitudinal data. *Biological Psychiatry Global Open Science*, 3(4), 912–918. https://doi.org/10.1016/j.bpsgos.2022.11.002.

Koterba, C. H., Considine, C. M., Becker, J. H., Hoskinson, K. R., Ng, R., Vargas, G., Basso, M. R., Puente, A. E., Lippa, S. M., & Whiteside, D. M. (2024). Neuropsychology practice guidance for the neuropsychiatric aspects of long COVID. *The Clinical Neuropsychologist*, 1–29. Advance online publication. https://doi.org/10.1080/13854046.2024.2392943.

Koterba, C. H., Hoskinson, K. R., Vargas, G., & Ng, R. (2024). *The impact of COVID-19 on children: Pediatric neuropsychological considerations in severe acute illness and Long COVID.* [Paper presentation], American Academy of Clinical Neuropsychology, Scottsdale, AZ.

Koterba, C. H., Vargas, G., Ng, R., & Hoskinson, K. R. (2023). Neuropsychological impact of COVID-19 on children and adolescents. *Journal of Pediatric Neuropsychology*, 10(1), 20–29. https://doi.org/10.1007/s40817-023-00151-7.

Liu, C. H., Smiley, P. A., Vicman, J. M., Wong, G. T. F., & Doan, S. N. (2022). The roles of life stress and preventative health behaviors on parent mental health during the COVID-19 pandemic. *Journal of Health Psychology*, 27(6), 1470–1483. https://doi.org/10.1177/13591053211026742.

Lopez-Leon, S., Wegman-Ostrosky, T., Ayuzo del Valle, N. C., Perelman, C., Sepulveda, R., Rebolledo, P. A., Cuapio, A., & Villapol, S. (2022). Long-COVID in children and adolescents: A systematic review and meta-analyses. *Scientific Reports*, 12(1), 9950. https://doi.org/10.1038/s41598-022-13495-5.

Lu, X., Zhang, L., Du, H., Zhang, J., Li, Y. Y., Qu, J., Zhanf, W., Wang, Y., Bao, S., Li, Y., Wu, C., Liu, H., Liu, D., Shao, J., Peng, X., Yang, Y., Liu, Z, Xiang, Y., Zhang, F., … & Wong, G. W. (2020). SARS-CoV-2 infection in children. *New England Journal of Medicine*, 382(17), 1663–1665. doi:10.1016/j.immuni.2022.01.014.

Luedke, J. C., Vargas, G., Jashar, D. T., Malone, L. A., Morrow, A., & Ng, R. (2024). Neuropsychological functioning of pediatric patients with long COVID. *The Clinical Neuropsychologist*, 1–18. https://doi.org/10.1080/13854046.2024.2344455.

Mainali, S. & Darsie, M. (2021, January). Neurologic manifestations and associations of COVID-19. *Practical Neurology*, 42–47.

Monje, M. & Iwasaki, A. (2022). The neurobiology of long COVID. *Neuron*, 110 (21), 3484–3496. doi:10.1016/j.neuron.2022.10.006.

Nalbandian, A., Sehgal, K., Gupta, A., Madhavan, M. V., McGroder, C., Stevens, J. S., Cook, J. R., Nordvig, A. S., Shalev, D., Sehrawat, T. S., Ahluwalia, N., Bikdeli, B., Dietz, D., Der-Nigoghossian, C., Liyanage-Don, N., Rosner, G. F., Bernstein, E. J., Mohan, S., Beckley, A. A., Seres, D. S., … & Wan, E. Y. (2021). Post-acute COVID-19 syndrome. *Nature Medicine*, 27(4), 601–615. https://doi.org/10.1038/s41591-021-01283-z.

National Academies of Science, Engineering, and Medicine (2024). *A long COVID definition: A chronic, systemic disease state with profound consequences.* The National Academies Press. https://doi.org/10.17226/27768.

Panda, P. K., Sharawat, I. K., Panda, P., Natarajan, V., Bhakat, R., & Dawman, L. (2021). Neurological complications of SARS-CoV-2 infection in children: A systematic review and meta-analysis. *Journal of Tropical Pediatrics*, 67(3). https://doi.org/10.1093/tropej/fmaa070.

Patel J. M. (2022). Multisystem Inflammatory Syndrome in Children (MIS-C). *Current Allergy and Asthma Reports*, 22(5), 53–60. https://doi.org/10.1016/j.prrv.2020.08.001.

Powell, A. A., Dowell, A. C., Moss, P., & Ladhani, S. N. (2024). Current state of COVID-19 in children: 4 years on. *Journal of Infection*, 88(5). DOI.org/10.1016/j.jinf.2024.106134.

Premraj, L., Kannapadi, N. V., Briggs, J., Seal, S. M., Battaglini, D., Fanning, J., Suen, J., Robba, C., Fraser, J., & Cho, S. M. (2022). Mid- and long-term neurological and neuropsychiatric manifestations of post-COVID-19 syndrome: A meta-analysis. *Journal of Neurological Sciences*, 434, 120162. doi:10.1016/j.jns.2022.120162.

Radtke, T., Ulyte, A., Puhan, M. A., & Kriemler, S. (2021). Long-term symptoms after SARS-CoV-2 infection in school children: Population-based cohort with 6-months follow-up. *JAMA*, 326(9), 869–871. https://doi.org/10.1101/2021.05.16.21257255.

Reiss A. B., Greene, C., Dayaramani, C., Rauchman, S. H., Stecker, M. M., De Leon, J., & Pinkhasov, A. (2023). Long COVID, the brain, nerves, and cognitive function. *Neurology International*, 15(3), 821–841. https://doi.org/10.3390/neurolint15030052.

Serrano Del Pueblo, V. M., Serrano-Heras, G., Romero Sánchez, C. M., Piqueras Landete, P., Rojas-Bartolome, L., Feria, I., Morris, R. G. M., Strange, B., Mansilla, F., Zhang, L., Castro-Robles, B., Arias-Salazar, L., López-López, S., Payá, M., Segura, T., & Muñoz-López, M. (2024). Brain and cognitive changes in patients with long COVID compared with infection-recovered control subjects. *Brain*, 147(10), 3611–3623. https://doi.org/10.1093/brain/awae101.

Stafstrom, C. E. (2022). Neurological effects of COVID-19 in infants and children. *Developmental Medicine & Child Neurology*, 64(7), 818–829. https://doi.org/10.1111/dmcn.15185.

Taruffi, L., Muccioli, L., Mitolo, M., Ferri, L., Descovich, C., Mazzoni, S., Michelucci, R., Lodi, R., Liguori, R., Cortelli, P., Tonon, C., & Bisulli, F. (2023). Neurological manifestations of long COVID: A single-center one-year experience. *Neuropsychiatric Disease and Treatment*, 19, 311–319. https://doi.org/10.2147/NDT.S387501.

Thaweethai, T., Jolley, S. E., & Karlson, E. W. (2023). Development of a definition of postacute sequelae of SARS-CoV-2 infection. *JAMA*. 329(22), 1934–1946. doi:10.1001/jama.2023.8823.

Vaes, A. W., Goërtz, Y. M. J., Van Herck, M., Machado, F. V. C., Meys, R., Delbressine, J. M., Houben-Wilke, S., Gaffron, S., Maier, D., Burtin, C., Posthuma, R., van Loon, N. P. H., Franssen, F. M. E., Hajian, B., Simons, S. O., Job, F. M., van Boven, F. A. K., Klok, F. A., Spaaetgens, B., Pinxt, C. M. H., ... & Spruit, M. A. (2021). Recovery from COVID-19: A sprint or marathon? 6-month follow-up data from online long COVID-19 support group members. *ERJ Open Research*, 7(2). doi:10.1183/23120541.00141-2021.

Valderas, C., Méndez, G., Echeverría, A., Suarez, N., Julio, K., & Sandoval, F. (2022). COVID-19 and neurologic manifestations: A synthesis from the child neurologist's corner. *World Journal of Pediatrics*, 18(6), 373–382. https://doi.org/10.1007/s12519-022-00550-4.

Whiteside, D. M., Naini, S. M., Basso, M. R., Waldron, E. J., Holker, E., Porter, J., Niskanen, N., Melnik, T. E., & Taylor, S. E. (2022). Outcomes in post-acute sequelae of COVID-19 (PASC) at 6 months post-infection. Part 2: Psychological functioning. *The Clinical Neuropsychologist*, 36(4), 829–847. https://doi.org/10.1080/13854046.2022.2030411.

Zachariah, P. (2022). COVID-19 in children. *Infectious Disease Clinics*, 36(1), 1–14. doi:10.1016/j.idc.2021.11.002.

10 Autoimmune Disorders

Pediatric Myalgic Encephalomyelitis/ Chronic Fatigue (ME/CFS), Pediatric Guillain-Barré Syndrome (GBS), and Juvenile Fibromyalgia Syndrome (JPFS)

Alicia M. Jones and Denise E. Maricle

Introduction

Autoimmune disorders (AIDs) constitute the 3rd most prevalent disease category, with approximately 50 million Americans suffering from autoimmune-related conditions (National Institute of Environmental Health Sciences; NIH, 2024). There are over 80 known autoimmune diseases and an unknown number of possible autoimmune disorders yet to be identified. An autoimmune disorder (AID) occurs when the body's immune system attacks its own cells, tissues, and organs. Data suggest that the incidence of AIDs has been increasing in both adults and children over the last 30 years, with some estimates suggesting a 3% to 12% annual increase in the incidence of various autoimmune disorders (Miller, 2023). Estimates of yearly increases in the overall worldwide incidence and prevalence of autoimmune diseases are 19.1% and 12.5%, respectively (Miller; Lerner et al., 2016). Of significant note is that AIDs in children are thought to have nearly doubled from 10.4% in 2010 to 20.8% today (Murray, 2024).

AIDs are usually chronic, with their severity ranging from mild to disabling, depending on the body systems affected and the damage generated over the course of the disease. The cause for many AIDs is unknown. Genes, infection, and environment have all been proposed to be contributing factors. There is generally no cure for autoimmune diseases, although treatments have been identified for some that may help manage symptoms. Most AIDs are chronic and require life-long treatment.

Although this chapter could focus on multiple autoimmune disorders impacting children, three autoimmune disorders: pediatric myalgic encephalomyelitis/chronic fatigue (ME/CFS), pediatric Guillain-Barré syndrome (GBS), and juvenile fibromyalgia syndrome (JPFS), previously thought to only affect adults, are now being identified more frequently in children and adolescents and so were chosen to be discussed. Other autoimmune-related disorders, such as Type 1 diabetes (Chapter 14), juvenile

DOI: 10.4324/9781032703923-12

arthritis (Chapter 11) and demyelinating disorders (Chapter 24) are the focus of additional chapters within this text.

Pediatric Myalgic Encephalomyelitis/Chronic Fatigue Syndrome (ME/CFS)

Little is known about pediatric myalgic encephalomyelitis/chronic fatigue syndrome (ME/CFS). It has only been in the last 25 years that clinicians and researchers have understood that ME/CFS exists in children and adolescents. Prior, it was thought to occur only in adults, and even then, numerous professionals considered it a psychiatric or somatic illness, rather than a physical disease. Consequently, the research on pediatric ME/CFS is quite limited. Initially, ME/CFS was thought to present similarly irrespective of age (Loades et al., 2021; Rowe, 2023), but research has shown slight differences in children, adolescents, and adults.

ME/CFS is a complex, multisystemic, debilitating illness characterized by severe and medically unexplained fatigue lasting longer than three months (duration is six months in adults). Fatigue is the universal symptom in pediatric ME/CFS, which is usually sufficient (in combination with other symptoms) to lead to marked functional impairment (Crawley, 2017). Post exertional malaise (PEM) is widely considered to be a common feature of ME/CFS and is characterized by the exacerbation of symptoms like fatigue, lightheadedness, pain, or generally feeling ill after even minor physical, cognitive, or emotional effort. Additionally, over 43% of children and 30% of adolescents display orthostatic intolerance (OI) or issues with orthostatic symptoms, and 9% to 20% experience significant or unrelenting chronic pain. Orthostatic intolerance is the umbrella term for a range of different conditions that result in difficulty with upright posture, particularly standing. The most dramatic problem people with orthostatic intolerance suffer is fainting, but in between fainting episodes they may have difficulty with orthostatic symptoms such as feeling weak, lightheaded, experiencing palpitations or abnormal sweating, feeling nauseated or experiencing problems with concentration. Unrefreshing sleep and sleep disturbances are common (reported prevalence is approximately 84% to 96%) and may include insomnia, sleep cycle disturbances, and excessive sleeping. Over 40% of children and adolescents with ME/CFS report gastrointestinal concerns, such as nausea, and a significant proportion develop eating problems as a result. Neurocognitive manifestations are commonly reported in children and adolescents with ME/CFS. For example, difficulty maintaining attention, especially switching or dividing attention; poor endurance for tasks that involve thinking and difficulty staying on task (task performance tends to deteriorate as fatigue levels increase); and lack of mental stamina that leads to difficulty in completing or finishing tasks. In general, they have difficulty concentrating, thinking, and remembering, and complain of "brain fog" type symptoms (76% of children and 86% of adolescents). ME/CFS appears to typically present with a triad of primary symptoms: persistent fatigue, unexplainable pain, and impaired thinking (Young, 2020). Almost a third of children and adolescents with CFS/ME appear to develop comorbid anxiety or depression (Crawley).

The reported prevalence of pediatric ME/CFS ranges dramatically from 0.11% to 4% and appears dependent on criteria being used to define ME/CFS (Crawley, 2017). Loades and colleagues (2021) cite an estimated prevalence of 0.89% and Rowe (2023) provides a prevalence rate of 0.1–1.9% of adolescents in the USA. Jason and colleagues (2020) reported an overall or average prevalence rate of 0.75% with substantially higher rates for females, ethnic/racial minorities, and older children. Post-pandemic there has been an emergence of a subset of individuals diagnosed with long COVID who display co-morbid ME/CFS (approximately 10% to 30% of long COVID patients). There are no apparent gender differences during childhood but beginning in adolescence and extending into adulthood, ME/CFS is 2 to 3 times more common in females. No genetic correlations have yet been found, but recent infection or illness is a known risk factor and may be a common trigger. ME/CFS has been associated with the Epstein Barr virus. Other common co-morbid disorders include fibromyalgia, irritable bowel syndrome (IBS), Danlos-Ehlers syndrome (EDS) and migraines.

Pediatric ME/CFS can have either an acute or gradual onset. There appears to be three phenotypes in the pediatric population: a polysymptomatic phenotype, a sore throat–painful lymph node phenotype, and a musculoskeletal phenotype (Crawley). Individuals with ME/CFS usually experience a prolonged, and often frustrating path toward diagnosis. The median time from the start of symptoms to diagnosis ranges from 8 to 17 months. No definitive treatments have been determined, and there are no known predictors for recovery. Long-term studies suggest that some individuals will report improvement within 10 years; however, a large proportion (20% to 25%) still exhibit reduced functionality 10 years post-illness (Rowe). Pediatric ME/CFS is best viewed as a chronic illness that impacts all aspects of the individual's life.

Pediatric Guillain-Barré Syndrome (GBS)

Pediatric Guillain-Barré syndrome (GBS) is a very rare autoimmune disorder that affects the nerves and can cause acute motor paralysis. It is a form of peripheral neuropathy (Schonbeck & Blake, 2020) and is one of the most common causes of acute flaccid paralysis in healthy children. Few validated large-scale population-based data are available concerning pediatric GBS, including incidence, risk factors, and initial clinical characteristics (Levinson et al., 2020).

Pediatric GBS is usually a short-term (but can be life-threatening) disorder that causes muscle weakness, pain, and temporary paralysis of the muscles in the face, chest, and legs. The child may experience tingling or pain in the extremities, or weakness and pain in their legs, making it difficult to walk. Schonbeck and Blake (2020) suggest onset is often characterized by tingling, burning, or numbing sensations in toes and feet, with symptoms progressing to lower legs, trunk, arms, hands, and fingers, resulting in severe discomfort and/or sharp jabs of pain. Paralyzed chest and swallowing muscles can lead to breathing issues, choking, and death if not treated.

Korinthenberg and colleagues (2020) report that pediatric GBS can be subclassified into a number of variants, depending on clinical presentation and electrophysiological findings. Acute demyelinating inflammatory polyneuropathy (AIDP) and acute motor axonal neuropathy (AMAN) are identified as the most common variants. They are characterized by rapidly progressing, ascending symmetrical weakness, with attenuation or loss of proprioceptive reflexes in the muscles. As the disease progresses and peaks, 75% can no longer walk unaided, 30% are tetraparetic (3 or more affected limbs), 35% to 50% show cranial nerve involvement, and 15% to 20% have respiratory failure and/or autonomic dysfunction. Up to 70% report neuropathic pain, which can be severe, and occasionally occurs as the very first symptom expressed. Two localized variants that are extremely rare in childhood include Miller Fisher syndrome (MFS: cranial nerve affection and ataxia, areflexia) and the pharyngeal-cervical-brachial variant (predominantly bulbar and neck weakness).

The prevalence rate for pediatric GBS ranges from 0.5 to 1.5 cases per 100,000. Levinson and colleagues (2020) estimate a world-wide incidence rate of 1 to 2 per 100,000. Males appear to be at greater risk than females. Younger children tend to be more vulnerable with an average age of onset of 4–8 years. The mortality rate is estimated to be 5%.

The exact cause of GBS is unknown, but it is considered an autoimmune disorder in which the body's immune system attacks the nervous system, as it sometimes develops after a viral infection, surgery, injury, or in extremely rare cases as a reaction to a vaccine. Acute infections before the onset of GBS are reported in 50% to 82% children (Levison et al.). Schonbeck & Blake (2020) identify other potential contributors, including other autoimmune disorders (lupus, rheumatoid arthritis), exposure to toxic substances, chronic liver or kidney disease, hormonal imbalances (such as thyroid), or cancer.

Children diagnosed with GBS usually need to be hospitalized for care, but most recover fully with no complications. The most effective treatment is intravenous immunoglobulin (IVIG), but plasmapheresis (the removal of plasma and antibodies that are then replaced with other fluids) may be used if IVIG is ineffective or intolerable. Recovery appears to depend on how serious the nerve damage is and often takes up to 2 months although full recovery may take 1 to 2 years. Korinthenberg and colleagues (2020) suggest that the overall long-term prognosis for children with GBS is more favorable than that of adults. The majority of children regain motor function; however, even after years, it is not uncommon to uncover mild to moderate neurological and neuropsychiatric deficits such as fatigue and paresthesia (abnormal skin sensations like tingling or numbness), as well as poor motor coordination and concentration difficulties. Limited information exists about the factors that could serve as predictors for recovery.

Juvenile Fibromyalgia Syndrome (JPFS)

Pediatric fibromyalgia, also known as juvenile primary fibromyalgia syndrome (JPFS), is a chronic condition that causes widespread pain and stiffness in the muscles, joints, and other soft tissues. It is often accompanied by fatigue, sleep disorders, chronic headaches, irritable bowel syndrome, and subjective soft tissue swelling (Vincenzo et al., 2019). Symptoms seen in JPFS include:

- Pain (described as dull ache, burning, shooting, or throbbing)
- Pain occurring on both sides of the body and throughout entire body
- Acute tenderness (tender to even slight touch). Individuals experience pain in numerous tender points on their body such as neck, shoulders, elbows, chest, lower back, or knees (Webb & Culvert, 2018)
- Frequent headaches
- Fatigue and sleep problems, such as non-restorative sleep, waking up tired, or having trouble falling asleep
- Pain or cramping in the lower abdomen
- Swelling or numbness
- Cognitive impairment, or feeling "foggy"
- Depression or anxiety

Chronic widespread pain is the primary symptom in JPFS. The other symptoms of fatigue, sleep disturbance, cognitive changes, and mood disturbances vary in severity. JPFS pain is described as being diffuse, deep, and continuous often with periods of exacerbation. Symptoms may be modulated by various factors including psychological stress, excessive physical activity, viral infections, and fatigue. This results in the clinical presentation of JPFS being quite diverse with some areas of the body more painful than others, fluctuations in intensity of pain, and variable intensity of other associated symptoms. Patients also differ considerably in terms of severity of functional impairment.

Chronic pain (persistent and recurrent pain) is a significant problem in pediatric populations. Conservatively, chronic pain is estimated to affect 20% to 35% of children (especially adolescents) worldwide (Chambers et al., 2024; Vincenzo et al., 2019). Clinically, pain is usually categorized into three overlapping types including *nociceptive or peripheral pain* (results from damaged tissues via trauma or inflammation); *neuropathic pain* (associated with damage to the peripheral or central nervous system); and *centralized pain*, which has no identifiable nerve or tissue damage and is thought to result from persistent neuronal dysregulation, overactive ascending pain pathways, or a deficiency of descending inhibitory pain pathways (Vincenzo et al.). In JPFS, research suggests acute pain activates the somatosensory, insular, and cingulate cortical areas, but that chronic pain preferentially activates the prefrontal and limbic cortical areas.

JPFS is an idiopathic disorder (of unknown cause) with no identified etiology. It sometimes develops in children who have experienced physical trauma (surgery, infection) or a major psychological stressor, but generally there is no obvious trigger. Current evidence suggests a combination of genetic predisposition and extrinsic stressors or triggers. Clinically, it is considered a pain processing disorder (Webb & Culvert, 2018), and possibly a neuroendocrine illness (due to abnormal hormonal/chemical levels associated with processing pain). The CDC describes it as a type of polyarthritis, and some have considered it a disorder affecting connective tissues. As a pain processing disorder, it appears to involve a process known as "central sensitization of the CNS." Central sensitization occurs when the patient's nervous system is persistently in a high activity state, which decreases sensitivity to the firing of action potentials. When this happens, the peripheral nervous system provides limited input, and the central nervous system responds as if there has been a high level of painful stimuli. An increase in the action potential firing leads to amplified neural signaling. Patients become hypersensitive to pain. Even innocuous non-nociceptive stimuli are perceived as painful and the perception of noxious stimuli is exaggerated, prolonged, and widespread. The pain in JPFS is not caused by local inflammation but seems to be due to abnormal functioning of pain receptors in the brain. However, inflammatory processes may play a significant role in the pathogenesis of JPFS. There is a subset of individuals that test positive for antinuclear antibody (ANA) and have symptoms that resemble early lupus, indicating that JPFS may be an autoimmune disease.

There are no tests to confirm a diagnosis of JPFS (Matallana & Bradley, 2009). Prevalence rates are scant. In the USA, the incidence is about 1% at age 5–9, 2.6% for ages 10–14 and about 6% for adolescents aged 15–19 (Vincenzo et al., 2019). JPFS occurs more commonly in girls than boys, usually affecting children during adolescence or late childhood. Most pediatric patients are diagnosed between ages 13–15 and adolescent girls are 6 times more likely to be diagnosed than boys. JPFS is a chronic disease, with 70% diagnosed in childhood continuing to meet criteria into adulthood.

Implications for Schools: Assessment, Diagnosis, and Intervention

Assessment

A school-based assessment for a child or adolescent diagnosed with ME/CFS, GBS, or JPFS should begin with a **comprehensive clinical and developmental history interview** with the parents/caretakers, the child, and involved school personnel. Appropriate consent releases should be obtained to share information with outside treatment providers and to encourage interdisciplinary collaboration. Given the complexity of these disorders, it is important for the child's overall health and well-being that school professionals be aware of and consider the prognosis for the child's particular disorder, the potential for adverse impact on the child's learning and behavior, and the mediating impact of any treatments being provided from outside sources (e.g., medication, occupational, or physical therapies). A child with ME/CFS, GBS, or JPFS should be offered a **comprehensive neuropsychological evaluation** to obtain information as to their neurocognitive and neuropsychological status, academic functioning, linguistic abilities, motor/physical skills, as well as adaptive and social-emotional or behavioral functioning.

School assessment professionals should be prepared to modify general assessment processes and procedures to accommodate for symptoms that may impact performance (e.g., fluctuating energy levels, fatigue, pain, memory lapses, disorganized thinking or brain fog, shortened attention span, or fine motor/gross motor mobility limitations). If school assessment professionals lack familiarity or expertise in the evaluation of pain, fatigue, or symptoms such as post exertional malaise (PEM), they will need to be prepared to seek consultation or recommend an external evaluation. School professionals may need to rely on outside professionals or experts for some assessments of more challenging symptomology such as PEM, or orthostatic intolerance (OI). Because debilitating pain and fatigue are prominent symptoms in these disorders, evaluation of pain and fatigue should be part of an ongoing (daily) assessment of functioning. Few resources are available for assessing symptoms like pain and fatigue, but some instruments have been validated for use with ME/CFS and might be useful to both the clinical and school psychologist. The DePaul Symptom Questionnaire (DSQ: Landgraf et al., 1996), the Autonomic Symptom Checklist (Sletten et al., 2012), and the Fatigue Severity Scale (Krupp et al., 1989) all show some validity with pediatric ME/CFS patients. Although not validated for use with JPFS or GBS, they may still be an applicable way to gather information about the child's experiences.

Qualification for Special Education and Supportive Services

School personnel are not likely to be involved in the diagnosis of these three conditions, whereas a pediatric neuropsychologist may, particularly if they are working in a multidisciplinary children's hospital, medical center, or specialty practice clinic. However, school personnel are likely to play a primary role in determining if a child meets criteria for educational supports and services in the public-school setting. Children or adolescents with ME/CFS, GBS, or JPFS will likely qualify for either special education supports and services under the IDEA or accommodations and supportive services under Section 504 of the Rehabilitation Act of 1973. The most appropriate IDEA classification is likely to be Other Health Impairment (OHI) as all three disorders (ME/CFS, GBS, and JPFS) are considered chronic health conditions which affect the individual's strength, vitality, or alertness, and create functional impairment and significant disruption in the child's daily life, including learning and school attendance. In rare situations, the psychological toll of the disorder, or paralyzing anxiety and/or depression, may warrant a classification of emotional disturbance (ED).

Interventions

There is clear evidence that ME/CFS, GBS, and JPFS disrupt normal childhood activities and daily life, and adversely impact educational and social development. Each child is affected differently and may experience differing symptoms or duration of symptoms. Their symptoms may change from day to day or week to week. This can affect the individual's ability to participate in activities of daily living such as attending school. Interventions should be designed to address the primary difficulties being displayed by each specific child, but in general, the clinician or school professional may want to address the major symptom areas: fatigue, sleep disturbance, pain, PEM or OI, neurocognitive challenges such as brain fog or cognitive endurance, and comorbid psychiatric difficulties (depression or anxiety), in addition to considering appropriate modifications or accommodations for daily living, school, and social challenges.

School attendance is often a major issue with affected children. Historically, these children may have been viewed as "lazy" "school avoidant" or "school phobic" and labeled as "truant" or "school refusers" or even erroneously thought to be "malingering." In addition to the physical toll of living with ME/CFS, GBS, or JPFS, the psychological and mental toll can be just as daunting to manage given the "invisible" nature of the disorders. Psychoeducation is often needed to convince school personnel that the child's physical health and well-being are compromised despite no visible disease process, and that the child is not attention-seeking or avoidant (Abril & Bruce, 2019).

Schools may need to be prepared to consider alternatives to typical school attendance, ranging from altering attendance requirements or exempting the student from absenteeism penalties, to modifying the school day or course schedule of the child, or to offering homebound instruction or additional home-based tutoring. Exemptions from graduation requirements may be needed for some children. Additionally, it may be necessary to consider alterations to work completion requirements, and alternatives to homework completion for more advanced students. Consider ways to reduce information and work overload for the individual (e. g., provide notes rather than expecting the adolescent to take notes; break larger projects into single steps completed one piece at a time), prioritize some courses (e.g., exempt student from electives) or areas of emphasis (e. g., focus on reading and math), provide additional time for work completion or test taking, or schedule rest periods throughout the day.

Activity management can be a useful approach in addressing fatigue, pain, and symptoms such as PEM. For example, it is important for the child with ME/CFS or JPFS to develop balance and pace rest and activity to avoid PEM. Any activity or exercise plan needs to be carefully designed with input from the individual child or adolescent. Trying to find the balance between doing nothing and lots of activity can be tricky. It may mean a new way of thinking about daily activities. For example, daily chores and school activities may need to be broken down into smaller steps. Exemptions for physical education classes and outdoor recess may need to be considered, or adaptive PE provided. An adaptive PE professional may be able to offer a graded aerobic exercise program, which has been found to be useful in increasing activity and engagement. Participation in after-school activities (if tolerated) can support social development and should be considered even if the child is not able to attend school despite school rules relating to attendance and participation.

Adjusting to a chronic illness is challenging. Several approaches might be considered, both pharmacological and non-pharmacological. Medications are often prescribed for children and adolescents with these conditions. Schools may need to be prepared to allow medication to be administered during the school day, and the IEP team may need to develop an Education Health Care Plan (EHCP) or an Individualized Health Care Plan (IHP) for the child, educating personnel on the medications being taken, and the side effects most commonly seen or that would indicate toxicity. Exceptions to district policies for school administration (e.g., giving out certain medications such as opiates) or self-administration can be recorded on the EHCP or IHP.

Selective serotonin reuptake inhibitors (SSRIs) are often prescribed to alleviate pain, improve sleep, and boost mood. Anticonvulsants and dopamine agonists have been used to treat pain and neuropathy. Corticosteroids and non-steroidal anti-inflammatories (NSAIDs) may be used to address inflammation and pain. In severe cases, narcotics (such as OxyContin) may also be prescribed for the alleviation of pain. Some children may be on stimulant medication to assist with concentration problems, especially if they have a co-morbid ADHD diagnosis. Stimulants can help improve attention/concentration, but they can also lead to a "push and crash" cycle, which actually worsens the symptoms of ME/CFS or JPFS. A push and crash cycle occurs when the child is having a good day, so they do more than they normally would, which then results in a worsening of symptoms or a "crash" setting them back significantly.

Alternative interventions, such as acupuncture, massage, hydrotherapy, or movement therapies (such as yoga, pilates, tai chi) may be used. Some individuals find these useful in alleviating pain, improving mobility, and promoting relaxation (Cooksey & Mertz, 2020; Ford-Martin & Blake, 2020). Experimental methods such as repetitive transcranial magnetic stimulation (TMS) or vagus nerve stimulation (VNS) show some promise (Webb & Culvert, 2018). Behavior modification, biofeedback, cognitive behavioral therapy, and stress reduction techniques have also been found useful. Adolescents struggling with severe depression comorbid with ME/CFS, GBS, or JPFS regardless of psychiatric or therapeutic care, should also be monitored for suicidality.

Conclusion

This exploration of pediatric ME/CFS, GBS, and JPFS has made it clear that these conditions, though distinct in their manifestations, share common threads of complexity and profound impact on young patients and their families. ME/CFS and JPFS present significant challenges in diagnosis and management, often requiring a multidisciplinary approach to address the diverse symptoms and improve quality of life. Similarly, pediatric GBS, while acute and often severe, necessitates prompt intervention and supportive care to optimize recovery and mitigate long-term effects. Collectively, these disorders highlight the critical need for continued research to unravel their underlying mechanisms and develop more effective treatments. A compassionate, child-centered approach is essential, recognizing the unique physical and emotional struggles faced by children and their families. As understanding and treatment of these conditions advance, increased support systems and improved outcomes ultimately offer hope and resilience for those navigating the challenges of pediatric chronic illness.

For many reasons, resources for children, adolescents, and families dealing with ME/CFS, GBS, or JPFS are scarce, and many focus only on ME/CFS or chronic pain. Following are a few recent sources that might serve as a starting point for individuals, parents, and professionals working in this area.

Resources

Fisher, P. (2021). *Tired Teens: Understanding and Conquering Chronic Fatigue and POTS*. Mayo Clinic Press.

Young, J. (2020). *Understanding and Treating Chronic Fatigue: A Practical Guide for Parents, Families, and Practitioners*. Praeger.

The MEG Foundation in conjunction with the Society of Pediatric Pain Special Interest Group has developed some great resources for children and parents (megfoundationforpain.org) including *Chronic Pain and Daily Functioning*, *CBT for Chronic Pain, Chronic Pain and School*, and *Healthy Sleep for Kids and Teens with Chronic Pain.*

Fibromyalgia Care Society of America Youth Advocates Program (FYA): fibro.org

National Fibromyalgia Association: fmaware.org

Stop Childhood Pain: stopchildhoodpain.org

References

Abril, A. & Bruce, B. K., (2019). *Mayo clinic guide to fibromyalgia: Strategies to take back your life.* Mayo Clinic Press.

Chambers, C., Dol, J., Tutelman, P. R., Langley, C. L., Parker, J. A, Cormier, B. T., Macfarlane, G. J., Jones, G. T., Chapman, D., Proudfoot, N., Grant, A., & Marianayagam, J. (2024). The prevalence of chronic pain in children and adolescents: A systematic review update and meta-analysis. *Pain*, 10, 1097. | doi:10.1097/j.pain.0000000000003267.

Cooksey, G. & Mertz, L. (2020). Myotherapy. In D. S. Hiam (Ed.). *The Gale Encyclopedia of Alternative Medicine* (5th ed., Vol. 3), pp. 1861–1863. Gale.

Crawley, E. (2017). Pediatric chronic fatigue syndrome: Current perspectives. *Pediatric Health, Medicine and Therapeutics*, 9, 27–33. https://doi.org/10.2147/PHMT.S126253.

Ford-Martin, P. & Blake, S. (2020). Hydrotherapy. In D. S. Hiam (Ed). *The Gale Encyclopedia of Alternative Medicine* (5th ed., Vol. 3), pp. 1365–1379. Gale.

Jason, L. A., Katz, B. Z., Sunnquist, M., Torres, C., Cotler, J., & Bhatia S. (2020). The prevalence of pediatric myalgic encephalomyelitis/chronic fatigue syndrome in a community-based sample. *Child Youth Care Forum*, 49(4), 563–579. doi:10.1007/s10566-019-09543-3.

Korinthenberg, R., Trollmann, R., Felderhoff-Müser, U., Bernert, G., Hackenberg, A., Hufnagel, M., Pohl, M., Hahn, G., Mentzel, H. J., Sommer, C., Lambeck, J., Mecher, F., Hessenauer, M., Winterholler, C., Kempf, U., Jacobs, B. C., Rostasy, K., & Müller-Felber, W. (2020). Diagnosis and treatment of Guillain-Barré syndrome in childhood and adolescence: An evidence- and consensus-based guideline. *European Journal of Paediatric Neurology*, 25, 5–16. https://doi.org/10.1016/j.ejpn.2020.01.003.

Krupp, L. B., LaRocca, N. G., Muir-Nash, J., & Steinberg, A. D. (1989). The fatigue severity scale: Application to patients with multiple sclerosis and systemic lupus erythematosus. *Archives of Neurology*, 46, 1121–1123. doi:10.1001/archneur.1989.00520460115022.

Landgraf, J. M., Abetz, L., & Ware, J. E. (1996). *The child health questionnaire (CHQ): A user's manual.* The Health Institute, New England Medical Center.

Lerner, A., Jeremias, P., & Matthias, T. (2016) The world incidence and prevalence of autoimmune diseases is increasing. *International Journal of Celiac Disease*, 3, 151–155. doi:10.12691/ijcd-3-4-8.

Levison, L. S., Thomsen, R. W., Markvardsen, L. K., Christensen, D. H., Sindrup, S. H., & Andersen, H. (2020). Pediatric Guillain-Barré Syndrome in a 30-year nationwide cohort. *Pediatric Neurology*, 107, 57–63. https://doi.org/10.1016/j.pediatrneurol.2020.01.017.

Loades, M. E., Crawley, E., Chalder, T., & Flannery, H. (2021). Pediatric chronic fatigue syndrome: 25-year perspective. *Clinical Child Psychology and Psychiatry* 26(1), 8–17. doi:10.1177/1359104520978461.

Matallana, L., & Bradley, L. A. (2009). *The complete idiot's guide to fibromyalgia* (2nd ed.). Alpha Penguin Group.

Miller, F. W. (2023). The increasing prevalence of autoimmunity and autoimmune diseases: An urgent call to action for improved understanding, diagnosis, treatment, and prevention. *Current Opinion in Immunology*, 80, 102266. doi:10.1016/j.coi.2022.102266.

Murray, M. (2024). Guest Blog: A major health crisis: The alarming rise of autoimmune disorders. *National Health Council* [online]. Retrieved August 8, 2024, from www.https:nationalhealthcouncil.org/blog.

National Institute of Environmental Health Sciences (NIH, 2024, February 20). Autoimmune diseases. *Health and Education*. Retrieved March 15, 2024, from https://www.niehs.nih.gov/health/topics/conditions/autoimmune.

Rowe, K. (2023). Chronic fatigue syndrome/myalgic encephalomyelitis (CFS/ME) in adolescents: Practical guidance and management challenges. *Adolescent Health, Medicine and Therapeutics*, 14, 13–26. https://doi.org/10.2147/AHMT.S317314.

Schonbeck, J. & Blake, S. (2020). Peripheral neuropathy. In D. S. Hiam (Ed.), *The Gale encyclopedia of alternative medicine* (5th ed., Vol. 3), pp. 2062–2065. Gale.

Sletten, D. M., Suarez, G. A., Low, P. A., Mandrekar, J., & Singer, W. (2012, December). COMPASS 31: A refined and abbreviated composite autonomic symptom score. *Mayo Clinic Proceedings*, 87(12), 1196–1201. doi:10.1016/j.mayocp.2012.10.013.

Vincenzo, A., Ashraf, T. S., Nada, S., Bernadette, F., & Christos, K. (2019). The juvenile fibromyalgia syndrome (JFMS): A poorly defined disorder. *Acta Biomed: Atenei Parmensis*, 90(1), 134–148. doi:10.23750/abm.v90i1.8141.

Webb, M. R. & Culvert, L. L. (2018). Fibromyalgia. In J. L. Longe (Ed.) *The Gale encyclopedia of nursing and allied health (*4th ed. Vol. 3). pp. 1447–1452. Gale.

Young, J. (2020). *Understanding and treating chronic fatigue: A practical guide for parents, families, and practitioners.* Praeger.

11 Juvenile Arthritis

Kendra A. Hamilton

Introduction

Juvenile arthritis (JA) is an umbrella term utilized to describe a group of inflammatory diseases in child and adolescent populations. Dr. George Still, a British pediatrician, first shed light on this condition in the late 19th century. Dr. Still's work with children at the Hospital for Sick Children yielded 22 cases that demonstrated a chronic form of arthritis specifically in youth (Kim & Kim, 2010). Today, the disease he described in those 22 children is called juvenile idiopathic arthritis.

Juvenile idiopathic arthritis (JIA) is one of the most common forms of JA, which is an inflammatory disease that can affect any joint and can cause extra-articular inflammation in youth (Garner et al., 2021). There are several types of JIA: oligoarthritis, polyarticular (rheumatoid factor (RF) negative and RF positive), systemic, psoriatic, enthesitis-related, and undifferentiated arthritis. The most common form of JIA is oligoarthritis (National Institute of Arthritis and Muscoskeletal and Skin Diseases, 2021).

JIA is an autoimmune disease where the body's immune system fights itself by attacking healthy cells and tissues. In JIA, inflammation occurs around the lining of the joint, which is known as synovial tissue or synovium. When this lining is inflamed, it creates more fluid than normal, causing joints to swell (Ravelli & Martini, 2007). This can lead to pain in the joints as well as stiffness, causing issues with physical mobility.

Inside the synovium, there is a thickening of tissue, and as this synovial tissue thickens, it causes immunocompetent cells such as T-cells, B-cells, natural killers, neutrophils, macrophages, dendritic cells, and plasma cells to increase (Twilt et al., 2017). These cells pool around the thickened synovial tissue and continue to increase in number, causing the release of more chemicals that lead to further inflammation. In addition to swelling, pain, and stiffness, this internal process can lead to damage of the cartilage and bone.

DOI: 10.4324/9781032703923-13

Etiology

Presently, the cause of JIA is unclear (Horton & Shenoi, 2019). Genetic factors have been reported as contributors. In a twin study, the concordance rate for JIA ranged from 25% to 40% in monozygotic twins (Giancane, Alongi, & Ravelli, 2017). Environmental factors have also been considered as a potential cause, including fetal exposure to antibiotics where those newly diagnosed with JIA had increased bacteroidetes post antibiotic exposure (Stoll, Weiss et al., 2018; Tejesvi et al., 2016). Other risk factors include infectious agents, stress, and trauma (Rigante et al., 2015).

Epidemiology

JIA is the most prevalent rheumatic disease in the Western world (Thatayatikom, Modica, & De Leucio, 2023). The prevalence varies, ranging from 3.8 to 400 cases per 100,000 children (Thierry et al., 2014). Gender differences have been indicated, and JIA appears more prevalent in females than males (Cattalini et al., 2019). Racial differences were indicated, but as a whole, JIA is more prevalent among Caucasian children (Espinosa & Gottlieb, 2012). Subtypes also demonstrated differences with an increase in oligo-articular JIA in Caucasian children and RF positive polyarticular JIA in African American children (Espinosa & Gottlieb).

Diagnosis

For a diagnosis to occur, symptoms must be evident before the 16th birthday and persist for at least 6 weeks (Jacobson & Pham, 2018). There are several methods utilized in the diagnostic procedure. Discussion of medical history, clinical symptoms, and a physical examination are essential (Zaripova et al., 2021). Laboratory testing is a common method to determine any inflammation markers (Thatayatikom, Modica, & De Leucio, 2023). Imaging, such as radiography, ultrasound, and magnetic resonance imaging, may also be necessary to improve the certainty of a diagnosis and assess joint damage (Thatayatikom et al.). It is imperative to seek a timely diagnosis to decrease the likelihood of joint damage (Stoll, Kau, et al., 2018).

Characteristics Symptoms and Medical Complications

Typically, across most subtypes, a hallmark symptom is swollen, stiff, painful joints that appear red or feel warm and/or tender. Due to the impact of JIA on joints, physical movement can become restricted, contributing to a decrease in range of motion. Also, a condition known as morning stiffness, or gelling, can happen after extended periods of physical inactivity (Jacobson & Pham, 2018). A pink or red rash across the face and/or body may also be present. Other distinctive features that may be associated with specific subtypes include fever and enlarged lymph nodes (systemic), the presence of inflammation of tendons (enthesitis), and psoriasis (psoriatic) (Petty, 2001). Some subtypes have distinguishing features based on the number of joints they impact like oligoarthritis, which impacts four or fewer joints and polyarticular, which impacts five or more joints (Petty). Fatigue, loss of appetite, difficulties with weight gain and slowed growth can also occur depending on the subtype. It should be noted that each subtype may have other associated symptoms and can vary in severity.

Complications of JIA can occur, and internal organs can be impacted. Digestive issues can arise causing constipation, bloating, and other gastrointestinal issues due to inflammation. Lung-related issues, like shortness of breath, and heart complications, specifically palpitations, may also occur.

Treatments

Treatment for youth impacted by JIA should be conducted by a multidisciplinary team including a pediatric rheumatologist, ophthalmologist, orthopedist, specialist nurse, physical therapist, occupational therapist, and mental-health worker. Treatment plans may incorporate the use of both non-pharmacological and pharmacological interventions. Physical therapy and occupational therapy may be ideal non-pharmacological methods utilized to restore joint function and alignment (Häfner, Truckenbrodt, & Spamer, 1998). Orthotic devices may also be useful depending on severity and need. Pharmacological methods that address the symptoms of JIA include nonsteroidal anti-inflammatory drugs (NSAIDs). NSAIDs are the most common pharmacological method, but only a few are approved in children: naproxen, ibuprofen, and indomethacin (Giancane et al., 2016). Intra-articular corticosteroid (IAC) injections are used to treat synovitis and provide rapid relief (Cleary, Murphy, & Davidson, 2003; Scott et al., 2010). Disease-modifying antirheumatic drugs (DMARDs) may also be used as a pharmacological intervention when NSAIDs are ineffective. The most common and effective DMARD is methotrexate (Gutiérrez-Suárez & Burgos-Vargas, 2010; Ravelli & Martini, 2000).

Implications for School

Qualification for Special Education Services

Under the Individuals with Disabilities Education Act (IDEA), a child with JIA may qualify under the Other Health Impairment (OHI) classification due to its impact on strength, endurance, and stamina. They may also qualify under the Orthopedic Impairment (OI) classification pending the severity of physical impairment caused by JIA. In other instances, a child may only need services under Section 504 of the Rehabilitation Act. A child with JIA that is classified under IDEA or 504 may receive modifications for additional time as one travels the campus, specialized or adaptive technology, tools, or seating, various accommodations for the common symptoms of pain or fatigue, adaptive physical education (APE) or access to therapeutic services like occupational or physical therapy.

Assessment in Schools

For most children with JIA, the most chronic symptoms are joint pain, stiffness, and/or swelling. Pain should be assessed daily, and accommodations should be adjusted based on the child's self-report. Assessment of pain can be conducted using several tools (Lalloo et al., 2020). The Visual Analog Scale is used to assess pain intensity using one item to measure intensity while the FACES Pain Rating Scale uses facial expressions to represent varying levels of pain. A more complex tool is the Bath Adolescent Pain Questionnaire, which uses 61 items to assess how pain is impacting the child's overall quality of life. Another tool is the Pain Coping Questionnaire (PCQ). This tool was developed for children with arthritis and is designed to assess coping strategies for children dealing with pain (Reid et al., 1998). The Bath or the PCQ might be useful additions to multidisciplinary assessments and re-evaluations to track long-term coping and quality of life related to pain.

Since there are various symptoms associated with the different subtypes, students may experience other symptoms such as fatigue or loss of appetite. Many of these symptoms can impact a student's mental health, and psychological disorders, like depression and anxiety, are common co-occurring disorders in the JIA population (Fair et al., 2019). Screening should occur using pediatric measures of depression and anxiety.

School-Based Interventions and Accommodations to Consider

Most children with JIA can be included within regular education classrooms. However, accommodations may be necessary to address joint pain, swelling, and tenderness as well as fatigue. Students with JIA may experience pain or stiffness when engaging in any physical activity including sitting, walking, or carrying things. Physically, these students may benefit from additional time to move from class to class, assistance with carrying items, specialized seating, access to adaptive course like physical education, periods of rest, or time to visit with the school nurse to address their medical needs (Jordan et al., 2021). Accommodations for pain relief (e.g., allowing medication and self-administration) need to be considered.

During recess, pain can arise while engaging in activities like running or throwing. Weather conditions, like cold air, can trigger and even worsen pain. When the classroom teacher and other school staff are aware of these concerns, they can be attentive and proactive in addressing them.

Academically, pain can impact students within the classroom setting, causing issues with writing, and completing extended assignments and tasks. Teachers can convey flexibility and adaptability by being aware of the pain's impact. Teachers can provide additional time for coursework completion or allow larger academic tasks to be condensed into smaller ones (Jordan et al., 2021). Specialized writing tools or assistance with notetaking during academic assignments may also be beneficial.

Emotionally, students with JIA may struggle with anxiety and depression. Students that struggle with these mental disorders should be assessed and have consistent access to school-based mental health professionals. The parents of the student should regularly communicate with the teacher and school staff regarding any changes in symptoms and needs of the students (Jordan et al., 2021). Communication is critical in providing the school based supports the student needs.

A great resource is *Juvenile Arthritis: A Teacher's Guide*: https://www.arthritis.org/getmedia/4fee18c7-7c56-4bfa-8951-fccf7c16aad0/ja-teachers-guide-pdf.pdf

Other resources can be found below:

- National Institute of Arthritis and Musculoskeletal and Skin Disease: https://www.niams.nih.gov/health-topics/juvenile-arthritis
- American College of Rheumatology: https://rheumatology.org/patients/juvenile-arthritis

Juvenile Lupus

Juvenile lupus is an autoimmune disease also housed under the umbrella of JA. Like other forms of JA, juvenile lupus is a disease characterized by inflammation of skin, joints, and organs. The damage caused by lupus can lead to disability or even death in some instances (Charras, Smith, & Hedrich, 2021).

The history of lupus dates back centuries when cutaneous ulcers were first described by Hippocrates as herpes esthiomenos (Smith & Cyr, 1988). It was Robert Willan, an English physician of the late 1700s and early 1800s, who used lupus as the term to describe destructive and vesicular diseases of the face. In 1833, the first clear depiction of lupus erythematosus was made by Laurant-Theodore Biett. Later, in 1872, Moirz Kapozi divided lupus into discoid and systemic types (Smith & Cyr), ultimately laying the groundwork for the foundational classification of lupus today.

There are four types of lupus. Systemic lupus erythematosus (SLE) is the most common type. The other common form of lupus is cutaneous lupus erythematosus (CLE), and similar to its name, this form affects the skin through rashes and lesions. The last two types of lupus are fairly rare: neonatal lupus, a rare form of lupus that primarily affects infants of women with lupus, and drug-induced lupus which is a disease triggered by certain medications that cause symptoms similar to lupus. For the purpose of this chapter, the emphasis will be on juvenile systemic lupus erythematosus (jSLE) due to its prevalence.

The pathophysiological process of jSLE is complex and unknown with much of the pathophysiological research conducted in SLE among adult populations. While there are numerous contributors of SLE, two critical components have been consistently researched: T and B cells. Typically, SLE is triggered when there is an interaction of factors, such as a genetically susceptible individual and exposure to one or more environmental factors (Justiz Vaillant et al., 2023). These environmental factors lead to cell damage. The immune system is then activated including the activation of immunocompetent cells, such as T and B cells. In patients with lupus, T cells tend to display abnormalities, such as defects in their signaling and effector functions. Damaged T cells then contribute to the autoimmune response by creating a cyclical process where inflammatory T cells and dysregulated B cells continuously activate one another. In a healthy state, T cells can create homeostasis; however, in patients with SLE, the continuous activation of T and B cells leads to tissue damage in major organs of the body such as the kidneys and heart (Justiz Vaillant, Goyal, & Varacallo).

Etiology

The cause of lupus is unclear. Research highlights the contribution of genetic and environmental factors. The genetic basis appears strong with a 43% to 66% heritability estimate across the population (Chen et al., 2020; Wang et al., 2021). Various studies have identified other genetic contributions, such as genetic mutations or polymorphism, aneuploidy, and copy number variations (Charras et al., 2021). Environmental contributors include ultraviolet light exposure, smoking, silica exposure, exogenous hormone exposure, pollutant/chemical exposures, microbiome composition, and prior infection (Gulati & Brunner, 2018; Leffers et al., 2019; Parks et al., 2017).

Epidemiology

The prevalence rate of jSLE is 3.3 to 8.8 per 100,000 children (Kamphuis & Silverman, 2010). Prevalence rates are higher among females than males. Race has been identified as a risk factor; African Americans tend to have the highest rates. Asians and Hispanics are also impacted at higher frequencies than Caucasian counterparts (Justiz Vaillant et al., 2023).

Diagnosis

The diagnosis of jSLE can be difficult and requires a multi-measure diagnostic process. Typically, a physical examination is essential coupled with a discussion of symptomology and medical history. Laboratory testing is important and may include complete blood count, antinuclear antibody, anti-DNA, complement (C3 and C4), and c reactive protein (Justiz Vaillant et al., 2023). Urinalysis is helpful in identifying if lupus has affected the kidneys, and likewise, chest x-rays can be helpful in determining if lupus has impacted the heart (Justiz Vaillant et al.). Biopsies may also be critical in determining the impact of lupus on organs of the body. Lastly, diagnostic criteria for lupus were given by the American College of Rheumatology and at least four diagnostic criteria must be present for a diagnosis (Hochberg, 1997). Furthermore, a diagnosis of lupus may require additional time and effort due to its ability to mimic other autoimmune diseases like JIA; therefore, it is imperative to be evaluated by a pediatric rheumatologist to receive a timely and accurate diagnosis.

Characteristics Symptoms and Medical Complications

The hallmark symptom of jSLE is the malar rash with other common symptoms of extreme fatigue, fever, decrease in appetite, weight loss, and hair changes (Levy & Kamphuis, 2012). Additionally, pain or even swelling within the joints is another common symptom, and most with jSLE have arthritis similar to JIA. Lastly, muscle aches, ulcers in mouth/nose, and fingers that turn white or blue when under the duration of physical and mental stress are also common. These symptoms may wax and wane as symptoms flare or go into remission and may vary from child to child.

Medical complications often arise. Vital organs, such as the kidneys, heart, lungs, and brain, are commonly affected. Kidney inflammation can occur, causing lupus nephritis (kidney disease) and even kidney failure (Levy & Kamphuis, 2012). Shortness of breath and chest pain have also been indicated as common complications of the lungs while palpitations were identified as a common issue of the heart. Inflammation in the brain can lead to headaches, cognitive impairments such as memory issues, or even seizures in some instances. Gastrointestinal issues, including stomach pain and discomfort, are also prevalent.

Treatments

While there is no cure for jSLE, there are several treatment approaches to consider. A multidisciplinary team is essential and should consist of a rheumatologist, primary care physician, any specialists that may address specific complications (e.g., dermatologist, nephrologist, and cardiologist), the school nurse, and/or any therapeutic providers (e.g., physical therapists, occupational therapists) (Levy & Kamphuis, 2012).

Treatments for jSLE are categorized as non-pharmacological and pharmacological. The pharmacological methods are divided into two categories: non-immunosuppressants, which tend to be milder, provide relief, and have fewer side effects, and immunosuppressants, which are more powerful, regulate the immune system more, and have more significant side effects. One of the safest immunosuppressants is called *hydroxychloroquine*, which works for disease maintenance in mild conditions (Lee et al., 2011). NSAIDs, such as ibuprofen and naproxen, are also staple non-immunosuppressants administered for musculoskeletal symptoms. One of the more prevalent immunosuppressants administered is corticosteroids, as this drug works to suppress the immune system. Other immunosuppressants include steroid sparing therapies, biologics, and cytotoxins (Levy & Kamphuis, 2012). In instances when a child is suffering from additional medical complications, such as kidney or heart issues, the use of other pharmacological methods may be required.

Non-pharmacological methods may include physical or occupational therapy as these therapies can help to relieve pain and restore physical function and mobility. Other non-pharmacological methods that may reduce symptoms include liberal use of sunscreen, ensuring quality sleep, eating nutritious foods, minimizing stress, and treating any infections immediately.

Implications for the School

Qualification for Special Education Services

A child with jSLE may qualify under the Other Health Impairment (OHI) classification of the IDEA or under Section 504 of the Rehabilitation Act. A child with jSLE that is classified under IDEA or 504 may receive modifications for provision of health-related services by medical staff, additional time to rest, adaptive physical education (APE) or access to therapeutic services such as occupational or physical therapy.

Assessments in the Schools

Children with jSLE exhibiting symptoms, such as the malar rash, fever, weight changes, hair changes, and ulcers in mouth may need to be assessed by the school nurse or other medical professional/specialist. As the hallmark symptom, the malar rash can contribute to students experiencing feelings of low self-esteem regarding physical appearance. Some students may experience sadness about the disease and its impact on daily functioning as well as nervousness about the future. Anxiety and depression are prevalent in the jSLE population; therefore, screening for these disorders may be necessary.

Extreme fatigue is another common symptom in jSLE, and there are several measures that can be used to evaluate this symptom. These measures have been validated in children that experience chronic pain, specifically cancer, but not specifically in jSLE populations. The Childhood

Fatigue Scale (Hockenberry et al., 2003) is a 14-item measure that evaluates for any fatigue during the past week by having the child report with yes/no. There is also a Parent Fatigue Scale and Staff Fatigue Scale available that provides additional assessment of fatigue in a child. The Fatigue Scale Adolescent (Hinds et al., 2007) is another 14-item self-report measure to assess fatigue. Fatigue should be assessed daily and adjustments should be made based on these reports.

For symptoms such as joint pain, professional assessments should be completed to identify severity and impact on the child. If joint pain is a common symptom, it should be assessed daily. See previous subsection of this chapter on *Juvenile Idiopathic Arthritis, Implications for the School, Assessments in the Schools* for possible measures of pain.

School-Based Interventions and Accommodations to Consider

Most children with jSLE can be included within the regular education classrooms. Academically, jSLE students may struggle with extreme fatigue during academic activities; therefore, appropriate accommodations may include oral options for timed test/activities, use of computers and laptops for work, copies of notes and learning materials, and memory aids.

Physically, extreme fatigue and chronic pain can also impact the well-being and physical mobility of jSLE students. Teachers should be mindful of activity levels and tolerance, allowing students to sit, move, or rest as needed. Also, students may benefit from extra time to maneuver around the campus, as well as accommodations for mobility (such as using an elevator instead of stairs), and consideration of adaptive physical education in lieu of a typical PE class. There may be times when the student needs access to the nurse to address physical needs, pain, or fatigue. Services, like physical and occupational therapy, may also be crucial to increase physical mobility and range of motion. The malar rash is another symptom that can impact students physically, and since this rash is triggered by sun exposure, limiting classroom seating and school-based activities with sun exposure (such as recess) is essential.

Social and emotional aids may also be needed. Children with jSLE may struggle with the physical and mental impact of the malar rash and fatigue, as well as the mental load of having jSLE. Social-emotional support can occur through a campus support person for student check ins or via regular access to the campus mental-health provider.

Students with jSLE may also require time away from school due to hospitalization. The family of the student should communicate with the teacher and staff to discuss next steps regarding schooling and any emerging needs that require school-based supports.

Resources

A great resource is *Children's Health School Guide for Children with Lupus*: https://www.childrens.com/wps/wcm/connect/childrenspublic/826802b3-4671-4f10-bd70-3f03073b21d9/Lupus.pdf?MOD=AJPERES&CVID=np4rnBm.

Other resources:

- Children's Health Systemic Lupus: https://www.childrens.com/specialties-services/conditions/systemic-lupus-erythematosus
- Systemic Lupus Erythematosus in Children and Adolescents: https://www.ncbi.nlm.nih.gov/pmc/articles/*PMC3348509*/

References

Cattalini, M., Soliani, M., Caparello, M. C., & Cimaz, R. (2019). Sex differences in pediatric rheumatology. *Clinical Reviews in Allergy & Immunology*, 56(3), 293–307. https://doi.org/10.1007/s12016-017-8642-3.

Charras, A., Smith, E., & Hedrich, C. M. (2021). Systemic lupus erythematosus in children and young people. *Current Rheumatology Reports*, 23(3), 1–15. https://doi.org/10.1007%2Fs11926-021-00985-0.

Chen, L., Wang, Y-F., Liu, L., Bielowka, A., Ahmed, R., Zhang, H., Tombleson, P., Roberts, A. L., Odhams, C. A., Cunninghame Graham, D. S., Zhang, X., Yang, W., Vyse, T. J., & Morris, D. L. (2020). Genome-wide assessment of genetic risk for systemic lupus erythematosus and disease severity. *Human Molecular Genetics*, 29(10), 1745–1756. https://doi.org/10.1093/hmg/ddaa030.

Cleary, A. G., Murphy, H. D., & Davidson, J. E. (2003). Intra-articular corticosteroid injections in juvenile idiopathic arthritis. *Archives of Disease in Childhood*, 88(3), 192–196. https://doi.org/10.1136/adc.88.3.192.

Espinosa, M. & Gottlieb, B. S. (2012). Juvenile idiopathic arthritis. *Pediatrics in Review*, 33(7), 303–313. https://njaap.org/uploadfiles/documents/2015/AC/JIA Gottleib.pdf.

Fair, D. C., Rodriguez, M., Knight, A. M., & Rubinstein, T. B. (2019). Depression and anxiety in patients with juvenile idiopathic arthritis: Current insights and impact on quality of life, a systematic review. *Open Access Rheumatology*, 11, 237–252. https://doi.org/10.2147%2FOARRR.S174408.

Garner, A. J., Saatchi, R., Ward, O., & Hawley, D. P. (2021). Juvenile idiopathic arthritis: A review of novel diagnostic and monitoring technologies. *Healthcare*, 9(12), 1683. https://doi.org/10.3390%2Fhealthcare9121683.

Giancane, G., Alongi, A., & Ravelli, A. (2017). Update on the pathogenesis and treatment of juvenile idiopathic arthritis. *Current Opinion in Rheumatology*, 29 (5), 523–529. https://doi.org/10.1097/BOR.0000000000000417.

Giancane, G., Consolaro, A., Lanni, S., Davì, S., Schiappapietra, B., & Ravelli, A. (2016). Juvenile idiopathic arthritis: Diagnosis and treatment. *Rheumatology and Therapy*, 3(2), 187–207. https://doi.org/10.1007/s40744-016-0040-4.

Gulati, G. & Brunner, H. I. (2018). Environmental triggers in systemic lupus erythematosus. *Seminars in Arthritis and Rheumatism*, 47(5), 710–717. https://doi.org/10.1016/j.semarthrit.2017.10.001

Gutiérrez-Suárez, R. & Burgos-Vargas, R. (2010). The use of methotrexate in children with rheumatic diseases. *Clinical and Experimental Rheumatology*, 28(5 Suppl 61), S122–S127.

Häfner, R., Truckenbrodt, H., & Spamer, M. (1998). Rehabilitation in children with juvenile chronic arthritis. *Bailliere's Clinical Rheumatology*, 12(2), 329–361. https://doi.org/10.1016/s0950-3579(98)80022-80028.

Hinds, P. S., Hockenberry, M. J., Tong, X., Rai, S. N., Gattuso, J. S., McCarthy, K., & Srivastava D. K. (2007). Validity and reliability of a new instrument to measure cancer-related fatigue in adolescents. *Journal of Pain Symptom Management*, 34, 607–618. https://doi.org/10.1016/j.jpainsymman.2007.01.009.

Hochberg, M. C. (1997). Updating the American College of Rheumatology revised criteria for the classification of systemic lupus erythematosus. *Arthritis and Rheumatism*, 40(9), 1725. https://doi.org/10.1002/art.1780400928.

Hockenberry, M. J., Hinds, P. S., Barrera, P., Bryant, R., Adams-McNeill, J., Hooke, C., Rasco-Baggott, C., Patterson-Kelly, K., Gattuso, J. S., & Manteuffel, B. (2003). Three instruments to assess fatigue in children with cancer: The child, parent, and staff perspectives. *Journal of Pain and Symptom Management*, 25(4), 319–328. https://doi.org/10.1016/S0885-3924(02)680–682.

Horton, D. B. & Shenoi, S. (2019). Review of environmental factors and juvenile idiopathic arthritis. *Open Access Rheumatology: Research and Reviews*, 11, 253–267. https://doi.org/10.2147/OARRR.S165916.

Jacobson, J. L. & Pham, J. T. (2018). Juvenile idiopathic arthritis: A focus on pharmacologic management. *Journal of Pediatric Health Care*, 32(5), 515–528. https://doi.org/10.1016/j.pedhc.2018.02.005.

Jordan, A., Vasileiou, K., Brown, C., & Caes, L. (2021). Supporting primary school children with juvenile idiopathic arthritis: A qualitative investigation of teaching staff experiences. *Children*, 8(7), Article 555. https://doi.org/10.3390/children8070555.

Justiz Vaillant, A. A., Goyal, A., & Varacallo, M. (2023, August 4). *Systemic lupus erythematosus*. StatPearls Publishing. https://www.ncbi.nlm.nih.gov/books/NBK535405/.

Kamphuis, S. & Silverman, E. D. (2010). Prevalence and burden of pediatric-onset systemic lupus erythematosus. *Nature Reviews. Rheumatology*, 6(9), 538–546. https://doi.org/10.1038/nrrheum.2010.121.

Kim, K. H. & Kim, D. S. (2010). Juvenile idiopathic arthritis: Diagnosis and differential diagnosis. *Korean Journal of Pediatrics*, 53(11), 931–935. https://doi.org/10.3345%2Fkjp.2010.53.11.931.

Lalloo, C., Mesaroli, G., Makkar, M., & Stinson, J. (2020). Outcome measures for pediatric pain: Practical guidance on clinical use in juvenile arthritis. *Arthritis Care and Research*, 72(S10), 358–362. https://doi.org/10.1002/acr.24217.

Lee, S. J., Silverman, E., & Bargman, J. M. (2011). The role of antimalarial agents in the treatment of SLE and lupus nephritis. *Nature Reviews. Nephrology*, 7(12), 718–729. https://doi.org/10.1038/nrneph.2011.150.

Leffers, H. C. B., Lange, T., Collins, C., Ulff-Møller, C. J., & Jacobsen, S. (2019). The study of interactions between genome and exposome in the development of systemic lupus erythematosus. *Autoimmunity Reviews*, 18(4), 382–392. https://doi.org/10.1016/j.autrev.2018.11.005.

Levy, D. M. & Kamphuis, S. (2012). Systemic lupus erythematosus in children and adolescents. *Pediatric Clinics of North America*, 59(2), 345–364. https://doi.org/10.1016/j.pcl.2012.03.007.

National Institute of Arthritis and Muscoloskeletal and Skin Diseases (2021, May). *Juvenile idiopathic arthritis*. https://www.niams.nih.gov/health-topics/juvenile-arthritis.

Parks, C. G., de Souza Espindola Santos, A., Barbhaiya, M., & Costenbader, K. H. (2017). Understanding the role of environmental factors in the development of systemic lupus erythematosus. *Best Practice & Research. Clinical Rheumatology*, 31(3), 306–320. https://doi.org/10.1016/j.berh.2017.09.005.

Petty, R. E. (2001). Growing pains: The ILAR classification of juvenile idiopathic arthritis. *The Journal of Rheumatology*, 28(5), 927–928. https://www.jrheum.org/content/jrheum/28/5/927.full.pdf.

Ravelli, A. & Martini, A. (2000). Methotrexate in juvenile idiopathic arthritis: Answers and questions. *The Journal of Rheumatology*, 27(8), 1830–1833.

Ravelli, A. & Martini, A. (2007). Juvenile idiopathic arthritis. *Lancet*, 369(9563), 767–778. https://doi.org/10.1016/S0140-6736(07)60363–60368.

Reid, G. J., Gilbert, C. A., & McGrath, P. J. (1998). The Pain Coping Questionnaire: Preliminary validation. *Pain*, 76(1–2),83–96. https://doi.org/10.1016/s0304-3959(98)29–23.

Rigante, D., Bosco, A., & Esposito, S. (2015). The etiology of juvenile idiopathic arthritis. *Clinical Reviews in Allergy & Immunology*, 49(2), 253–261. https://doi.org/10.1007/s12016-014-8460-9.

Scott, C., Meiorin, S., Filocamo, G., Lanni, S., Valle, M., Martinoli, C., Martini, A., & Ravelli, A. (2010). A reappraisal of intra-articular corticosteroid therapy in juvenile idiopathic arthritis. *Clinical and Experimental Rheumatology*, 28(5), 774–781.

Smith, C. D. & Cyr, M. (1988). The history of lupus erythematosus. From Hippocrates to Osler. *Rheumatic Diseases Clinics of North America*, 14(1), 1–14. https://www.sciencedirect.com/science/article/abs/pii/S0889857X2100942X?via%3Dihub.

Stoll M. L., Kau C. H., Waite P. D., & Cron R. Q. (2018).Temporomandibular joint arthritis in juvenile idiopathic arthritis, now what? *Pediatric Rheumatology*, 16(32), 1–14. https://doi.org/10.1186/s12969-018-0244-y.

Stoll, M. L., Weiss, P. F., Weiss, J. E., Nigrovic, P. A., Edelheit, B. S., Bridges, S. L., Jr, Danila, M. I., Spencer, C. H., Punaro, M. G., Schikler, K., Reiff, A., Kumar, R., Cron, R. Q., Morrow, C. D., & Lefkowitz, E. J. (2018). Age and fecal microbial strain-specific differences in patients with spondyloarthritis. *Arthritis Research & Therapy*, 20(1), 1–10. https://doi.org/10.1186/s13075-018-1510-6.

Tejesvi, M. V., Arvonen, M., Kangas, S. M., Keskitalo, P. L., Pirttilä, A. M., Karttunen, T. J., & Vähäsalo, P. (2016). Faecal microbiome in new-onset juvenile idiopathic arthritis. *European Journal of Clinical Microbiology & Infectious Diseases: Official Publication of the European Society of Clinical Microbiology*, 35(3), 363–370. https://doi.org/10.1007/s10096-015-2548-x.

Thatayatikom, A., Modica, R., & De Leucio, A. (2023, January 16) *Juvenile idiopathic arthritis*. StatPearls Publishing. https://www.ncbi.nlm.nih.gov/books/NBK554605/.

Thierry, S., Fautrel, B., Lemelle, I., & Guillemin, F. (2014). Prevalence and incidence of juvenile idiopathic arthritis: A systematic review. *Joint Bone Spine*, 81 (2), 112–117. https://doi.org/10.1016/j.jbspin.2013.09.003.

Twilt, M., Pradsgaard, D., Spannow, A. H., Horlyck, A., Heuck, C., & Herlin, T. (2017). Joint cartilage thickness and automated determination of bone age and bone health in juvenile idiopathic arthritis. *Pediatric Rheumatology Online Journal*, 15(1),1–6. https://doi.org/10.1186/s12969-017-0194-9.

Wang, Y. F., Zhang, Y., Lin, Z., Zhang, H., Wang, T. Y., Cao, Y., Morris, D. L., Sheng, Y., Yin, X., Zhong, S. L., Gu, X., Lei, Y., He, J., Wu, Q., Shen, J. J., Yang, J., Lam, T. H., Lin, J. H., Mai, Z. M., Guo, M., … Yang, W. (2021). Identification of 38 novel loci for systemic lupus erythematosus and genetic heterogeneity between ancestral groups. *Nature Communications*, 12(1), 772. https://doi.org/10.1038/s41467-021-21049-y.

Zaripova, L. N., Midgley, A., Christmas, S. E., Beresford, M. W., Baildam, E. M., & Oldershaw, R. A. (2021). Juvenile idiopathic arthritis: From aetiopathogenesis to therapeutic approaches. *Pediatric Rheumatology Online Journal*, 19(1), 1–14. https://doi.org/10.1186/s12969-021-00629-8.

12 Postural Orthostatic Tachycardia Syndrome (POTS) and Ehlers Danlos Syndrome (EDS) in Pediatric Patients

Christina Kokorelis

Postural Orthostatic Tachycardia Syndrome (POTS)

POTS is a disorder of the autonomic nervous system (ANS) characterized by an abnormal increase in heart rate (HR) upon standing and the presence of chronic orthostatic symptoms. Despite documented accounts of POTS dating back to the 1800s (Da Costa, 1951), the term POTS was not firmly established as a unique clinical diagnosis until 1993 (Schondorf & Low, 1993); even so, a majority of providers continue to remain unaware of POTS and how to diagnose and treat the condition (Raj et al., 2021). On average, POTS patients report symptoms for over four years and have seen seven medical providers for their symptoms before receiving an actual diagnosis of POTS (Shaw et al., 2019).

While POTS can affect individuals of any age, it is predominantly found in females (80%) and disproportionately affects adolescents (Sheldon et al., 2015); in a large survey of over 4800 patients with self-reported POTS, the most common age at onset was 14 years (Shaw et al.). One study in China reported that 6.8% of adolescents met clinical criteria for POTS (Lin et al., 2014).

Diagnostic Criteria and Symptomatology

According to the 2019 National Institute of Health Expert Consensus Meeting, for those individuals between the ages of 12 and 19, the diagnostic criteria for POTS include (Vernino et al., 2021):

1 A sustained HR increase of at least 40 beats/minute (bpm) within 10 minutes of standing or during head-up tilt
2 An absence of orthostatic hypotension (i.e., no sustained systolic blood pressure (BP) drop of 20 mmHg or more)
3 Frequent orthostatic symptoms (e.g., lightheadedness, palpitations, blurry vision, and headache) during standing, with rapid improvement upon recumbency
4 Duration of symptoms for at least 3 months

DOI: 10.4324/9781032703923-14

5 Absence of other conditions that could explain the elevation in HR, such as dehydration, anorexia, hyperthyroidism, anemia, pain, infection, or primary anxiety disorder

Of note, the HR parameter remains undefined for patients under the age of 12, although many providers continue to use the 40 bpm parameter for patients younger than 12.

The most common symptoms of POTS include dizziness, fatigue, palpitations, visual disturbance, headache, nausea, and difficulty concentrating (Vernino et al., 2021). These symptoms are typically exacerbated by upright posture and tend to improve or resolve with recumbency. Other factors that can exacerbate POTS symptoms include heat, illness, stress, large meals, and menstruation. Although syncope, defined as a temporary loss of consciousness due to decreased blood flow to the brain, is a stereotypical feature of POTS, in actuality, it is not a predominant symptom; in fact, only ~20% to 30% of POTS patients experience syncope, and in most cases, the syncope is attributed to vasovagal syncope (Shen et al., 2017).

Clinicians often use a combination of clinical history, physical examination, and orthostatic vitals to establish the diagnosis of POTS. The standard test for diagnosis is the head-up tilt test with non-invasive beat-to-beat hemodynamic monitoring to measure HR and BP response (Fedorowski, 2019). The tilt test consists of at least 10 minutes of supine rest on the tilt table followed by a passive head-up tilt to a 70-degree angle for at least 10 minutes but up to 40 minutes depending on the protocol. The test ends prematurely in the event of syncope or at the patient's request. Throughout the duration of the test, HR and BP are documented in addition to the symptoms reported by the patient (Aponte-Becerra & Novak, 2021). A 10-minute passive standing test performed in a clinical setting is a similar but cheaper, more readily available alternative for measuring orthostatic vitals, and can also be used for diagnostic purposes (Roma, Marden, & Rowe, 2018). Diagnosing POTS in adolescents poses unique challenges due to the overlap of symptoms with normal adolescence, such as growth spurts and hormonal changes, in addition to the high prevalence of mood disorders in adolescents, which can complicate the diagnostic process.

The onset of POTS is not always but is often precipitated by a trigger, including viral infection, vaccination, trauma, pregnancy, surgery, or psychosocial stress (Fedorowski, 2019). A history of viral infection preceding the onset of POTS symptoms is most common and has been reported in 20% to 50% of POTS patients (Vernino et al., 2021). A variety of infections have been linked to POTS, including Epstein Barr virus (EBV), mycoplasma pneumoniae, and more recently, SARS-CoV-2 (Vernino et al.). It may be helpful to review past medical records and/or ask about a precipitating event when making a diagnosis of POTS, although at this time, the presence and type of trigger does not generally determine the treatment plan.

A heterogenous clinical picture, early age of onset, and presence of various triggers have led to the development of several different hypotheses regarding the origin of POTS (Fedorowski, 2019). Some of the proposed mechanisms for POTS described in the literature include autonomic denervation, deconditioning, hypovolemia, hyperadrenergic stimulation, and hypervigilance; likely, multiple mechanisms may be present in some patients (Safavi-Naeini & Razavi, 2020). Genetics may also contribute to the pathophysiology, with some cases of POTS showing a familial predisposition (Shannon et al., 2000).

In adolescent POTS patients, hypovolemia, defined as a decreased amount of blood circulating in the body, frequently plays a large role in the pathophysiology. It is known that the likelihood of POTS increases almost 4-fold if an adolescent's water intake is <800 mL daily; most individuals do not reach this daily amount (Chen, et al., 2020). In addition, low iron storage and/or anemia, resulting in low blood volume, has been shown to be more prevalent in pediatric POTS patients compared to healthy children (Blitshteyn, 2015). Furthermore, eating disorders and disordered eating are common causes of hypovolemia particularly in the adolescent female population, which can contribute to POTS or POTS-like symptoms. To avoid misdiagnosis, it is important to address these causes of hypovolemia prior to making a diagnosis of POTS.

Treatment Planning

The high prevalence of POTS following viral infection supports the argument for possible immune involvement in POTS. Other factors, such as the overwhelming preponderance of women with POTS (80%) and a reported 20% rate of comorbid autoimmune disorders in POTS patients, are further suggestive of an underlying immune etiology (Blitshteyn, 2015). Despite some studies noting increased concentrations of certain autoantibodies in POTS patients, currently very little conclusive evidence has emerged for autoimmune mechanisms in POTS (Blitshteyn). There are several ongoing trials looking into the efficacy of using intravenous immunoglobulin (IVIG) as a treatment for POTS.

Considering the pathophysiology of POTS is likely heterogeneous and incompletely understood, it is not surprising that there is very limited data on effective treatment options for POTS. Patient education is a key aspect of managing POTS, and in many cases, non-pharmacologic interventions are sufficient (Vernino et al., 2021). Patients should be instructed to avoid long periods of standing, sudden head-up postural changes, large meals, and warm environments, which can all aggravate symptoms (Shannon et al., 2000). Lifestyle modifications, including increasing fluid intake to three liters per day, avoiding caffeine and alcohol intake, and increasing sodium intake to 3–5 grams daily, along with a graduated exercise program, are commonly recommended. In addition, wearing compression stockings to reduce venous pooling can be helpful (Vernino et al.). An initial exercise program is typically restricted to non-upright exercises, such as rowing machine, recumbent cycling, and swimming, to mitigate the impact of symptoms during exercise (Sheldon et al., 2015).

While there are currently no FDA-approved medications for POTS, medications are often trialed to reduce POTS symptoms; however, non-pharmacologic interventions should always be attempted first. The medications most frequently used in the management of POTS include β-blockers to reduce heart rate, midodrine to increase vasoconstriction, and fludrocortisone to expand blood volume. Other medications prescribed include central sympatholytic agents like clonidine, pyridostigmine bromide, ivabradine, octreotide, and erythropoietin (Safavi-Naeini & Razavi, 2020). Increasing plasma volume with intravenous (IV) saline is another potential intervention. Although there may be a benefit to using IV saline as rescue therapy for acute decompensation, long-term infusions are generally not recommended due to complications associated with central line placement such as infection and blood clot (Hall et al., 2022). One study reported an 11% incidence of upper extremity deep vein thrombosis (DVT) in adolescent POTS patients who had a central line placed for chronic IV saline infusions (Moak et al., 2016).

POTS can significantly impact the quality of life of adolescents struggling with this condition; school attendance may be impacted, and participation in physical activities and extracurricular activities often becomes limited due to symptom burden. Thus, school-aged children diagnosed with POTS may be eligible for supports and services through the IDEA's other health impairment (OHI) classification or for supports, services, and accommodations via Section 504 of the Rehabilitation Act of 1973 as a child with a physical (medical) disability. Schools should be informed about the POTS diagnosis, and accommodations such as flexible schedules, easy access to water and salty snacks, and frequent bathroom and rest breaks, should be considered to ensure school success for adolescents with POTS. Consultation with physical therapy (PT), occupational therapy (OT), and adaptive PE professionals may be helpful in determining possible accommodations to physical education requirements and classes as well as the need for occupational and physical therapy services.

Social interactions and friendships may also be compromised in these patients, leading to feelings of isolation and depression. Psychosocial support, such as counseling, is often helpful, particularly for patients who feel that providers, family members, or friends have ignored, dismissed, or questioned their symptoms. In pediatric POTS patients, increased symptom burden has been linked to increased rates of depression and anxiety in patients and parents alike (Zhao et al., 2015).

Comorbid Conditions

Although the long-term outcome of POTS is not well-studied, around 50% of POTS patients may spontaneously recover within 1–3 years after symptom onset according to one study (Fedorowski, 2019). In a study of 172 adolescent POTS patients, 86% reported improved or resolved symptoms five years after diagnosis (Bhatia et al., 2016). Unfortunately, the presence of medical comorbidities can complicate or even serve as a barrier to the recovery process.

POTS is frequently co-morbid with other medical conditions, most commonly migraines, irritable bowel syndrome (IBS), myalgic encephalomyelitis/chronic fatigue syndrome (ME/CFS), and Ehlers Danlos syndrome (EDS) (Shaw et al., 2019). EDS, a group of heritable connective tissue disorders, is thought to be present in at least 25% of patients with POTS (Miller et al., 2020).

Ehlers Danlos Syndrome (EDS)

EDS Characteristics

EDS comprises a heterogeneous group of genetic disorders caused by mutations in genes involved in collagen synthesis and structure. Edvard Ehlers and Henri-Alexandre Danlos were dermatologists in the early twentieth century who first described the combination of joint hypermobility, excessive skin extensibility, easy bruising, and abnormal scarring as a clinical syndrome (Danlos, 1908; Ehlers, 1901). The updated 2017 International Classification of Diseases includes 13 subtypes of EDS, each with distinct clinical features (Malfait et al., 2017). The most common types include the hypermobile, classical, and vascular subtypes. For many decades, studies defined EDS as a rare disease and quoted an overall prevalence of 1 in 5000; however, a more recent study found a prevalence of 194.2 per 100,000 (0.19%) or 1 in 500 people in Wales with either hypermobile EDS (hEDS) or hypermobility spectrum disorder (HSD) (Demmler et al., 2019). HSD is a clinical spectrum ranging from asymptomatic joint hypermobility to hEDS. Aside from hEDS, the other types of EDS are rarer. Specifically, classical EDS has a prevalence of 1 in 20,000–40,000, vascular EDS has a prevalence of 1 in 100,000–200,000, and the other types of EDS are even less common (Malfait et al.).

Roughly 75% of patients with hEDS report experiencing symptoms by the age of 15 (Gazit, Jacob, & Grahame, 2016). The diagnosis is more frequently made in women than in men; however, it remains unclear whether the incidence truly differs among genders or whether women experience higher symptom burden and/or are more likely to report and investigate their symptoms compared to men. In contrast, the prevalence of the other types of EDS is equal among men and women (Malfait et al., 2020).

Diagnostic Characteristics

Establishing the diagnosis of hEDS and/or HSD is often a challenge for patients, with an average of 14 years elapsing between the first clinical manifestations and the actual diagnosis (Demmler et al., 2019). Most commonly, the diagnosis occurs after the patient has seen various providers; it is typically a lengthy process and is confirmed by a geneticist or rheumatologist. While genetic testing exists for the other subtypes, the diagnosis of hEDS/HSD remains a clinical diagnosis at this time as the etiology remains uncertain likely due to genetic heterogeneity. The lack of genetic testing often causes frustration among patients and providers alike, who are looking for a definitive diagnosis (Malfait et al., 2020). In cases of EDS where a specific genetic mutation is identified, genetic counseling is recommended to provide education regarding inheritance pattern, family planning, and potential risks for other family members. While hEDS is inherited in an autosomal dominant pattern, each subtype has its own inheritance pattern.

The clinical diagnosis of hEDS requires the simultaneous presence of criteria 1, 2, and 3 (Malfait et al., 2017):

1 Criteria 1 is generalized joint hypermobility, defined as a Beighton Score of ≥6 for prepubertal children and a score ≥5 for pubertal men and women ≥50 years. The 9-point Beighton score remains the most recognized tool for assessing hypermobility. There is some leniency with the cut-off of 5/9 depending on various factors, including sex, age, previous medical history, and co-morbidities.
2 Criteria 2 is the presence of two or more features (A–C):

    a Feature A: systemic manifestations of a more generalized connective tissue disorder (at least five must be present):

        i Unusually soft or velvety skin
        ii Mild skin hyperextensibility
        iii Unexplained striae
        iv Bilateral piezogenic papules of the heel
        v Recurrent or multiple abdominal hernia(s) (e.g., umbilical and inguinal)
        vi Atrophic scarring involving at least two sites
        vii Pelvic floor, rectal, and/or uterine prolapse in children, men, or nulliparous women
        viii Dental crowding and high or narrow palate
        ix Arachnodactyly (abnormally long and slender fingers)
        x Arm span-to-height ≥1.05
        xi Mitral valve prolapse (MVP) mild or greater based on strict echocardiographic criteria
        xii Aortic root dilatation with Z-score > +2

b Feature B: positive family history, with one or more first degree relatives also meeting the current criteria for hEDS.

c Feature C: musculoskeletal complications (must have at least one):

  i Musculoskeletal pain in two or more limbs, recurring daily for at least 3 months
  ii Chronic, widespread pain for ≥3 months

d Criteria 3 ~~iii~~ includes the following prerequisites:

  i Absence of unusual skin fragility, which should prompt consideration of other types of EDS
  ii Exclusion of other heritable and acquired connective tissue disorders, including autoimmune rheumatologic conditions
  iii Exclusion of alternative diagnoses that may also include joint hypermobility by means of hypotonia and/or connective tissue laxity

Diagnosing hEDS in adolescents is particularly challenging; namely, hypermobility and musculoskeletal symptoms may be mistakenly attributed to growth pains or sports-related injuries. In young children, there is a risk that unexplained bruising and joint dislocations secondary to EDS can be misdiagnosed as behavioral disorders, Munchausen by proxy, or even child abuse (Chopra et al., 2017).

While soft tissue injury, such as easy bruising and scarring, and joint instability, including joint subluxations and dislocations, are the hallmarks of hEDS/HSD, it has become increasingly apparent that the clinical features are multi-systemic. In fact, features can include cardiovascular dysfunction, gastrointestinal dysfunction, psychiatric and neurodevelopmental disorders, chronic pain syndromes, and allergy conditions such as mast cell activation syndrome (MCAS) (Demmler et al., 2019). It is estimated that two-thirds of individuals with hEDS suffer from orthostatic symptoms, with up to half of them having POTS (Roma et al., 2018). Many of the associated features, including sleep disturbance, fatigue, dysautonomia, depression, anxiety, and functional gastrointestinal disorders, can be more debilitating than the joint symptoms themselves (Malfait et al., 2017). Some subtypes of EDS, such as the vascular subtype, are associated with increased vulnerability to arterial and organ rupture, and thus require ongoing surveillance. Although there are no specific guidelines for hEDS patients, periodic (every 3–5 years) cardiac echocardiograms are generally recommended to monitor the valves and aortic diameters in these patients as well (Malfait et al., 2020).

Treatment Planning

Several studies have revealed that pain, fatigue, sleep disorders, and functional disability have a considerable effect on quality of life in pediatric patients with hEDS/HSD (Malfait et al., 2020). These patients may specifically face challenges in educational settings due to physical limitations and the need for accommodations. Schools should be informed about the condition, and individualized education plans (IEPs) or 504 plans may be necessary to address specific needs, such as modified physical activities or additional rest breaks. Symptoms of joint pain and fatigue may limit adolescents' ability to participate in physical activities, such as gym class and after school activities, thus leading to increased inactivity and isolation. In addition, these symptoms, while genuine, are typically invisible to others. Thus, these patients are at risk of being dismissed, not believed, or accused of making up their symptoms. Adequate psychosocial support, including counseling and support groups, is crucial to addressing the emotional aspects of living with an invisible, chronic illness.

Although chronic pain is widespread in the EDS population, both the mechanisms and treatment options for EDS-related pain are poorly understood. Most experts agree that there are both nociceptive and neuropathic components to the pain (Song et al., 2020). Other proposed mechanisms include connective tissue spasm, nerve entrapment, joint instability, central sensitization, generalized hyperalgesia, and chronic regional pain syndrome (Tinkle et al., 2017).

As EDS is a genetic condition, there is no cure per se; however, physical therapy (PT) plays a key role in managing the symptoms. Goals of PT include strengthening muscles, improving joint stability, reducing pain, and enhancing overall physical function. An ideal PT program should emphasize low resistance exercises and avoid high-impact activities for joint preservation; walking, cycling, and swimming are particularly well-tolerated forms of exercise for EDS patients (Song et al., 2020; Tinkle et al., 2017). Occupational therapy (OT) is also commonly prescribed for EDS-related pain, and utilizes splinting, bracing, and specific exercises to improve joint stability and proprioception (Malfait et al., 2020).

A comprehensive, patient-specific approach is commonly recommended to treat EDS-related pain; it often includes non-pharmacological interventions, like PT, acupuncture, heat, and massage, in addition to analgesic medications and/or interventional procedures if needed. One study found that 59% of EDS patients who underwent interventional procedures for their chronic pain experienced relief in their pain, with nerve blocks being the most efficacious intervention (Song et al., 2020).

The prognosis of EDS is variable based on the subtype. For hEDS specifically, patient education and measures for joint preservation may result in minimal long-term musculoskeletal morbidity; however, repeated joint injuries can lead to early-onset osteoarthritis and other orthopedic issues (Miklovic & Sieg, 2023). In general, hEDS does not impact mortality (Miklovic & Sieg).

Summary

In summary, POTS and EDS are two frequently co-morbid conditions that are underrecognized and often go undiagnosed for years. They often manifest during teenage years, making it difficult for patients to attend school and participate in activities. With a comprehensive treatment approach, both conditions have largely favorable outcomes over time.

References

Aponte-Becerra, L. & Novak, P. (2021). Tilt test: A review. *Journal of Clinical Neurophysiology*, 38(4), 279–286. doi:10.1097/WNP.0000000000000625.

Bhatia, R., Kizilbash, S. J., Ahrens, S. P., Killian, J. M., Kimmes, S. A., Knoebel, E. E., Muppa, P., Weaver, A. L., & Fischer, P. R. (2016). Outcomes of adolescent-onset postural orthostatic tachycardia syndrome. *The Journal of Pediatrics*, 173, 149–153. https://doi.org/10.1016/j.jpeds.2016.02.035.

Blitshteyn, S. (2015). Autoimmune markers and autoimmune disorders in patients with postural tachycardia syndrome (POTS). *Lupus*, 24(13), 1364–1369. https://doi.org/10.1177/0961203315587566.

Chen, G., Du, J., Jin, H., & Huang, Y. (2020). Postural tachycardia syndrome in children and adolescents: Pathophysiology and clinical management. *Frontiers in Pediatrics*, 8, 474. https://doi.org/10.3389/fped.2020.00474.

Chopra, P., Tinkle, B., Hamonet, C., Brock, I., Gompel, A., Bulbena, A., & Francomano, C. (2017, March). Pain management in the Ehlers-Danlos syndromes. In *American Journal of Medical Genetics Part C: Seminars in Medical Genetics*, 175 (1), 212–219. https://doi.org/10.1002/ajmg.c.31554.

Da Costa, J. M. (1951). On irritable heart: A clinical study of a form of functional cardiac disorder and its consequences. *The American Journal of Medicine*, 11(5), 559–567. https://doi.org/10.1016/0002-9343(51)90038-90031.

Danlos, H. (1908). Un cas de cutis laxa avec tumeurs par comtusion chronique des coudes et des genoux. *Bull Soc Franc Dermatol Syph*, 19, 70–72.

Demmler, J. C., Atkinson, M. D., Reinhold, E. J., Choy, E., Lyons, R. A., & Brophy, S. T. (2019). Diagnosed prevalence of Ehlers-Danlos syndrome and hypermobility spectrum disorder in Wales, UK: A national electronic cohort study and case-control comparison. *BMJ Open*, 9(11), e031365. https://doi.org/10.1136/bmjopen-2019-031365.

Ehlers, E. (1901). Cutis laxa, Neigung zu Hemorrhagien in der Haut, Lockerung mehrerer Artikulation. *Dermatologia*, 2, 173–174.

Fedorowski, A. (2019). Postural orthostatic tachycardia syndrome: Clinical presentation, aetiology and management. *Journal of Internal Medicine*, 285(4), 352–366. https://doi.org/10.1111/joim.12852.

Gazit, Y., Jacob, G., & Grahame, R. (2016). Ehlers-Danlos syndrome—hypermobility type: A much neglected multisystemic disorder. *Rambam Maimonides Medical Journal*, 7(4). doi:10.5041/RMMJ.10261.

Hall, J., Bourne, K. M., Vernino, S., Hamrefors, V., Kharraziha, I., Nilsson, J., Sheldon, R. S., Fedorowski, A., & Raj, S. R. (2022). Detection of G protein–coupled receptor autoantibodies in postural orthostatic tachycardia syndrome using standard methodology. *Circulation*, 146(8), 613–622. https://doi.org/10.1161/CIRCULATIONAHA.122.059971.

Lin, J., Han, Z., Li, X., Ochs, T., Zhao, J., Zhang, X., Yang, J., Xiong, Z., Gai, Y., Tang, C., Du, J., & Jin, H. (2014). Risk factors for postural tachycardia syndrome in children and adolescents. *PLoS One*, 9(12), e113625. https://doi.org/10.1371/journal.pone.0113625.

Malfait, F., Castori, M., Francomano, C. A., Giunta, C., Kosho, T., & Byers, P. H. (2020). The Ehlers-Danlos syndromes. *Nature Reviews Disease Primers*, 6(1), 64. https://doi.org/10.1038/s41572-020-0194-9.

Malfait, F., Francomano, C., Byers, P., Belmont, J., Berglund, B., Black, J., Bloom. L., Bowen, J. M., Brady, A. F., Burrows, N. P., Castori, M., Colombi, M., Demirdas, S., De Backer, J., De Paepe, A., Fournel-Gigleux, S., Frank, M., Ghali, N., Giunta, C., ... Tinkle, B. (2017, March). The 2017 international classification of the Ehlers-Danlos syndromes. *American Journal of Medical Genetics Part C: Seminars in Medical Genetics* 175(1), 8–26). https://doi.org/10.1002/ajmg.c.31552.

Miklovic, T. & Sieg, V. C. (2023). Ehlers-Danlos syndrome. In *StatPearls* [Internet]. StatPearls Publishing.

Miller, A. J., Stiles, L. E., Sheehan, T., Bascom, R., Levy, H. P., Francomano, C. A., & Arnold, A. C. (2020). Prevalence of hypermobile Ehlers-Danlos syndrome in postural orthostatic tachycardia syndrome. *Autonomic Neuroscience*, 224, 102637. https://doi.org/10.1016/j.autneu.2020.102637.

Moak, J. P., Leong, D., Fabian, R., Freedenberg, V., Jarosz, E., Toney, C., Hanumanthaiah, S., & Darbari, A. (2016). Intravenous hydration for management of medication-resistant orthostatic intolerance in the adolescent and young adult. *Pediatric Cardiology*, 37, 278–282. https://doi.org/10.1007/s00246-015-1274-6.

Raj, S. R., Bourne, K. M., Stiles, L. E., Miglis, M. G., Cortez, M. M., Miller, A. J., Freeman, R., Biaggioni, I., Rowe, P. C., Sheldon, R. S., Shibao, C. A., Diedrich, A., Systrom, D. M., Cook, G. A., Doherty, T. A., Abdallah, H. I., Grubb, B. P., Fedorowski, A, Stewart, J. M.... Vernino, S. (2021). Postural orthostatic tachycardia syndrome (POTS): Priorities for POTS care and research from a 2019 National Institutes of Health Expert Consensus Meeting–Part 2. *Autonomic Neuroscience*, 235, 102836. https://doi.org/10.1016/j.autneu.2021.102836.

Roma, M., Marden, C. L., De Wandele, I., Francomano, C. A., & Rowe, P. C. (2018). Postural tachycardia syndrome and other forms of orthostatic intolerance in Ehlers-Danlos syndrome. *Autonomic Neuroscience*, 215, 89–96. https://doi.org/10.1016/j.autneu.2018.02.006.

Roma, M., Marden, C. L., & Rowe, P. C. (2018). Passive standing tests for the office diagnosis of postural tachycardia syndrome: New methodological considerations. *Fatigue: Biomedicine, Health & Behavior*, 6(4), 179–192. https://doi.org/10.1080/21641846.2018.1512836.

Safavi-Naeini, P. & Razavi, M. (2020). Postural orthostatic tachycardia syndrome. *Texas Heart Institute Journal*, 47(1), 57–59. https://doi.org/10.14503/THIJ-19-7060.

Schondorf, R. & Low, P. A. (1993). Idiopathic postural orthostatic tachycardia syndrome: An attenuated form of acute pandysautonomia? *Neurology*, 43 (1_part_1), 132. https://doi.org/10.1212/WNL.43.1_Part_1.132.

Shannon, J. R., Flattem, N. L., Jordan, J., Jacob, G., Black, B. K., Biaggioni, I., Blakely, R. D., & Robertson, D. (2000). Orthostatic intolerance and tachycardia associated with norepinephrine-transporter deficiency. *New England Journal of Medicine*, 342(8), 541–549. doi:10.1056/NEJM200002243420803.

Shaw, B. H., Stiles, L. E., Bourne, K., Green, E. A., Shibao, C. A., Okamoto, L. E., Garland, E. M., Gamboa, A., Diedrich, A., Raj, V., Sheldon, R. S., Biaggioni, I., Robertson, D., & Raj, S. R. (2019). The face of postural tachycardia syndrome–insights from a large cross-sectional online community-based survey. *Journal of Internal Medicine*, 286(4), 438–448. https://doi.org/10.1111/joim.12895.

Sheldon, R. S., GrubbII, B. P., Olshansky, B., Shen, W.-K., Calkins, H., Brignole, M., Raj, S. R., Krahn, A. D., Morillo, C. A., Stewart, J. M., Sutton, R., Sandroni, P., Friday, K. J., Tessariol Hachul, D., Cohn, M. I., Lou, D. H., Mayuga, K. A., Moak, J. P., Sandhu, R. K., & Kanjwal, K. (2015). 2015 heart rhythm society expert consensus statement on the diagnosis and treatment of postural tachycardia syndrome, inappropriate sinus tachycardia, and vasovagal syncope. *Heart Rhythm*, 12(6), e41–e63. https://doi.org/10.1016/j.hrthm.2015.03.029.

Shen, W. K., Sheldon, R. S., Benditt, D. G., Cohen, M. I., Forman, D. E., Goldberger, Z. D., Grubb, B. P., Hamdan, M. H., Krahn, A. D., Link, M. S., Olshansky, B., Raj, S. R., Sandhu, R. K., Soraija, D., Sun, B. C., & Yancy, C. W. (2017). 2017 ACC/AHA/HRS guideline for the evaluation and management of patients with syncope: A report of the American College of Cardiology/American Heart Association Task Force on Clinical Practice Guidelines and the Heart Rhythm Society. *Journal of the American College of Cardiology*, 70(5), e39–e110.

Song, B., Yeh, P., Nguyen, D., Ikpeama, U., Epstein, M., & Harrell, J. (2020). Ehlers-Danlos syndrome: An analysis of the current treatment options. *Pain Physician*, 23(4), 429.

Tinkle, B., Castori, M., Berglund, B., Cohen, H., Grahame, R., Kazkaz, H., & Levy, H. (2017, March). Hypermobile Ehlers–Danlos syndrome (aka Ehlers-Danlos syndrome Type III and Ehlers-Danlos syndrome hypermobility type): Clinical description and natural history. *American Journal of Medical Genetics Part C: Seminars in Medical Genetics*, 175(1), 48–69. https://doi.org/10.1002/ajmg.c.31538.

Vernino, S., Bourne, K. M., Stiles, L. E., Grubb, B. P., Fedorowski, A., Stewart, J. M., Arnold, A. C., Pace, L. A., Axelsson, J., Boris, J. R., Moak, J. P., Goodman, B. P., Chemoli, K. R., Chung, T. H., Goldstein, D. S., Diedrich, A., Miglis, M. G., Cortez, M. M., Millker, A. J., … Raj, S. R. (2021). Postural orthostatic tachycardia syndrome (POTS): State of the science and clinical care from a 2019 National Institutes of Health Expert Consensus Meeting-Part 1. *Autonomic Neuroscience*, 235, 102828. https://doi.org/10.1016/j.autneu.2021.102828.

Zhao, J., Han, Z., Zhang, X., Du, S., Liu, A. D., Holmberg, L., Li, X., Lin, J., Xiong, Z., Gai, Y., Yang, J., Liu, P., Tang, C., Du, J., & Jin, H. (2015). A cross-sectional study on upright heart rate and BP changing characteristics: Basic data for establishing diagnosis of postural orthostatic tachycardia syndrome and orthostatic hypertension. *BMJ Open*, 5(6). https://doi.org/10.1136/bmjopen-2014-007356.

Section III

Medically Complex Disorders

13 Epilepsy and Seizures in Children and Adolescents

Nadine Ndip

Introduction

Epilepsy is one of the most common neurological disorders affecting children and adolescents. To effectively plan healthcare services and allocate appropriate resources, it is imperative to understand the prevalence of epilepsy in children and adolescents, which varies across different regions and populations. According to the latest estimates from the Centers for Disease Control and Prevention (CDC), approximately 0.6% of children and adolescents aged 0–17 years have active epilepsy (Zack, 2017). Moreover, an estimated 20,000 to 45,000 children are newly diagnosed with seizures each year, with the median age of onset occurring between 5 and 6 years of age. Research indicates that individuals in early childhood have a higher risk compared to individuals in middle childhood, with another peak emerging during adolescence (Aaberg et al., 2017).

Defining Epilepsy and Seizures

The International League Against Epilepsy (ILAE), defines seizures as single events brought on by abnormal electrical activity in the brain that can cause temporary changes in body movement or function, sensation, behavior, and/or awareness (Berg et al. 2010). Traditionally, epilepsy (i.e., seizure disorder) was described as a chronic neurological condition characterized by two or more unprovoked seizures separated by at least 24 hours. However, in 2014, the ILAE redefined epilepsy to expand beyond the traditional requirement of two or more unprovoked seizures. Under new guidelines, an individual is considered to have epilepsy if they meet either of the following conditions: a single seizure, combined with a high likelihood of future seizures, or the diagnosis of a specific epilepsy syndrome (Fisher et al., 2014). Broadening the definition of epilepsy not only acknowledges the diverse presentations of the disorder, but also allows for timely intervention and management, particularly in children and adolescents with specific epilepsy syndromes.

DOI: 10.4324/9781032703923-16

International League Against Epilepsy (ILAE) Classification System

Children and adolescents with epilepsy experience diverse seizure types categorized using the evolving ILAE system. This system classifies seizures based on clinical features and brain activity and also offers insights into potential future seizure types, triggers, and long-term risks. Additionally, the classification system assists in guiding treatment planning, including the selection of the most appropriate anti-epileptic medications. ILAE's classification system has three levels (seizure type, epilepsy type, and epilepsy syndrome). The first level of classification pertains to the clinical and electroencephalographic features of the seizures (i.e., Seizure Type; Scheffer et al., 2017). Seizures are categorized into three main types: focal onset, generalized onset, and unknown onset. For children and adolescents, the primary types of seizures relevant to the ILAE classification system include focal seizures and generalized seizures. Focal seizures, (previously called partial seizures), originate in specific regions of the brain and lead to symptoms and experiences related to the affected area (Sirven, 2015). Focal seizures can be further classified into focal aware seizures (previously referred to as simple partial seizures) and focal impaired awareness seizures (previously referred to as complex partial focal seizures). Focal aware seizures typically involve alterations in sensory perception or motor activity without loss of consciousness. In contrast, focal impaired awareness seizures are characterized by altered consciousness or awareness.

Generalized seizures involve widespread electrical activity in both hemispheres of the brain, impacting the entire body and consciousness (Sirven, 2015). There are several subtypes of generalized seizures, including absence seizures, tonic-clonic seizures (previously referred to as grand mal seizures), tonic seizures, clonic seizures, myoclonic seizures, and atonic seizures. Each subtype presents distinct clinical features and patterns of motor activity. Absence seizures are characterized by brief lapses of consciousness, often lasting seconds, during which an individual can appear blank and unresponsive. Tonic-clonic seizures involve loss of consciousness, muscle stiffening, jerking movements, and postictal confusion. Myoclonic seizures are characterized by brief, sudden muscle jerks involving one or more parts of the body. Finally, atonic seizures involve the sudden loss of muscle tone causing falls.

The second level of classification pertains to the origin of the seizures (i.e., Epilepsy Type; Scheffer et al., 2017). Within this level there are four categories: focal epilepsy, generalized epilepsy, combined generalized and focal epilepsy, and unknown epilepsy. Finally, the third level of classification pertains to the specific diagnosis based on a group of features, such as seizure type, diagnostic imaging and electroencephalogram (EEG) findings, and age of onset (i.e., Epilepsy Syndrome; Scheffer et al.). These syndromes vary in age of onset, seizure types, and diagnostic imaging findings, necessitating tailored approaches to diagnosis and treatment for affected children and adolescents (see Table 13.1).

Table 13.1 Common Epilepsy Syndromes in Children and Adolescents

Epilepsy Syndrome	*Onset Age Range*	*Characteristics*
Childhood Absence Epilepsy (CAE)	4–10 years	Brief staring spells or "absences"; EEG typically shows 3 Hz spike-and-wave discharges
Juvenile Myoclonic Epilepsy (JME)	12–18 years	Myoclonic jerks often upon awakening; may involve generalized tonic-clonic seizures and absences
Benign Rolandic Epilepsy (BRE/RE)	3–13 years	Twitching or numbness on one side of the face or mouth, often during sleep
Lennox-Gastaut Syndrome (LGS)	1–8 years	Multiple seizure types including tonic, atonic, and atypical absence seizures; associated with cognitive impairment and developmental delays
Dravet Syndrome	Infancy	Prolonged seizures often triggered by fever (febrile seizures); associated with developmental delays and intellectual disability
West Syndrome (Infantile Spasms)	First year	Clusters of spasms or seizures consisting of sudden flexion or extension of the body; associated with developmental regression and intellectual disability
Landau-Kleffner Syndrome (LKS)	2–7 years	Loss of language skills and seizure activity, often focal seizures or atypical absence seizures

Note: Adapted from Howell et al., 2021; Shbarou & Mikati, 2016.

Diagnosing Epilepsy in Children and Adolescents

Diagnosing epilepsy in children and adolescents requires a comprehensive multidisciplinary approach. The initial step involves obtaining a detailed clinical history, which includes gathering information about the individual's developmental history (e.g., prenatal, perinatal, and postnatal factors that could contribute to seizures) and medical history (e.g., past illnesses, injuries, medications, and family history of neurological disorders). Additionally, specific details about the semiology of seizures, such as onset, duration, frequency, and associated symptoms, are crucial for accurate diagnosis and treatment planning.

Following the clinical history, thorough neurological and general physical examinations are conducted to identify any neurological abnormalities potentially linked to seizures or signs suggestive of underlying conditions. Neuroimaging studies play an important role in epilepsy diagnosis by identifying structural abnormalities (e.g., lesions, tumors, or malformations of cortical development) that may be causing seizures (Fine & Wirrell, 2020). Magnetic resonance imaging (MRI) scans are considered the gold standard imaging tool for diagnosing epilepsy in children and adolescents.

Additionally, electroencephalogram (EEG) is essential for capturing abnormal electrical activity in the brain, even during interictal (i.e., between seizure) periods. Prolonged EEG monitoring, including video-EEG, may be necessary to capture seizures and determine their localization and lateralization, further aiding in accurate diagnosis and treatment planning. Finally, other tests, such as blood tests and lumbar puncture, may be used in specific situations to identify underlying metabolic imbalances or infections which may be contributing to seizures.

Differential Diagnosis

It is important to recognize that various other conditions can mimic epilepsy, making misinterpretations and misdiagnoses frequent. Psychogenic non-epileptic seizures (PNES) are one such example. These events, often triggered by emotional stress or trauma, mimic epileptic seizures in appearance but lack the characteristic brain electrical activity (Alsaadi & Marquez, 2005; Jafari et al., 2020; Takasaki et al., 2016). Distinguishing PNES requires a multi-step approach: detailed history to identify potential psychological triggers, witness accounts for event characteristics, and video-EEG monitoring to confirm normal brain activity during episodes. Diagnosing PNES can take on average 7 years from when an individual first experiences symptoms to receiving a confirmed diagnosis. This delay can sometimes lead to misdiagnosis and unnecessary treatments, such as medications typically prescribed for epilepsy, emergency room visits, or even hospital admissions (Alsaadi & Marquez; Jafari et al.; Takasaki et al.).

Beyond PNES, other conditions warrant consideration. Syncope, characterized by a temporary loss of consciousness due to decreased blood flow to the brain, presents with symptoms like paleness and lightheadedness. Unlike epileptic seizures, however, syncope lacks jerking movements or postictal (post-seizure) confusion. EEG findings in syncope are also usually normal. Some migraines can be preceded by an aura, which is a sensory disturbance like flashing lights or tingling sensations. While these sensory disturbances can resemble focal seizures, the specific features of the aura as well as the individual's history of migraines usually aid in differentiation. Certain movement disorders, such as dystonia or tremors, can mimic seizure-like movements. A thorough neurological examination, potentially supplemented by MRI scans, helps distinguish these movement disorders from epilepsy.

For children and adolescents, various non-epileptic conditions further complicate the diagnosis (Benbadis, 2009). Tics, common between ages 5 and 10, are distinguishable from seizures by their non-episodic nature and the presence of premonitory urges. Shuddering attacks, often seen in older infants, may resemble seizures but lack associations with increased morbidity and occur predominantly while awake. Breath-holding spells, typically affecting children aged 6 months to 5 years, can be confused with seizures but are distinguished by their occurrence during crying spells and the subsequent cyanosis. Differential diagnosis is a crucial step in accurately identifying epilepsy or its counterparts in order to formulate appropriate treatment plans.

Coexisting Conditions in Children and Adolescents with Epilepsy

Children and adolescents diagnosed with epilepsy face a myriad of additional challenges stemming from coexisting conditions or "comorbidities." These encompass various mental health concerns, learning difficulties, and other physical health issues. It is important to emphasize that while epilepsy may exacerbate these conditions, they are typically not directly caused by the epilepsy itself, but rather by shared underlying factors contributing to both epilepsy and the comorbidities. While precise estimates of risk vary, research suggests that a significant proportion of children with epilepsy contend with at least one comorbidity. A comprehensive study involving over a million children unveiled that nearly 80% of those diagnosed with epilepsy had at least one additional condition (Aaberg et al., 2016). These comorbidities often fall into distinct categories: medical conditions impacting general health (e.g., respiratory or digestive issues), neurological conditions impacting the nervous system (e.g., learning disabilities or attention-deficit/hyperactivity disorder), and developmental/psychiatric conditions (e.g., depression, anxiety, or autism spectrum disorder; Russ et al., 2012). Research indicates that children and adolescents with more complex forms of epilepsy are at an elevated risk of experiencing multiple comorbidities (Aaberg et al.). Even individuals diagnosed with seemingly uncomplicated epilepsy face a significant risk of developing coexisting medical and/or psychiatric conditions. This increased vulnerability can be attributed to several factors.

The seizures themselves, particularly if frequent or severe, can disrupt developing neural networks crucial for cognitive and emotional function. Additionally, medications used to control seizures have their own side effects, potentially exacerbating existing difficulties or leading to new ones. The psychosocial challenges associated with epilepsy, including stigma, social isolation, and limitations in daily activities, can contribute to the development of anxiety and depression. Early identification and appropriate management of these comorbidities are essential for ensuring comprehensive care and optimizing the well-being of children and adolescents with epilepsy.

The Role of Neuropsychological Assessment in Epilepsy

The impact of epilepsy goes beyond the seizures themselves, with impacts on an individual's cognitive, emotional, behavioral, academic, and social functioning. The utilization of neuropsychological assessment is a valuable tool in identifying strengths and weaknesses in children and adolescents with epilepsy, especially during the initial stages of the condition (Fastenau et al., 2009). A thorough assessment makes it possible to understand the cognitive and behavioral aspects of the individual, which can aid in devising effective treatments. Additionally, neuropsychological assessment can inform educational planning by determining the appropriate placement and allocation of educational resources in individualized educational plans.

Common Findings in Neuropsychological Assessments

Research indicates that cognitive and behavioral difficulties are more prevalent in children and adolescents with epilepsy (Fastenau et al., 2009). Cognitive difficulties may precede the onset of the first seizure, highlighting the need for early intervention and support. Although some individuals with epilepsy may demonstrate normal cognitive functioning, a significant proportion of children and adolescents with epilepsy experience cognitive impairments. Neuropsychological assessment of children and adolescents with epilepsy often reveals deficits across various cognitive domains, including intelligence, memory, attention, executive functioning, and language (Kernan et al., 2012; MacAllister & Sherman, 2015). These difficulties can persist even after the remission of seizures, underscoring the long-lasting effects of epilepsy on cognitive functioning. In fact, research has shown that even "benign" pediatric epilepsies, such as benign childhood occipital epilepsy and benign childhood epilepsy with centrotemporal spikes, are associated with higher rates of cognitive difficulties (Garcia-Ramos et al., 2015). For example, children and adolescents with these benign epilepsies may experience ongoing issues with attention and executive functioning.

Children and adolescents with epilepsy are also at increased risk for academic difficulties. While they may not always meet the strict criteria for learning disabilities, they often experience challenges that make learning difficult (Pastor et al., 2015; Russ et al., 2012). For example, difficulties in reading, writing, or math skills may be mild, but other factors, such as seizures and the postictal state (often characterized by fatigue and/or confusion) can lead to disruptions in learning that persist for minutes or hours. Additionally, interictal activity (i.e., epileptiform discharges between seizures) has also been found to interfere with learning and may account for variability in academic performance.

In the case of a child or adolescent who experiences seizures, implementing accommodations and specialized instruction is crucial to mitigate the impact of lapses in consciousness and post-seizure fatigue. Providing multiple presentations of material, offering extra practice opportunities, and supplying study guides beforehand can facilitate information consolidation. Recording interrupted material for reteaching and employing frequent checks for understanding with constructive feedback can further support learning. Access to lecture notes beforehand can assist in following along, while reviewing notes and creating summaries soon after can strengthen memory retention. Regarding memory challenges, incorporating contextual learning approaches with rich examples and visual aids is recommended to enhance encoding and retrieval. Mnemonic devices and memory training tools can further support retention, while modified testing formats, such as providing word banks or segmenting assessments, can accommodate potential limitations in memory capacity and retrieval. By implementing these recommendations, educators can work towards optimizing students' academic experiences and fostering success despite the challenges presented by epilepsy.

Children and adolescents with epilepsy have an increased risk of developing comorbid conditions, such as attention-deficit/hyperactivity disorder (ADHD), anxiety, and depression (Russ et al., 2012). The relationship between epilepsy and ADHD is particularly noteworthy, with several factors contributing to their co-occurrence, including the chronic impact of seizures, effects of antiepileptic medications, underlying brain pathology, genetic predisposition, noradrenergic system dysregulation, and psychosocial factors (Dunn et al., 2003). The presence of comorbid conditions can complicate the management of epilepsy and may require additional interventions and support services. Beyond its emotional and behavioral challenges, epilepsy can also significantly impact psychosocial well-being and overall quality of life of children and adolescents. By understanding the factors contributing to social difficulties, clinicians are better equipped to develop tailored interventions that support the social and emotional development of children and adolescents with epilepsy.

Treatment and Management of Epilepsy in Children and Adolescents

Managing epilepsy in children and adolescents involves a multifaceted approach, with various treatment options available to address individual needs and specific seizure characteristics. Following is an overview of some of the key options, such as antiepileptic drugs (AEDs), surgical interventions, dietary therapy, and neuromodulation techniques such as vagus nerve stimulation (VNS).

Pharmacological Interventions

Antiepileptic drugs (AEDs) serve as the primary treatment modality, aiming to regulate abnormal electrical activity in the brain and prevent seizures. Different AEDs work through diverse mechanisms, and the choice of medication is carefully selected based on the type of seizure, age, and other individual factors. Medication adherence is important in the management of epilepsy, as consistent and timely administration of antiepileptic drugs is crucial for seizure control and optimizing treatment outcomes. Non-adherence to medication regimens can lead to breakthrough seizures, worsening of symptoms, and increased risk of complications. It is essential for healthcare providers to educate patients and their families about the importance of medication adherence and to address any barriers or concerns that may impact adherence. Additionally, it is important to monitor for potential side effects of antiepileptic drugs, which can include dizziness, drowsiness, cognitive impairment, mood changes, and gastrointestinal disturbances. Regular monitoring and adjustments to medication regimens may be necessary to minimize side effects and ensure optimal tolerability.

Other Medical Interventions

In cases where AEDs cannot provide adequate seizure control, surgical intervention may become an option. Surgical interventions involve precisely targeting and removing the area of the brain responsible for initiating seizures (epileptogenic focus) or disrupting the abnormal electrical pathways involved. Specialized diets can also significantly reduce seizure frequency, especially in children and adolescents with specific epilepsy syndromes and other forms resistant to medication (Kossoff et al., 2003; Kossoff, 2012; Sharma & Jain, 2014). Finally, vagus nerve stimulation (VNS) is a minimally invasive procedure that involves implanting a device that delivers electrical stimulation to the vagus nerve, which indirectly influences brain activity and potentially reduces seizure frequency and severity.

Psychosocial Interventions

In managing epilepsy in children and adolescents, incorporating psychosocial interventions alongside medical treatment can significantly enhance overall well-being. Among these interventions, cognitive behavioral therapy (CBT) offers a range of techniques tailored to address the specific challenges faced by children and adolescents (Leeman-Markowski & Schachter, 2017; Li et al., 2023). CBT focuses on the interconnectedness of thoughts, emotions, and behaviors. Relaxation training can equip young individuals with tools to manage stress, a known trigger for seizures in some cases. Psychoeducation is another crucial component, providing children, adolescents, and their families with comprehensive knowledge about epilepsy, its various aspects, and potential management strategies.

Family therapy can be immensely beneficial in strengthening communication and fostering a supportive environment within the family unit. Support groups offer another valuable resource, connecting individuals and families with others in similar situations. Sharing experiences, fostering a sense of community, and receiving encouragement from peers can contribute significantly to emotional well-being and coping with the specific challenges associated with epilepsy.

It is vital to emphasize the importance of a team approach in managing epilepsy effectively. This typically involves collaboration between various professionals, including neurologists, social workers, neuropsychologists, therapists, and educators. This collaborative approach ensures holistic care, addressing not only the seizures themselves but also the potential cognitive, social-emotional, and educational needs of children and adolescents living with epilepsy.

Developmental Considerations for Children and Adolescents with Epilepsy

While epilepsy affects children and adolescents similarly, the specific challenges and considerations vary significantly across different age groups. Tailoring treatment and management approaches to address these unique concerns is crucial for optimal outcomes.

Early Childhood

Identifying seizures in toddlers can be particularly challenging due to subtle presentations and ongoing developmental changes. Careful observation and collaboration between caregivers and healthcare professionals are essential for accurate diagnosis and timely intervention. Early and frequent seizures can significantly impact language, motor, and cognitive development, therefore early intervention programs are important in minimizing the long-term consequences of epilepsy on these critical developmental domains. Medication adherence can also be difficult within this age group. Creative strategies, such as using flavored medications or incorporating medication administration into daily routines, are often required.

Middle Childhood

As children enter their preteen years, seizures and epilepsy management can become a source of anxiety and/or social isolation. Addressing these concerns through peer support groups and fostering open communication within the family is important for children's emotional well-being. Cognitive and academic difficulties associated with epilepsy can become more pronounced during this critical academic period. The utilization of special education services and accommodations is likely to be important for success within the classroom environment.

Adolescence

Puberty, a period of significant hormonal change, presents unique challenges for individuals with epilepsy. Fluctuations in hormone levels may lead to increased seizure frequency or changes in seizure patterns (Verrotti et al., 2008). Additionally, hormonal changes can affect how the body absorbs and utilizes antiepileptic drugs, altering their effectiveness and potentially increasing the risk of side effects. Therefore, during puberty, healthcare professionals must carefully monitor seizure activity and medication response.

This may involve adjusting medication dosages or switching medications entirely to ensure optimal seizure control and minimize side effects.

Epilepsy can also add an additional layer of complexity to the already challenging process of adolescent identity exploration and formation. Understanding and adhering to driving restrictions based on seizure control is essential for adolescent safety. Many jurisdictions have specific regulations regarding epilepsy and driving, requiring individuals to be seizure-free for a certain period before obtaining or maintaining a driver's license. Healthcare providers play a crucial role in assessing driving eligibility, providing guidance to patients and families, and facilitating compliance with regulatory requirements. As adolescents transition towards adulthood, planning for independent healthcare management, including medication adherence and future treatment decisions, becomes increasingly important to empower them to take ownership and navigate the healthcare system effectively.

Prognosis for Children and Adolescents with Epilepsy

While epilepsy presents challenges, the long-term outlook for children and adolescents is generally positive, though the experience of epilepsy varies greatly across individuals. Factors influencing outcomes include seizure control, the underlying cause of epilepsy (etiology), how well medications are taken (adherence), and the presence of other conditions (Devinsky et al., 2018). Research suggests that a large proportion of children and adolescents achieve seizure freedom with medication, and some may even outgrow epilepsy entirely (Sirven, 2015). Others continue to experience seizures in adulthood. Refractory epilepsy, where seizures are difficult to control, can have a significant impact on various aspects of life.

Healthcare providers play a central role in coordinating care, providing education and counseling, and addressing the complex medical, psychosocial, and educational needs of children and adolescents with epilepsy and their families. By understanding the unique long-term experiences surrounding epilepsy in children and adolescents, emphasizing ongoing management and support, and accessing relevant resources, healthcare professionals and support networks can empower individuals to live fulfilling and productive lives despite the challenges posed by epilepsy.

Conclusion

Epilepsy significantly impacts children and adolescents. Diagnosis involves a comprehensive approach to differentiate from other conditions. Comorbidities are common, requiring holistic management of general health, neurological functioning, and mental health. Neuropsychological assessment reveals cognitive and academic challenges, highlighting the need for tailored educational support. Treatment options include medications, surgery, diet, and psychotherapy. With appropriate intervention, many achieve seizure control and lead fulfilling lives. Collaboration among healthcare providers, families, and support networks is crucial for their success. Numerous resources are available for families and professionals seeking information and support related to epilepsy:

- Patient advocacy groups (Epilepsy Foundation, Child Neurology Foundation) provide resources, support, and advocacy.
- Online portals (National Institute of Neurological Disorders and Stroke and the American Epilepsy Society) offer evidence-based information and resources for professionals and families.

References

Aaberg, K. M., Bakken, I. J., Lossius, M. I., Søraas, C. L., Håberg, S. E., Stoltenberg, C., Surén, P., & Chin, R. (2016). Comorbidity and childhood epilepsy: A nationwide registry study. *Pediatrics*, 138(3), e20160921. https://doi.org/10.1542/peds.2016-0921.

Aaberg, K. M., Gunnes, N., Bakken, I. J., Lund Søraas, C., Berntsen, A., Magnus, P., Lossius, M. I., Stoltenberg, C., Chin, R., & Surén, P. (2017). Incidence and prevalence of childhood epilepsy: A nationwide cohort study. *Pediatrics*, 139(5), e20163908. https://doi.org/10.1542/peds.2016-3908.

Alsaadi, T. M. & Marquez, A. V. (2005). Psychogenic nonepileptic seizures. *American Family Physician*, 72(5), 849–856.

Benbadis S. (2009). The differential diagnosis of epilepsy: A critical review. *Epilepsy & Behavior*, *15*(1), 15–21. https://doi.org/10.1016/j.yebeh.2009.02.024.

Berg, A. T., Berkovic, S. F., Brodie, M. J., Buchhalter, J., Cross, J. H., Van Emde Boas, W., Engel, J., French, J., Glauser, T. A., Mathern, G. W., Moshé, S. L., Nordli, D., Plouin, P., & Scheffer, I. E. (2010), Revised terminology and concepts for organization of seizures and epilepsies: Report of the ILAE Commission on Classification and Terminology, 2005–2009. *Epilepsia*, 51(4), 676–685. https://doi.org/10.1111/j.1528-1167.2010.02522.x.

Devinsky, O., Vezzani, A., O'Brien, T. J., Jette, N., Scheffer, I. E., de Curtis, M., & Perucca, P. (2018). Epilepsy. *Nature Reviews. Disease Primers*, 4, 18024. https://doi.org/10.1038/nrdp.2018.24.

Dunn, D. W., Austin, J. K., Harezlak, J., & Ambrosius, W. T. (2003). ADHD and epilepsy in childhood. *Developmental Medicine and Child Neurology*, 45(1), 50–54. https://doi.org/10.1017/S0012162203000094.

Fastenau, P. S., Johnson, C. S., Perkins, S. M., Byars, A. W., DeGrauw, T. J., Austin, J. K., & Dunn, D. W. (2009). Neuropsychological status at seizure onset in children: Risk factors for early cognitive deficits. *Neurology*, 73(7), 526–534. https://doi.org/10.1212/WNL.0b013e3181b23551.

Fine, A. & Wirrell, E. C. (2020). Seizures in children. *Pediatrics in Review*, 41(7), 321–347. https://doi.org/10.1542/pir.2019-0134.

Fisher, R. S., Acevedo, C., Arzimanoglou, A., Bogacz, A., Cross, J. H., Elger, C. E., Engel, J., Jr, Forsgren, L., French, J. A., Glynn, M., Hesdorffer, D. C., Lee, B. I., Mathern, G. W., Moshé, S. L., Perucca, E., Scheffer, I. E., Tomson, T., Watanabe,

M., & Wiebe, S. (2014). ILAE official report: A practical clinical definition of epilepsy. *Epilepsia*, 55(4), 475–482. https://doi.org/10.1111/epi.12550.

Garcia-Ramos, C., Jackson, D. C., Lin, J. J., Dabbs, K., Jones, J. E., Hsu, D. A., Stafstrom, C. E., Zawadzki, L., Seidenberg, M., Prabhakaran, V., & Hermann, B. P. (2015). Cognition and brain development in children with benign epilepsy with centrotemporal spikes. *Epilepsia*, 56(10), 1615–1622. https://doi.org/10.1111/epi.13125.

Howell, K. B., Freeman, J. L., Mackay, M. T., Fahey, M. C., Archer, J., Berkovic, S. F., Chan, E., Dabscheck, G., Eggers, S., Hayman, M., Holberton, J., Hunt, R. W., Jacobs, S. E., Kornberg, A. J., Leventer, R. J., Mandelstam, S., McMahon, J. M., Mefford, H. C., Panetta, J., … Harvey, A. S. (2021). The severe epilepsy syndromes of infancy: A population-based study. *Epilepsia*, 62(2), 358–370. https://doi.org/10.1111/epi.16810.

Jafari, A., Tavirani, M. R., Hamrah, M. P., Karvigh, S. A., & Fakhar, H. B. Z. (2020). Psychogenic non-epileptic seizures: A narrative review. *Archives of Academic Emergency Medicine*, 8(1), e10.

Kernan, C. L., Asarnow, R., Siddarth, P., Gurbani, S., Lanphier, E. K., Sankar, R., & Caplan, R. (2012). Neurocognitive profiles in children with epilepsy. *Epilepsia*, 53(12), 2156–2163. https://doi.org/10.1111/j.1528-1167.2012.03706.x.

Kossoff, E. H. (2012). Efficacy of ketogenic dietary therapy: What is the evidence? In: E. Neal (Ed.), *Dietary Treatment of Epilepsy: Practical implementation of ketogenic therapy* (pp. 24–33). Wiley-Blackwell.

Kossoff, E. H., Krauss, G. L., McGrogan, J. R., & Freeman, J. M. (2003). Efficacy of the Atkins diet as therapy for intractable epilepsy. *Neurology*, 61(12), 1789–1791. https://doi.org/10.1212/01.wnl.0000098889.35155.72.

Leeman-Markowski, B. A. & Schachter, S. C. (2017). Cognitive and behavioral interventions in epilepsy. *Current Neurology and Neuroscience Reports*, 17, 1–11. https://doi.org/10.1007/s11910-017-0752-z.

Li, D., Song, Y., Zhang, S., Qiu, J., Zhang, R., Wu, J., Wu, Z., Wei, J., Xiang, X., Zhang, Y., Yu, L., Wang, H., Niu, P., Fan, C., & Li, X. (2023). Cognitive behavior therapy for depression in people with epilepsy: A systematic review and meta-analysis. *Epilepsy & Behavior*, 138, 109056. https://doi.org/10.1016/j.yebeh.2022.109056.

MacAllister, W. S. & Sherman, E. M. S. (2015). Evaluation of children and adolescents with epilepsy. In W. B. Barr & C. Morrison (Eds.), *Handbook on the Neuropsychology of Epilepsy* (pp. 37–62). Springer Science + Business Media.

Pastor, P. N., Reuben, C. A., Kobau, R., Helmers, S. L., & Lukacs, S. (2015). Functional difficulties and school limitations of children with epilepsy: Findings from the 2009–2010 National Survey of Children with Special Health Care Needs. *Disability and Health Journal*, 8(2), 231–239. https://doi.org/10.1016/j.dhjo.2014.09.002.

Russ, S. A., Larson, K., & Halfon, N. (2012). A national profile of childhood epilepsy and seizure disorder. *Pediatrics*, 129(2), 256–264. https://doi.org/10.1542/peds.2010-1371.

Scheffer, I. E., Berkovic, S., Capovilla, G., Connolly, M. B., French, J., Guilhoto, L., Hirsch, E., Jain, S., Mathern, G. W., Moshé, S. L., Nordli, D. R., Perucca, E., Tomson, T., Wiebe, S., Zhang, Y. H., & Zuberi, S. M. (2017). ILAE classification of the epilepsies: Position paper of the ILAE Commission for Classification and Terminology. *Epilepsia*, 58(4), 512–521. https://doi.org/10.1111/epi.13709.

Sharma, S. & Jain, P. (2014). The modified Atkins diet in refractory epilepsy. *Epilepsy Research and Treatment, 2014*, 404202. https://doi.org/10.1155/2014/404202.

Shbarou, R. & Mikati, M. A. (2016, May). The expanding clinical spectrum of genetic pediatric epileptic encephalopathies. *Seminars in Pediatric Neurology*, 23 (2), 134–142. https://doi.org/10.1016/j.spen.2016.06.002.

Sirven J. I. (2015). Epilepsy: A spectrum disorder. *Cold Spring Harbor Perspectives in Medicine*, 5(9), a022848. https://doi.org/10.1101/cshperspect.a022848.

Takasaki, K., Stransky, A. D., & Miller, G. (2016). Psychogenic nonepileptic seizures: Diagnosis, management, and bioethics. *Pediatric Neurology*, 62, 3–8. https://doi.org/10.1016/j.pediatrneurol.2016.04.011.

Verrotti, A., Manco, R., Scardapane, A., & Chiarelli, F. (2008). Adolescents and epilepsy: Hormonal aspects. *Minerva Pediatrica*, 60(4), 417–428.

Zack, M. M. (2017). National and state estimates of the numbers of adults and children with active epilepsy—United States, 2015. *MMWR. Morbidity and Mortality Weekly Report*, 66(31), 821–825. https://doi.org/10.15585/mmwr.mm6631a1.

14 Evaluation and Management of Neurocognitive Dysfunction in Children and Adolescents with Type 1 Diabetes

David D. Schwartz

Introduction

Type 1 diabetes (T1D) is a common chronic condition in which the immune system destroys pancreatic beta cells that produce the hormone insulin. Insulin facilitates transport of blood sugars across the cell membrane, providing the body's primary energy source. As beta cell destruction progresses, insulin production eventually ceases, causing a build-up of glucose in the bloodstream that can damage the eyes, kidneys, peripheral nerves, cardiovascular system, and brain. T1D differs from type 2 diabetes where cells become insulin-resistant and the pancreas cannot produce enough insulin to compensate. This chapter focuses on T1D, as it accounts for most cases of childhood diabetes.

People with T1D rely on lifelong administration of insulin to stay alive, either through daily injections or via an insulin pump. The goal of diabetes management is to maintain glucose homeostasis, which requires ensuring that the right amount of insulin is delivered at the right time so that blood sugars stay within a tight range (90–130 milligrams per deciliter [mg/dL] of blood; American Diabetes Association; ADA, 2024). High blood sugars (*hyperglycemia*) and low blood sugars (*hypoglycemia*) can lead to acute and chronic health complications, some of which are life-threatening.

To walk this tightrope between high and low blood sugars, people with diabetes track their carbohydrate intake and regularly check their blood sugars and based on these data calculate the appropriate dose of insulin to take. They have to do this multiple times per day with tools that are not nearly as effective as a normally functioning pancreas. The need to keep balanced glucose levels, and the challenges of doing so, can place a huge amount of stress on individuals with diabetes and their families, leading to significant distress and burnout.

Managing T1D effectively is a complex and unremitting job that places a substantial burden on mental health and on a person's cognitive and organizational skills. Moreover, if not well managed, diabetes can have deleterious effects on cognitive and executive functioning, potentially

DOI: 10.4324/9781032703923-17

resulting in a vicious cycle in which neurocognitive deficits compromise diabetes management, leading to worsening glycemic levels and progressive cognitive decline over time.

Pathophysiology

T1D is believed to result from an interaction between genetic susceptibility and as-yet-unknown environmental factors. T1D is a polygenic disorder with studies implicating genetic variants that play a role in immune function (Redondo et al., 2018). Suspected triggers include viruses that may elicit an autoimmune reaction, including SARS-CoV-2; other possible triggers include vitamin D deficiency, cold climates, and environmental pollutants (Zorena et al., 2022).

Onset of T1D progresses through a series of three stages (Insel et al., 2015). Stages 1 and 2 are pre-symptomatic. It is not known how long they last, but they represent a time during which the child is exposed to heightened levels of blood glucose that may make the brain more vulnerable to subsequent insult (Ryan et al., 2016). Stage 3 represents the onset of symptomatic T1D. As the family does not yet know the child has diabetes, the illness may progress to a dangerous state before medical attention is sought.

Measures of Blood Glucose

Acute blood sugar levels are measured in mmol/L (millimoles per liter) or mg/dL (milligrams per deciliter) of blood. Hemoglobin A1c (HbA1c) represents the percent concentration of glucose adhering to hemoglobin in red blood cells, providing an approximate measure of average blood sugars over the past 2–3 months. For children with T1D, it is recommended that HbA1c be kept below 7%, though the average HbA1c for youth with T1D in the U.S. is well above this range; for example, in the large SEARCH for Diabetes in Youth study (N=6369), mean HbA1c was 8.8 ± 0.04% (Malik et al., 2022).

A newer measure is time-in-range (TIR), which refers to the percentage of time blood sugars fall within the range of 70–180 mg/dL. TIR has become available with increasing use of continuous glucose monitors (CGMs). The more time a person with diabetes spends in-range, the lower their risk for long-term complications.

Mechanisms and Risk Factors for Cognitive Dysfunction

T1D is distinguished by dramatic fluctuations in blood glucose throughout the day. Out-of-range blood sugars can acutely affect cognition, and when they persist over time, they can also have more chronic effects.

Acute Cognitive Dysfunction

Several studies have found acute hypoglycemia and hyperglycemia are both associated with slower processing speed (Hawks et al., 2024). Effects on attention are less clear, with some studies showing reduced attention (Sattar et al., 2017) and others finding no effect (Hawks et al.). Behaviorally slower processing speed can mimic inattention in daily life.

Chronic Hyperglycemia

Hyperglycemia is the defining clinical characteristic of T1D. Children with T1D may spend as much as half of each day in hyperglycemia (Tansey et al., 2016). A mean blood glucose in the hyperglycemic range (>180 mg/dL) translates to a HbA1c of 8%, and as noted, the majority of youth with T1D in the U.S. have an average HbA1c higher than this. Chronic hyperglycemia has a deleterious effect on white matter (Barnea-Goraly et al., 2014), particularly in frontal and parietal-occipital regions. A recent longitudinal study found reduced white, gray, and total brain matter volumes in children with T1D compared to age-matched controls, a difference that increased from age 6 to 12 years (Mauras et al., 2021).

Chronic hyperglycemia appears to be the primary cause of cognitive dysfunction in T1D (Jaser & Jordan, 2021), resulting in a profile of slower information processing speed and psychomotor efficiency (Tonoli et al., 2014). Longitudinal studies suggest increased declines in processing speed over the lifespan in individuals with a greater burden of hyperglycemia (Jacobson et al., 2011); conversely, processing speed may improve with lower blood sugars (Kirchhoff et al., 2017). Meta-analyses have shown moderate effects of hyperglycemia on selective attention, sustained attention (Brands et al., 2005; Gaudieri et al., 2008; Naguib et al., 2009), and executive function (Broadley et al., 2017). Executive function (EF) is of particular relevance to managing T1D, with studies finding an association between EF, regimen adherence, and glycemic control (Ding et al., 2021). Hyperglycemia also appears to have downstream effects on IQ, possibly mediated by processing-level deficits.

Hypoglycemia

Mild-to-moderate hypoglycemia is common in T1D. Severe hypoglycemia, defined by the need for immediate assistance, is much less common, but potentially life-threatening. Severe hypoglycemia was previously thought to be the primary risk factor for cognitive dysfunction in T1D but is now considered less relevant than hyperglycemia (Jaser & Jordan, 2021). This is likely because acute hypoglycemia must be treated immediately, making it rare for it to persist long enough to permanently damage the brain. Still, hypoglycemia does appear to have an impact on cognition in individuals with *early onset of disease* (EOD; onset of T1D in the first five to seven years of life; Gaudieri et al., 2008). Severe hypoglycemia can have damaging effects on the hippocampus and associated areas such as the thalamus (Seaquist, 2015). Studies show an association between severe hypoglycemia and deficits in learning and memory, but only in individuals with EOD (Blasetti et al., 2011; Gaudieri et al.; Tonoli et al., 2014).

Diabetic Ketoacidosis

Diabetic ketoacidosis (DKA) is an acute metabolic crisis that results from lack of insulin. Between 30% and 40% of children present in DKA at diagnosis (Dabelea et al., 2014). In youth with established T1D, DKA is most commonly the result of under-dosing or omitting insulin (Wolfsdorf et al., 2009). DKA can cause cerebral swelling that at its most severe results in coma and death, but even milder DKA is often associated with subclinical edema (Glaser et al., 2006) that can have neurocognitive consequences.

Neuroimaging studies have shown brain changes subsequent to DKA, including reduced white matter volume in frontal, temporal, and parietal regions and reduced neuronal density in frontal gray matter at the time of diagnosis (Cameron et al., 2014), abnormal gray and white matter 18 months post-diagnosis (Aye et al., 2019), and changes in the thalamus associated with recurrent DKA (Antenor-Dorsey et al., 2013). DKA at diagnosis has been found to be associated with acute deficits in attention and memory that persisted 6 months later in patients with baseline changes in white and gray matter (Ghetti et al., 2020). Studies have found associations between DKA and memory, especially in patients with EOD (Cameron et al.; Ghetti et al.). Other research has shown effects on EF, especially in individuals with a history of chronic hyperglycemia (Cato et al., 2016), and decrements in IQ, especially in more severe DKA (Aye et al.; Ghetti et al.).

Cognitive Outcomes in T1D

Compared to children without diabetes, children with T1D are more likely to show slower processing speed and psychomotor deficits, attention problems, and deficits in EF. Problems in these areas are more likely among children with a history of chronic hyperglycemia and DKA, and in children with EOD.

Memory deficits are seen only in children with EOD or a history of DKA. DKA is an independent risk factor for memory deficits, but these problems are exacerbated in EOD. Children with severe hypoglycemia in the context of EOD are also at greater risk for memory dysfunction.

Lower IQ scores are reported in T1D, and again, the effects are magnified in EOD. Meta-analyses indicate a small (2–3 point) decrement in IQ in children with T1D (Gaudieri et al. 2008; Naguib et al. 2009) that may become larger (e.g., 6–12 points) in adults (Brands et al., 2005). These findings suggest there is a cumulative effect on IQ over time, likely associated with chronic dysglycemia and DKA (Cato et al., 2016), and possibly secondary to earlier-emerging deficits in attention, processing speed, and memory (Blasetti et al., 2011).

In general, language appears intact, though some children with a history of severe hypoglycemia may experience subtle language problems. There is also some evidence of academic difficulties in children with EOD, though reported differences are generally small (Gaudieri et al.; Naguib et al.).

Neuropsychological Assessment

Not everyone with T1D requires a neuropsychological assessment. In general, children with T1D should be referred for evaluation if:

1. They present with cognitive concerns in the context of one or more diabetes-related risk factors (EOD, chronic hyperglycemia, DKA, severe hypoglycemia).
2. There is a question of whether cognitive and/or executive functioning may be contributing to suboptimal diabetes management.
3. They have a history of repeat DKA, or DKA with verified cerebral edema.
4. They have a history of severe hypoglycemia, especially in the context of chronic hyperglycemia, or a history of hypoglycemic seizures.
5. There is a question of ADHD.

Clinical Interview

As part of the psychological diagnostic interview, it is important to get a good diabetes history. Variables to consider include age at diagnosis, most recent HbA1c and trends in blood glucose levels, history of complications and diabetes-related hospitalizations, who is responsible for which parts of diabetes care, and challenges with diabetes management (e.g., forgetfulness, arguing, lying about blood sugar values, sneaking food). It is also important to ask children if they feel overwhelmed or burned out by having diabetes, and if they feel they receive enough support. Adolescents should be asked if they ever take less insulin than prescribed, which can be a dangerous way to manage weight (Goebel-Fabbri, 2009). There are numerous standardized proxy-report and self-report measures to help answer these questions (see below); for more detailed discussion of psychosocial screening of children and youth with T1D, see Anderson and Schwartz (2014).

Assessment Batteries

An appropriate test battery for children with T1D should include measures of intellectual functioning/IQ, attention, memory (especially verbal memory), processing speed, fine-motor and visuomotor skills, and functional academic skills necessary for following a medical regimen (e.g., sentence comprehension, math calculation). Caregiver rating scales are crucial for evaluating attention and EF in daily life, as performance-based measures tend to measure efficiency of cognitive abilities, whereas rating scales measure aspects of real-world, goal-directed behavior (Toplak et al., 2013), which may be of greater relevance for managing T1D.

Based on findings from the clinical interview, clinicians may also add some diabetes-specific measures. Scales to consider include:

1 A measure of diabetes management, such as the Diabetes Behavior Rating Scale (DBRS; Iannotti et al., 2006) or the Self-Management of Type 1 Diabetes in Adolescence (SMOD-A; Schilling et al., 2009).
2 A measure documenting responsibility for diabetes self-care tasks, such as the Diabetes Family Responsibility Questionnaire (DFRQ; Anderson et al., 1990).
3 A measure of diabetes distress, such as the Problem Areas in Diabetes Survey (PAID), which has versions for teens (PAID-T; Weissberg-Benchell et al., 2011) and younger children (PAID-Peds; Markowitz et al., 2015).
4 A measure of family conflict (e.g., Diabetes Family Conflict Scale–Revised, DFCS-R; Hood et al., 2007), which is another major predictor of diabetes-related outcomes.

Comorbidity Screening

T1D is associated with mental health comorbidities that can affect diabetes management and cognitive functioning. Screening for symptoms of depression, anxiety, and disordered eating is recommended as part of standard clinical guidelines for all individuals with T1D (ADA, 2024). It is also important to assess for ADHD, which is associated with problematic diabetes management (Dehnavi et al., 2024). Positive screens should involve referral to a mental health professional familiar with diabetes when indicated.

Neuropsychological Testing

Before starting testing, it is important to ascertain current blood sugar levels to ensure the child is well enough to proceed. We typically report blood glucose data and use it when evaluating the validity of the assessment, interpreting findings, and justifying recommendations such as having the child check blood sugars before taking a test in school.

For children who have a CGM, it is recommended that blood sugars be checked at the start of testing and every hour thereafter. If the child does not have a CGM, we suggest checking at the beginning and end of testing, unless there is a clinical need to re-check. If blood sugars are low, testing cannot begin until the low is managed. It is then often possible to start in 15–30 minutes with a return to normoglycemia. High blood sugars should also be managed, but do not prevent testing; we typically proceed as long as blood glucose is <240 mg/dL and the child does not feel ill; after all, the majority of children with T1D referred for evaluation have chronically high blood sugars. Moreover, stress can elevate blood sugars, and it is not uncommon for a child to be nervous about the evaluation. If blood sugars are >240 mg/dL, we ask the family to manage high blood sugars as they normally would; if blood sugars remain high, assessment may be deferred to another day.

Timing of meals is also an important consideration. If the child ate right before arriving, it might be sensible to add an additional blood sugar check half an hour into testing. Similar considerations pertain if they are given a snack or a drink other than water during the evaluation.

Management Recommendations

School Supports

Children with TID may be eligible for services under either the Individuals with Disabilities Education Act (IDEA) or Section 504 of the Rehabilitation Act of 1973 under an Other Health Impairment (OHI) classification. At a minimum we recommend asking the school to develop a Section 504 Plan to mitigate the impact of diabetes on the child's educational opportunity (similar plans can be developed at private schools). To ensure that diabetes is managed appropriately at school, children with T1D should have a Diabetes Medical Management Plan (DMMP) developed by the child's healthcare providers. A DMMP is similar to, or can be used in lieu of, an Education Health Care Plan (EHCP) or Individualized Health Care Plan (IHP). Other common 504 recommendations include:

1. Accommodations for inattention and slower processing speed, which can fluctuate with acute changes in blood sugars (even when teachers do not observe overt inattention).
2. Checking blood sugars before tests (by the child or trained school personnel), and if they are out-of-range, deferring the test until blood sugars are back in-range. The exact ranges should be determined through consultation with the child's healthcare providers.
3. Accommodations for absences due to illness and medical appointments, so the child is not penalized for missing class or late work.

It is also important to ensure that the child is not sent home for most high and low blood sugars, which should be managed at school per the DMMP. If a child is being sent home frequently for out-of-range blood sugars, the family should discuss the issue with the school and their diabetes healthcare provider.

Psychosocial supports should also be considered, including educating teachers about T1D; educating other students about the child's diabetes (if the child and family approve); monitoring for and preventing bullying, which is common for children with T1D (Andrade & Alves, 2019); and provision of in-school counseling as needed.

The American Diabetes Association has an extensive website dedicated to helping children with T1D at school; see https://diabetes.org/advocacy/safe-at-school-state-laws/position-statements. For up-to-date guidelines, see March et al. (2023), Jackson et al. (2015), and Lawrence et al. (2022).

Diabetes Management

Youth with neurocognitive and executive dysfunction can have difficulty initiating self-care tasks, staying organized, planning ahead, stopping an activity to manage blood sugars, and remembering to check blood sugars or take insulin at appropriate times. They may also be more likely to take risks with their diabetes, for example skipping a dose of insulin rather than interrupt an activity (Wasserman et al., 2017). We therefore recommend close parent involvement in all diabetes management tasks. Parent monitoring and oversight can buffer youth against declines in blood sugar levels (Young et al., 2014), and families who share responsibility have better diabetes outcomes (Marker et al., 2018). Parents may counter that their child knows how to manage diabetes but having knowledge and using it to guide day-to-day behaviors are very different things, especially when children have executive dysfunction. It is important to explain that many youths benefit from extra support for managing diabetes, and that increasing parent involvement is not an indication of failure or meant to be punitive. If conflict results from more active parent involvement, working with a psychologist on reducing conflict and fostering communication and collaboration around diabetes care can be beneficial.

Finally, use of technology can help youth keep track of diabetes care. Smartphones can be particularly helpful tools for older adolescents. There are many apps available such as One Drop (https://onedrop.today/) and Glooko (https://www.glooko.com/) to help manage diabetes. The family might ask their healthcare team about preferred apps, as some diabetes centers are now integrating these apps into standard care.

Summary

Diabetes-related dysglycemia can have deleterious effects on cognitive development and functioning in children with T1D. Overall, the impact is generally modest, with small effect sizes reported in children and moderate effect sizes in adults, though even small effects can have a large functional impact (Schwartz et al., 2014). When weighing the effect of T1D on cognition, one should consider that:

- Certain groups are at greater risk for cognitive dysfunction. These include individuals with EOD, and those who experience repeated acute complications or complications in the context of chronic hyperglycemia.
- Neurocognitive deficits that affect adherence can lead to further worsening of cognition.
- The impact of T1D on cognition tends to accumulate over the lifespan.

Maintaining blood sugars in recommended ranges and preventing acute diabetes-related events has substantial potential for improving the health and well-being of individuals with T1D. Psychologists can play an important role in supporting children with T1D and their families in managing this complex illness and its associated stresses and comorbidities. A number of professional resources were listed within this chapter to assist pediatric specialists working with children and adolescents living with T1D.

References

American Diabetes Association (ADA) (2024). Children and adolescents: Standards of care in diabetes-2024. *Diabetes Care*, 47 (Supplement_1), S258–S281. https://doi.org/10.2337/dc24-S014.

Anderson, B. J., Auslander, W. F., Jung, K. C., Miller, J. P., & Santiago, J. V. (1990). Assessing family sharing of diabetes responsibilities. *Journal of Pediatric Psychology*, 15(4), 477–492. https://doi.org/10.1093/jpepsy/15.4.477.

Anderson, B. J. & Schwartz, D. D. (2014). Psychosocial and family issues in children with type 1 diabetes. In G. Umpierrez, (Ed.) *Therapy for Diabetes Mellitus and Related Disorders* (6th ed.). American Diabetes Association.

Andrade, C. J. D. N. & Alves, C. A. D. (2019). Relationship between bullying and type 1 diabetes mellitus in children and adolescents: A systematic review. *Jornal de Pediatria*, 95(5), 509–518. https://doi.org/10.1016/j.jped.2018.10.003.

Antenor-Dorsey, J. A. V., Meyer, E., Rutlin, J., Perantie, D. C., White, N. H., Arbalaez, A. M., Shimony, J. S., & Hershey, T. (2013). White matter microstructural integrity in youth with type 1 diabetes. *Diabetes*, 62(2), 581–589. https://doi.org/10.2337/db12-0696.

Aye, T., Mazaika, P. K., Mauras, N., Marzelli, M. J., Shen, H., Hershey, T., Cato, A., Weinzimer, S. A., White, N. H., Tsalikian, E., Jo, B., Riess, A. L., & Diabetes Research in Children Network Study Group. (2019). Impact of early diabetic ketoacidosis on the developing brain. *Diabetes Care*, 42(3), 443–449. https://doi.org/10.2337/dc18-1405.

Barnea-Goraly, N., Raman, M., Mazaika, P., Marzelli, M., Hershey, T., Weinzimer, S. A., Aye, T., Buckingham, B., Mauras, N., White, N. H., Fox, L. A., Tansey, M., Beck, R. W., Ruedy, K. J., Kollman, C., Cheng, P., Reiss, A. L., & Diabetes Research in Children Network (2014). Alterations in white matter structure in young children with type 1 diabetes. *Diabetes Care*, 37(2), 332–340. https://doi.org/10.2337/dc13-1388.

Blasetti, A., Chiuri, R. M., Tocco, A. M., Di Giulio, C., Mattei, P. A., Ballone, E., Chiarelli, F., & Verrotti, A. (2011). The effect of recurrent severe hypoglycemia on cognitive performance in children with type 1 diabetes: A meta-analysis. *Journal of Child Neurology*, 26(11), 1383–1391. https://doi.org/10.1177/0883073811406730.

Brands, A. M., Biessels, G. J., De Haan, E. H., Kappelle, L. J., & Kessels, R. P. (2005). The effects of type 1 diabetes on cognitive performance: A meta-analysis. *Diabetes Care*, 28(3), 726–735. https://doi.org/10.2337/diacare.28.3.726.

Broadley, M. M., White, M. J., & Andrew, B. (2017). A systematic review and meta-analysis of executive function performance in type 1 diabetes mellitus. *Psychosomatic Medicine*, 79(6), 684–696. doi:10.1097/PSY.0000000000000460.

Cameron, F. J., Scratch, S. E., Nadebaum, C., Northam, E. A., Koves, I., Jennings, J., Finney, K., Neil, J. L., Wellard, R. M., Mackay, M., Inder, T. E., & DKA Bran Injury Study Group (2014). Neurological consequences of diabetic ketoacidosis at initial presentation of type 1 diabetes in a prospective cohort study of children. *Diabetes Care*, 37(6), 1554–1562. https://doi.org/10.2337/dc13-1904.

Cato, M. A., Mauras, N., Mazaika, P., Kollman, C., Cheng, P., Aye, T., Ambrosino, J., Beck, R. W., Ruedy, K. J., Reiss, A. L., Tansey, M., White, N. H., & Hershey, T. (2016). Longitudinal evaluation of cognitive functioning in young children with type 1 diabetes over 18 months. *Journal of the International Neuropsychological Society*, 22(3), 293–302. doi:10.1017/S1355617715001289.

Dabelea, D., Rewers, A., Stafford, J. M., Standiford, D. A., Lawrence, J. M., Saydah, S, Imperatore, G., D'Agostino, R. B., Mayer-Davis, E. J., & Pihoker, C., & SEARCH for Diabetes in Youth Study Group (2014). Trends in the prevalence of ketoacidosis at diabetes diagnosis: The SEARCH for diabetes in youth study. *Pediatrics*, 133(4), e938–945 https://doi.org/10.1542/peds.2013-2795.

Dehnavi, A. Z., Elmitwalli, I., Alsharif, H. O. H., Razavi, A. S., Gumpel, T. A., Smith, A., Weinstock, R. S., Faraone, S. V., & Zhang-James, Y. (2024). Effects of ADHD and ADHD treatment on glycemic management in type 1 diabetes: A systematic review and meta-analysis of observational studies. *Diabetes Research and Clinical Practice*, 209, 111566. https://doi.org/10.1016/j.diabres.2024.111566.

Ding, K., Reynolds, C. M., Driscoll, K. A., & Janicke, D. M. (2021). The relationship between executive functioning, type 1 diabetes self-management behaviors, and glycemic control in adolescents and young adults. *Current Diabetes Reports*, 21(3), 1–13. https://doi.org/10.1007/s11892-021-01379-3.

Gaudieri, P. A., Chen, R., Greer, T. F., & Holmes, C. S. (2008). Cognitive function in children with type 1 diabetes: A meta-analysis. *Diabetes Care*, 31(9), 1892–1897. https://doi.org/10.2337/dc07-2132.

Ghetti, S., Kuppermann, N., Rewers, A., Myers, S. R., Schunk, J. E., Stoner, M. J., Garro, A., Quayle, K. S., Brown, K. M., Trainor, J. L., Tzimenatos, L., DePiero, A. D., McManemy, J. K., Nigrovic, L. E., Kwok, M. Y., Perry, C. S.III., Olsen, C. S., Casper, T. C., Glaser, N. S., & Pediatric Emergency Care Applied Research Network (PECARN) DKA FLUID Study Group. (2020). Cognitive function following diabetic ketoacidosis in children with new-onset or previously diagnosed type 1 diabetes. *Diabetes Care*, 43(11), 2768–2775. https://doi.org/10.2337/dc20-0187.

Glaser, N. S., Wootton-Gorges, S. L., Buonocore, M. H., Marcin, J. P., Rewers, A., Strain, J., DiCarlo, J., Neely, E. K., Barnes, P., & Kuppermann, N. (2006). Frequency of sub-clinical cerebral edema in children with diabetic ketoacidosis. *Pediatric Diabetes*, 7(2), 75–80. https://doi.org/10.1111/j.1399-543X.2006.00156.x.

Goebel-Fabbri, A. E. (2009). Disturbed eating behaviors and eating disorders in type 1 diabetes: Clinical significance and treatment recommendations. *Current Diabetes Reports*, 9(2), 133–139. https://doi.org/10.1007/s11892-009-0023-8.

Hawks, Z. W., Beck, E. D., Jung, L., Fonseca, L. M., Sliwinski, M. J., Weinstock, R. S., Grinspoon, E., Xu, I., Strong, R. W., Singh, S., Van Dongen, H. P. A., Frumkin, M. R., Bulger, J., Cleveland, M. J., Janess, K., Kudva, Y. C., Pratley, R., Rickels, M. R., Rizvi, S. R., … Germine, L. T. (2024). Dynamic associations between glucose and ecological momentary cognition in type 1 diabetes. *NPJ Digital Medicine*, 7(1), 59. https://doi.org/10.1038/s41746-024-01036-5.

Hood, K. K., Butler, D. A., Anderson, B. J., & Laffel, L. M. (2007). Updated and revised diabetes family conflict scale. *Diabetes Care*, 30(7), 1764–1769. https://doi.org/10.2337/dc06-2358.

Iannotti, R. J., Nansel, T. R., Schneider, S., Haynie, D. L., Simons-Morton, B., Sobel, D. O., Zeitzoff, L., Plotnick, L. P., & Clark, L. (2006). Assessing regimen adherence of adolescents with type 1 diabetes. *Diabetes Care*, 29(10), 2263–2267. https://doi.org/10.2337/dc06-0685.

Insel, R. A., Dunne, J. L., Atkinson, M. A., Chiang, J. L., Dabalea, D., Gottlieb, P. A., Greenbaum, C. J., Herold, K. C., Krischer, J. P., Lernmark, A., Ratner, R. E., Rewers, M. J., Schatz, D. A., Skyler, J. S., Sosenko, J. M., & Ziegler, A. G. (2015). Staging presymptomatic type 1 diabetes: A scientific statement of JDRF, the Endocrine Society, and the American Diabetes Association. *Diabetes Care*, 38(10), 1964–1974. https://doi.org/10.2337/dc15-1419.

Jackson, C. C., Albanese-O'Neill, A., Butler, K. L., Chiang, J. L., Deeb, L. C., Hathaway, K., Kraus, E., Weissberg-Benchell, J., Yatvin, A. L., & Siminerio, L. M. (2015). Diabetes care in the school setting: A position statement of the American Diabetes Association. *Diabetes Care*, 38(10), 1958–1963. doi:10.2337/dc15-1418.

Jacobson, A. M., Ryan, C. M., Cleary, P. A., Waberski, B. H., Weinger, K., Musen, G., Dahms, W. & DCCT/EDIC Research Group (2011). Biomedical risk factors for decreased cognitive functioning in type 1 diabetes: An 18-year follow-up of the diabetes control and complications trial (DCCT) cohort. *Diabetologia*, 54, 245–255. https://doi.org/10.1007/s00125-010-1883-9.

Jaser, S. S. & Jordan, L. C. (2021). Brain health in children with type 1 diabetes: Risk and protective factors. *Current Diabetes Reports*, 21(4), 1–10. https://doi.org/10.1007/s11892-021-01380-w.

Kirchhoff, B. A., Jundt, D. K., Doty, T., & Hershey, T. (2017). A longitudinal investigation of cognitive function in children and adolescents with type 1 diabetes mellitus. *Pediatric Diabetes*, 18(6), 443–449. https://doi.org/10.1111/pedi.12414.

Lawrence, S. E., Albanese-O'Neill, A., Besançon, S., Black, T., Bratina, N., Chaney, D., Cogen, F. R., Cummings, E. A., Moreau, E., Pierce, J. S., Richmond, E., & Mahmud, F. H. (2022). ISPAD Clinical practice consensus guidelines 2022: Management and support of children and adolescents with diabetes in school. *Pediatric Diabetes*, 23(8), 1478–1495. doi:10.1111/pedi.13432.

Malik, F. S., Sauder, K. A., Isom, S., Reboussin, B. A., Dabelea, D., Lawrence, J. M., Roberts, A., Mayer-Davis, E. J., Marcovina, S., Dolan, L., Igudesman, D., Pihoker, C., & SEARCH for Diabetes in Youth Study (2022). Trends in glycemic control among youth and young adults with diabetes: The SEARCH for diabetes in youth study. *Diabetes Care*, 45(2), 285–294. https://doi.org/10.2337/dc21-0507.

March, C., Sherman, J., Bannuru, R. R., Fischer, A., Gabbay, R. A., Rodriguez, H., Rodriguez, J., Weissberg-Benchell, J., Woodward, C., & ElSayed, N. A. (2023). Care of young children with diabetes in the childcare and community setting: A statement of the American Diabetes Association. *Diabetes Care*, 46 (12), 2102–2111. https://doi.org/10.2337/dci23-0083.

Marker, A. M., Noser, A. E., Clements, M. A., & Patton, S. R. (2018). Shared responsibility for Type 1 diabetes care es associated with glycemic variability and risk of glycemic excursions in youth. *Journal of Pediatric Psychology*, 43(1), 61–71. https://doi.org/10.1093/jpepsy/jsx081.

Markowitz, J. T., Volkening, L. K., Butler, D. A., & Laffel, L. M. (2015). Youth-perceived burden of type 1 diabetes: Problem areas in diabetes survey-pediatric version (PAID-Peds). *Journal of Diabetes Science and Technology*, 9(5), 1080–1085. https://doi.org/10.1177/1932296815583506.

Mauras, N., Buckingham, B., White, N. H., Tsalikian, E., Weinzimer, S. A., Jo, B., Cato, A., Fox, L. A., Aye, T., Arbelaez, A. M., Hershey, T., Tansey, M., Tamborlane, W., Foland-Ross, L. C., Shen, H., Englert, K., Mazaika, P., Marzelli, M., Reiss, A. L., & Diabetes Research in Children Network (2021). Impact of type 1 diabetes in the developing brain in children: A longitudinal study. *Diabetes Care*, 44(4), 983–992. https://doi.org/10.2337/dc20-2125.

Naguib, J. M., Kulinskaya, E., Lomax, C. L., & Garralda, M. E. (2009). Neurocognitive performance in children with type 1 diabetes: A meta-analysis. *Journal of Pediatric Psychology*, 34(3), 271–282. https://doi.org/10.1093/jpepsy/jsn074.

Redondo, M. J., Steck, A. K., & Pugliese, A. (2018). Genetics of type 1 diabetes. *Pediatric Diabetes*, 19(3), 346–353. https://doi.org/10.1111/pedi.12597.

Ryan, C. M., van Duinkerken, E., & Rosano, C. (2016). Neurocognitive consequences of diabetes. *American Psychologist*, 71(7), 563–576. https://doi.org/10.1037/a0040455.

Sattar L., Renneboog B., & Decaux, G. (2017). Hyperglycemia induces attention and gait deficits in diabetic mellitus patients. *Acta Diabetologica*, 54, 953–959. https://doi.org/10.1007/s00592-017-1034-6.

Schilling, L. S., Dixon, J. K., Knafl, K. A., Lynn, M. R., Murphy, K., Dumser, S., & Grey, M. (2009). A new self-report measure of self-management of type 1 diabetes for adolescents. *Nursing Research*, 58(4), 228–236. doi:10.1097/NNR.0b013e3181ac142a.

Schwartz, D. D., Wasserman, R., Powell, P. W., & Axelrad, M. E. (2014). Neurocognitive outcomes in pediatric diabetes: A developmental perspective. *Current Diabetes Reports*, 14, 1–10. https://doi.org/10.1007/s11892-014-0533-x.

Seaquist, E. R. (2015). The impact of diabetes on cerebral structure and function. *Psychosomatic Medicine*, 77, 616–621. doi:10.1097/PSY.0000000000000207.

Tansey, M., Beck, R., Ruedy, K., Tamborlane, W., Cheng, P., Kollman, C., Fox, L., Weinzimer, S., Mauras, N., White, N. H., Tsalikian, E., & Diabetes Research in Children Network. (2016). Persistently high glucose levels in young children with type 1 diabetes. *Pediatric Diabetes*, 17(2), 93–100. https://doi.org/10.1111/pedi.12248.

Tonoli, C., Heyman, E., Roelands, B., Pattyn, N., Buyse, L., Piacentini, M. F., Berthoin, S., & Meeusen, R. (2014). Type 1 diabetes-associated cognitive decline: A meta-analysis and update of the current literature. *Journal of Diabetes*, 6(6), 499–513. https://doi.org/10.1111/1753-0407.12193.

Toplak, M. E., West, R. F., & Stanovich, K. E. (2013). Practitioner review: Do performance-based measures and ratings of executive function assess the same construct? *Journal of Child Psychology and Psychiatry*, 54(2), 131–143. https://doi.org/10.1111/jcpp.12001.

Wasserman, R., Anderson, B. J., & Schwartz, D. D. (2017). Illness-specific risk-taking in adolescence: A missing piece of the nonadherence puzzle for youth with type 1 diabetes? *Diabetes Spectrum*, 30(1), 3–10. https://doi.org/10.2337/ds15-0060.

Weissberg-Benchell, J. & Antisdel-Lomaglio, J. (2011). Diabetes-specific emotional distress among adolescents: Feasibility, reliability, and validity of the problem areas in diabetes-teen version. *Pediatric Diabetes*, 12(4 Pt 1), 341–344. doi:10.1111/j.1399-5448.2010.00720.x.

Wolfsdorf, J., Craig, M. E., Daneman, D., Dunger, D., Edge, J., Lee, W., Rosenbloom, A., Sperling, M., & Hanas, R. (2009). Diabetic ketoacidosis in children and adolescents with diabetes. *Pediatric Diabetes*, 10(Suppl 12), 118–133. doi:10.1111/j.1399-5448.2009.00569.x.

Young, M. T., Lord, J. H., Patel, N. J., Gruhn, M. A., & Jaser, S. S. (2014). Good cop, bad cop: Quality of parental involvement in type 1 diabetes management in youth. *Current Diabetes Reports*, 14(11), 1–12. https://doi.org/10.1007/s11892-014-0546-5.

Zorena, K., Michalska, M., Kurpas, M., Jaskulak, M., Murawska, A., & Rostami, S. (2022). Environmental factors and the risk of developing type 1 diabetes-old disease and new data. *Biology*, 11(4), 608. https://doi.org/10.3390/biology11040608.

15 Pediatric Stroke/Cardiovascular Accident (CVA)

Jennifer N. Longoria and Rachel M. Bridges

Introduction

The cerebrovascular system is a complex network of arteries, veins, and capillaries that is responsible for circulating blood throughout the brain. Although the brain comprises 2% of volume in the human body, it demands 20% of the body's available oxygen supply. Oxygen binds to hemoglobin molecules in red blood cells and is transported in the carotid and vertebral arteries to the brain. Once oxygen is absorbed and depleted, cerebral veins transport red blood cells back to the heart and lungs for replenishment and recirculation. Oxygen is essential to neuronal health and function. Given that neurons have limited ability to store oxygen reserves, these cells rely on constant rejuvenation from cerebrovascular arteries. Increased neuronal activity, as required for complex cognitive activities, generates increased demand for cerebral perfusion. Neurons are highly sensitive to fluctuations in oxygen saturation and cerebral blood flow. Hypoxic brain injuries occur when there is a decline in available oxygen (e.g., ischemic stroke or cardiac arrest) and anoxic injuries follow a complete lack of oxygen in the brain (e.g., suffocation, carbon monoxide poisoning). Cellular death in the brain can occur rapidly, within approximately three to four minutes after anoxia onset (Puig et al., 2018).

An ischemic stroke is a CVA that occurs when there is a change in cerebral perfusion (i.e., blood flow) to a specific part of the brain. Ischemic strokes typically generate immediate neurobehavioral and motor changes. Border zones in the brain that are between major arteries, such as the anterior cerebral and middle cerebral arteries, are particularly susceptible to stroke since this brain tissue does not receive as high of volume of oxygen rich blood from either artery. Watershed areas in the brain (e.g., lenticulostriate arteries) are also vulnerable to ischemic stroke given the distance from a singular cerebral artery that is the primary source of oxygenated blood. In some instances, there can be a change in cerebral perfusion that does not generate real-time neurobehavioral or motor change (s). These ischemic events are known as silent cerebral infarcts (SCI). SCI remain undetected after onset and are normally identified during routine

DOI: 10.4324/9781032703923-18

magnetic resonance imaging (MRI). SCI most commonly impact white matter in the frontal and parietal lobes (DeBaun et al., 2012).

Hemorrhagic stroke represents another type of CVA that occurs when there is a rupture within an artery or vein. Ruptures can be precipitated by traumatic or nontraumatic circumstances. In cases where there is a blunt force injury to the brain, blood vessels may tear and pooled blood (i.e., hematoma) can lead to increased intracranial pressure and herniation. Nontraumatic hemorrhagic strokes are typically associated with the rupture of an aneurysm. These events are not precipitated by blunt force injury to the head but are typically accompanied by a sudden and catastrophic headache. Regardless of the cause, hemorrhagic strokes require immediate medical attention to prevent serious injury or death. Arterial veinous malformations (AVM) reflect a distinct type of rupture caused by increased pressure within irregular cerebrovascular networks. In this congenital condition, some blood vessels are tangled and the normal flow of blood between arteries and veins is disrupted. AVM typically remains undetected and asymptomatic until the time of rupture.

Perinatal stroke is a specific CVA that occurs after the 20th week of gestation through the first 28 days after delivery (Raju et al., 2007). Perinatal strokes may be ischemic, hemorrhagic, or both. Intraventricular hemorrhage is common at the germinal matrix, a highly vascularized zone near the ventricles that proliferates neurons and glial cells. The timing of perinatal stroke can lead to significant disruptions in neuronal migration, connectivity, and maturation. The impact of stroke in this critical period of cerebral development can lead to long-term neurodevelopmental differences.

Epidemiology

The risk for perinatal stroke in term infants is 1:1100 and estimated to be near 7:1000 for preterm infants (Dunbar et al., 2020; Srivastava et al., 2022). Infants born preterm are most at risk for intraventricular hemorrhage in the parietal lobe or ischemic stroke in the left middle cerebral artery (Roy et al., 2022). For full-term infants, ischemic stroke most commonly involves the middle cerebral arteries.

The annual incidence rate of pediatric stroke is estimated to be 1.6 to 2.4 per 100,000 (Agrawal et al., 2009; Mallick et al., 2014). Risk is greatest for males and Black children, even after accounting for sickle cell disease (SCD) and head trauma (Fullerton et al., 2003). Pediatric stroke is a leading cause of mortality among children. The incidence of ischemic and hemorrhagic stroke is roughly equivalent in children, whereas ischemic stroke is more common in adults due to lifestyle factors that impact integrity of cerebral arteries (e.g., plaque buildup due to high cholesterol).

Children born with SCD are at increased risk for ischemic stroke and SCI. In SCD, inefficient transport of oxygen throughout the body is caused by mutations on the hemoglobin molecule, which creates an environment of vascular instability within major organs, particularly the brain. SCI are the most common vascular event in SCD, with nearly 40% of children exhibiting a silent infarct by age 14. The risk for ischemic stroke in children with SCD is greatest before age 10 (Ohene-Frempong et al., 1998). Ischemic stroke rates have declined greatly over the past two decades after transcranial doppler (TCD) ultrasound, a procedure which measures cerebrovascular velocity, became integrated in the care pathway. Chronic blood transfusions mitigate stroke risk for patients with abnormal TCD findings by infusing healthy red blood cells into the body, thus improving transportation and availability of oxygen within the brain.

There are several other complex medical conditions that place children at increased risk for stroke. Approximately 10% to 15% of children with congenital heart disease will have a stroke. See Cassidy et al. (2018) for a primer on congenital heart disease in pediatric patients. The rate of stroke in AVM spans 0.06–0.11 in children and represents the greatest risk for spontaneous intracranial hemorrhage in childhood (El-Ghanem et al., 2016). Children with human immunodeficiency virus (HIV) and clotting disorders (e.g., hemophilia) are also at increased risk for stroke.

Diagnosis

Early identification of stroke is essential for treatment and future stroke prevention. Stroke and SCI are confirmed via neuroimaging techniques, including computed tomography (CT) or magnetic resonance imaging (MRI). Workup for children presenting to the emergency department with stroke symptoms typically includes a physical exam, blood tests, and neuroimaging. Ultrasounds and echocardiograms can be used to identify abnormalities in the carotid arteries and/or heart that may have contributed to stroke. Neurological exams are used to identify deficits with sensory and motor functioning and typically include evaluation of cranial nerves, upper and lower motor tracts, and brief cognitive skills (e.g., comprehension, memory). Assessment of cognitive skills during a neurological exam is brief and similar to an abbreviated mental status exam but without the use of standardized paper-and-pencil measures. These findings can be used to quickly identify areas of sensory, motor, or cognitive functioning that may have been impacted by stroke.

Characteristic Symptoms and Medical Complications

Ischemic stroke is generally localized to one hemisphere of the brain. The anterior and middle cerebral arteries cover vast territory, which include the most common locations for ischemic stroke. Clinical presentation during stroke is typically marked by rapid onset of behavioral changes, including hemiparesis (i.e., weakness on one side of the body), imbalance, hemisensory deficits (e.g., visual field changes, numbness in extremities), and difficulty with speech and language. Stroke onset can also include seizures, a severe headache, and vomiting.

Damage to the sensory and motor cortices, basal ganglia, and thalamus will produce contralateral motor deficits. For example, a stroke in the right hemisphere will impact motor functioning on the left side of the body. Onset of sensory and motor impact occurs during the stroke and typically persists to some degree after the event. Stroke symptoms localized in the fronto-temporal lobe in the left hemisphere will generate language deficits, including problems with comprehension, naming, repetition, and fluency. Right hemisphere strokes are associated with hemineglect, visuospatial deficits, and difficulty processing nonverbal elements of speech and language. Stroke in the cerebellum will generate ipsilateral motor deficits, including ataxia, dysmetria, and tremor.

Trauma is the leading cause of hematoma in children and may include motor vehicle accidents, falls, or abusive head trauma. After experiencing a blunt force injury, an individual with a hematoma may present with a period of typical functioning for several hours. However, as the hematoma increases in size, intracranial pressure will rise rapidly and can cause midline shift. During this period of increased intracranial pressure, the onset of cognitive changes is likely to be quick. Without immediate medical attention, the hematoma may spur herniation and death.

Children who experience perinatal stroke are at increased risk of cerebral palsy, a group of motor disorders caused by brain damage in early childhood (see Chapter 23, Cerebral Palsy). Ischemic strokes in the perinatal period are most likely to impact the pyramidal system, resulting in a spastic presentation due to injuries in upper motor neurons. In addition to muscle tension, pyramidal lesions tend to impact cognitive functioning and are localized to specific regions of impact (e.g., frontal or temporal lobes). For instance, a left anterior cerebral artery perinatal ischemic stroke may impact the right leg and executive functioning skills, such as working memory. Stroke in the extrapyramidal regions (e.g., basal ganglia, cerebellum, and brainstem) is rarer and tends to impact balance, coordination, and fine tuning of motor movements while typically sparing cognitive functioning.

Treatment

Brisk identification and management of stroke is essential for optimal cognitive outcomes. Although tissue plasminogen activator (tPA) is commonly used to dissolve thrombotic or embolic clots in adults, use in children is not integrated in the care pathway due to insufficient evidence of efficacy (Rivkin et al., 2015). Therefore, its use is inconsistent and sometimes controversial. For additional information on pediatric stroke management, see guidelines from the American Heart Association/American Stroke Association (Ferriero et al., 2019).

Rehabilitation services are essential for restoring functioning post-stroke. Inpatient rehabilitation is often initiated within days of the stroke and includes multidisciplinary collaboration among occupational therapy, physical therapy, speech therapy, and sometimes neuropsychology. Cognitive rehabilitation services offered by neuropsychology tend to emphasize regaining skills that have been impacted (e.g., language, memory, executive functioning), strengthening abilities that have been spared to prompt the use of compensatory strategies, and addressing concerns with adaptive living skills. Some settings will also offer academic rehabilitation support through licensed teachers who work in the hospital setting. Typically, the most recovery in functioning occurs within nine months of a stroke or CVA. During this time, revascularization is occurring at the site of the lesion and functioning can be restored with repetition of cognitive and physical activities.

Implications for the School

While some children demonstrate no apparent impairment following a stroke, the nature and severity of neurocognitive sequelae depend on the size and region of the lesion, age at stroke, and presence of coexisting medical conditions (Fuentes et al., 2016; Lo & Heyer, 2012). Survivors of pediatric stroke often require additional support in the educational environment for weaknesses across a wide range of cognitive domains. Deficits are common across vision, fine and gross motor skills, language, memory, attention and executive functioning, processing speed, behavior and emotional health, and activities of daily living (Jacomb et al., 2018). As a result, survivors are vulnerable to academic deficits and face unique academic challenges compared to their peers, including difficulty with tasks involving phonology, reading comprehension, and mathematical computation (Champigny et al., 2020). Given these risk factors, survivors of pediatric stroke require neuropsychological assessment and monitoring to inform educational supports and related interventions.

Assessment

Stroke survivors should receive comprehensive neuropsychological care from a clinical neuropsychologist with expertise in pediatrics. Careful assessment of patterns in cognitive functioning, accurate differential diagnosis, and monitoring of neurocognitive changes over time is particularly important due to the variability of neurocognitive sequelae following pediatric stroke. In addition to neuropsychological assessment, stroke survivors often require targeted physical, occupational, and speech-language therapy evaluations. Together, neuropsychological and related service evaluations serve as a basis for designing interventions, developing recommendations for school programming based on specific cognitive needs, and monitoring intervention efficacy. These evaluations are often completed or scheduled by the time the child is discharged from inpatient medical care and returns to school.

Neuropsychological evaluations from the clinical setting should be shared directly with the school team, followed by ongoing communication between medical providers, school personnel, and the family. Communication and access can be facilitated by parents through a release of information request at the facility that managed the child's stroke care. School psychologists should take care to request and review previous neuropsychological assessment findings, as this helps avoid unnecessary re-evaluations within a short period of time. Risks of repeating an evaluation for a child who has already been assessed by another professional include practice effects (which can skew data and limit interpretation), missed instructional time, and unnecessary fatigue for the child. In some situations, add-on testing by the school can be considered to enhance existing clinical evaluation data (e.g., administering select academic subtests to clarify specific reading or mathematics skills that are necessary to qualify the child for services).

Qualification for Special Education and Related Services

Research has demonstrated that roughly half of children who suffer a stroke require formalized educational programming (O'Keeffe et al., 2017). A child with history of stroke will likely qualify under the Other Health Impairment (OHI) classification of the Individuals with Disabilities Education Act (IDEA). Given that survivors of stroke are at increased risk for diagnoses of specific learning disability and sensory and/or motor impairments, additional areas of IDEA eligibility should be considered when appropriate.

The child's medical team will provide guidance on medical symptom management and/or monitoring, as well as any restrictions via a health plan tailored to the student's specific needs. A formalized health plan should be included within the child's individual education plan (IEP) to provide standardized guidelines for safely handling medical related concerns that may arise during the school day. For example, a child's health plan may include guidance on medication administration or when the child should be sent home due to fatigue or headache. Common health plans for survivors of pediatric stroke include care planning for signs and symptoms of stroke, seizure action plans, headache management plans, and activity restrictions (D'Achille & Bloom, 2018).

In addition to medical related supports within the school setting, the educational team will determine targeted school-based recommendations and related services guided by a child's specific neurocognitive profile and situational factors. A full review of recommendations for the school setting is beyond this chapter's scope; however, common considerations pertinent to pediatric stroke are discussed in the following sections.

Recovery and return to school

The process and timing of a child returning to school after a stroke will vary based on the severity of injury (D'Achille & Bloom, 2018). The medical team will provide guidelines as to when the child is medically stable and safe to return to school. During the initial recovery period, homebound instruction may be required. When deemed medically able to return to the classroom, the child may need to exert increased energy to accomplish routine activities and will be susceptible to increased fatigue. During this transition period, temporary modifications may be required such as a reduced course load and/or modified school schedule (e.g., half days, every other day). School personnel should take care when designing the secondary students' class schedules to avoid grouping multiple demanding courses back-to-back and/or postponing highly demanding courses until after the window of recovery. A child's school plan should include guidelines for handling work missed before their return to school. Additionally, the potential for future absences and associated missed work should be considered proactively. Considerations include the amount of missed work that will be required to be made up (e.g., emphasis on quality over quantity) and the approved time for completing work.

Safety

Survivors of stroke are at increased risk of injuries from falls or other accidents. Children with residual weakness, ataxia, visual loss, or inattention/impulsivity are particularly vulnerable (Lo & Heyer, 2012). The school team must consider a child's specific risk factors and associated safety concerns when developing educational supports. It may be helpful for the team to consider the child's immediate classroom environment, transitional and common spaces (e.g., hallways, cafeteria), and transportation between school and home when planning. Additionally, the school team should consider a child's use of supportive equipment (e.g., wheelchairs, orthotic devices) and how this will impact their ability to navigate the classroom and school building. Safety needs will likely change over time, particularly as a child recovers (e.g., improved mobility) or progresses to higher grade levels (e.g., transition to environments with increased independence). Thus, supports should be regularly reviewed and revised to ensure maximum access to the educational environments.

Vision

Childhood stroke can result in a variety of visual impairments, including visual field defects, nystagmus, and abnormal eye movements. It is important for school teams to consider the presence of visual impairments and the potential impact on the educational environment to inform tailored supports. A review indicated that visual field deficits are the most reported visual abnormality in children with stroke history (Crawford & Golomb, 2018). Survivors who demonstrate visual field cuts will require unique structuring of the educational environment to ensure academic content is presented within the line of vision. For example, children who experience visual field cuts should be placed near the front of the classroom on the side where vision was affected and the child's "center placement" for work should align with the unaffected visual field shoulder.

Speech and Language

Speech and language weaknesses are common during the acute phase of pediatric stroke, and can include dysphagia, oral motor difficulty, and deficits in receptive/expressive language (Sherman et al., 2021). Long-term, language-related difficulty may also occur in processing, verbal fluency, organization of ideas, and synthesis of information. School teams should work with the child's medical team to determine the presence of swallowing difficulty (e.g., dysphagia) and develop relevant safety plans, as necessary. In addition to outpatient speech-language therapy (SLT) services, children may benefit from a school-based evaluation to determine the educational impact of speech–language weaknesses, guide interventions, and inform classroom supports. SLT for pediatric patients often targets deficits in motor speech function or basic language skills. Within the classroom, students with weaknesses in basic speech–language domains may benefit from extended time when providing oral responses or the use of electronic communication tools (based on impairment severity). Children who have difficulty with higher-order aspects of language may benefit from the use of graphic organizers, questions provided one at a time, pairing of vocabulary words with visuals, and written/visual cues to accompany verbal information.

Motor

Motor weakness, dystonia, and spasticity are common manifestations of childhood stroke (Lo & Heyer, 2012). In addition to outpatient therapies, school-based physical therapy (PT) and/or occupational therapy (OT) evaluations can help determine the educational impact of motor impairment, as well as guide therapeutic interventions, inform classroom supports, and identify safety needs. Survivors of stroke with mobility difficulties may struggle with movement around the classroom (e.g., transitions from sitting to standing) or throughout the school (e.g., carrying books, navigating hallways, using the stairs; D'Achille & Bloom, 2018). They may also more easily lose balance and/or fatigue. Supports for mobility concerns include placing a student's desk closer to frequently accessed locations in the classroom, 1:1 adult aid or peer buddy, elevator access, use of a second set of books, and leaving class early to avoid crowded hallways. Fine motor deficits may manifest as not anchoring the paper when writing, poor handwriting, difficulty with copying information, and slow production of written work. Children with these weaknesses may benefit from accommodations related to typing or use of voice-to-text programs, copies of notes or study guides, or use of wide-ruled paper or clipboard. Related service professionals can also support activities of daily living (ADLs) within the school environment. Motor impact on ADLs within the school environment can include putting on a coat, tying shoes, using the bathroom, and opening food containers.

Social, Emotional, Behavioral

A variety of social, emotional, and behavioral changes can occur in survivors of pediatric stroke. Depression and psychiatric dysfunction are relatively common, as well as flat affect, emotional lability, and sleep difficulty. Psychiatric concerns in stroke survivors result largely from stroke-induced brain changes or an exacerbation of preexisting symptoms. These concerns may be further compounded by the emotional impact of coping with a serious medical event and residual symptoms. School teams should consider the need for a positive behavior support plan if disruptions occur within the classroom. Additionally, students with emotional concerns may benefit from school-based counseling or social skills groups.

Conclusion

Stroke and CVA are neurological emergencies for children who carry risk for future disruptions in sensory and motor functioning, cognition, and academic achievement. Severity of injury and optimization of future outcomes is subject to timing, location, and etiology of the stroke. Perinatal strokes are particularly disruptive given the damage to the developing brain, which can lead to lifelong differences in cognitive and developmental functioning. Some medical conditions predispose children to enhanced risk of stroke or CVA, including SCD, AVM, and congenital heart disease. Children who experience stroke or CVA typically receive multi-disciplinary services through the treatment center overseeing their care, including neuropsychological assessment, cognitive remediation services, and/or therapies for speech, motor, and occupational needs. School psychologists are well positioned to help children transition back to school post-stroke by tailoring educational supports to meet their evolving needs, including safety, vision, motor, and speech and language.

Resources

- American Stroke Association: www.strokeassociation.org
- Brain Aneurysm Foundation: www.bafound.org
- Children's Hemiplegia and Stroke Association (CHASA): www.chasa.org
- International Alliance for Pediatric Stroke— Family Tool Kit: https://iapediatricstroke.org/family-resources/
- International Pediatric Stroke Organization (IPSO): https://community.internationalpediatricstroke.org/

References

Agrawal, N., Johnston, S. C., Wu, Y. W., Sidney, S., & Fullerton, H. J. (2009). Imaging data reveal a higher pediatric stroke incidence than prior US estimates. *Stroke*, 40(11), 3415–3421. https://doi.org/10.1161/STROKEAHA.109.564633.

Cassidy, A. R., Ilardi, D., Bowen, S. R., Hampton, L. E., Heinrich, K. P., Loman, M. M., Sanz, J. H., & Wolfe, K. R. (2018). Congenital heart disease: A primer for the pediatric neuropsychologist. *Child Neuropsychology*, 24(7), 859–902. https://doi.org/10.1080/09297049.2017.1373758.

Champigny, C. M., Deotto, A., Westmacott, R., Dlamini, N., & Desrocher, M. (2020). Academic outcome in pediatric ischemic stroke. *Child Neuropsychology*, 26(6), 817–833. https://doi.org/10.1080/09297049.2020.1712346.

Crawford, L. B. & Golomb, M. R. (2018, Apr). Childhood Stroke and Vision: A Review of the Literature. *Pediatric Neurology*, 81, 6–13. https://doi.org/10.1016/j.pediatrneurol.2017.11.007.

D'Achille, E. A. & Bloom, J. (2018). Educational needs of a child/adolescent following a stroke. In H. L. Atkinson, Nixon-Cave, K., & Smith, S. E. (Eds), *Pediatric stroke rehabilitation: An interprofessional and collaborative approach* (pp. 227–254). SLACK, Incorporated.

DeBaun, M. R., Armstrong, F. D., McKinstry, R. C., Ware, R. E., Vichinsky, E., & Kirkham, F. J. (2012). Silent cerebral infarcts: A review on a prevalent and progressive cause of neurologic injury in sickle cell anemia. *Blood, The Journal of the American Society of Hematology*, 119(20), 4587–4596. https://doi.org/10.1182/blood-2011-02-272682.

Dunbar, M., Mineyko, A., Hill, M., Hodge, J., Floer, A., & Kirton, A. (2020). Population based birth prevalence of disease-specific perinatal stroke. *Pediatrics*, 146(5). https://doi.org/10.1542/peds.2020-013201.

El-Ghanem, M., Kass-Hout, T., Kass-Hout, O., Alderazi, Y. J., Amuluru, K., Al-Mufti, F., Prestigiacomo, C. J., & Gandhi, C. D. (2016). Arteriovenous malformations in the pediatric population: Review of the existing literature. *Interventional Neurology*, 5(3–4), 218–225. https://doi.org/10.1159/000447605.

Ferriero, D. M., Fullerton, H. J., Bernard, T. J., Billinghurst, L., Daniels, S. R., DeBaun, M. R., deVeber, G., Ichord, R. N., Jordan, L. C., Massicontte, P., Meldau, J., Roach, E. S., Smith, E. R., & American Heart Association Stroke Council and Council on Cardiovascular and Stroke Nursing (2019). Management of stroke in neonates and children: A scientific statement from the American Heart Association/American Stroke Association. *Stroke*, 50(3), e51–e96. https://doi.org/10.1161/STR.0000000000000183.

Fuentes, A., Deotto, A., Desrocher, M., deVeber, G., & Westmacott, R. (2016). Determinants of cognitive outcomes of perinatal and childhood stroke: A review. *Child Neuropsychology*, 22(1), 1–38. https://doi.org/10.1080/09297049.2014.969694.

Fullerton, H. J., Wu, Y. W., Zhao, S., & Johnston, S. C. (2003). Risk of stroke in children: Ethnic and gender disparities. *Neurology*, 61(2), 189–194. https://doi.org/10.1212/01.WNL.0000078894.79866.95.

Jacomb, I., Porter, M., Brunsdon, R., Mandalis, A., & Parry, L. (2018, Apr). Cognitive outcomes of pediatric stroke. *Child Neuropsychology*, 24(3), 287–303. https://doi.org/10.1080/09297049.2016.1265102.

Lo, W. D. & Heyer, G. L. (2012). Treatment of pediatric stroke. In E. S. Roach, Lo, W. D., & Heyer, G. L. (Eds), *Pediatric stroke and cerebrovascular disorders*, (3rd ed., pp. 321–340). Springer Publishing Company, Incorporated.

Mallick, A. A., Ganesan, V., Kirkham, F. J., Fallon, P., Hedderly, T., McShane, T., Parker, A. P., Wassmer, E., Wraige, E., & Amin, S. (2014). Childhood arterial ischaemic stroke incidence, presenting features, and risk factors: A prospective population-based study. *The Lancet Neurology*, 13(1), 35–43. doi:10.1016/S1474-4422(13)70290-4.

Ohene-Frempong, K., Weiner, S. J., Sleeper, L. A., Miller, S. T., Embury, S., Moohr, J. W., Wethers, D. L., Pegelow, C. H., Gill, F. M., & Cooperative Study of Sickle Cell Disease (1998). Cerebrovascular accidents in sickle cell disease: Rates and risk factors. *Blood, The Journal of the American Society of Hematology, 91*(1), 288–294. https://doi.org/10.1182/blood.V91.1.288.

O'Keeffe, F., Stark, D., Murphy, O., Ganesan, V., King, J., & Murphy, T. (2017). Psychosocial outcome and quality of life following childhood stroke: A systematic review. *Developmental Neurorehabilitation*, 20(7), 428–442. https://doi.org/10.1080/17518423.2017.1282052.

Puig, B., Brenna, S., & Magnus, T. (2018, Sep 19). Molecular communication of a dying neuron in stroke. *International Journal of Molecular Sciences*, 19(9). https://doi.org/10.3390/ijms19092834.

Raju, T. N., Nelson, K. B., Ferriero, D., Lynch, J. K., & NICHD-NINDS Perinatal Stroke Workshop Participants (2007). Ischemic perinatal stroke: Summary of a workshop sponsored by the National Institute of Child Health and Human Development and the National Institute of Neurological Disorders and Stroke. *Pediatrics*, 120(3), 609–616. https://doi.org/10.1542/peds.2007-0336.

Rivkin, M. J., deVeber, G., Ichord, R. N., Kirton, A., Chan, A. K., Hovinga, C. A., Gill, J. C., Szabo, A., Hill, M. D., Scholz, K., & Amlie-Lefond, C. (2015). Thrombolysis in pediatric stroke study. *Stroke*, 46(3), 880–885. https://doi.org/10.1161/strokeaha.114.008210.

Roy, B., Walker, K., Morgan, C., Finch-Edmondson, M., Galea, C., Epi, M., Badawi, N., & Novak, I. (2022). Epidemiology and pathogenesis of stroke in preterm infants: A systematic review. *Journal of Neonatal-Perinatal Medicine*, 15 (1), 11–18. https://doi.org/10.3233/NPM-200597.

Sherman, V., Martino, R., Bhathal, I., DeVeber, G., Dlamini, N., MacGregor, D., Pulcine, E., Beal, D. S., Thorpe, K. E., & Moharir, M. (2021). Swallowing, oral motor, motor speech, and language impairments following acute pediatric ischemic stroke. *Stroke*, 52(4), 1309–1318. https://doi.org/doi:10.1161/STROKEAHA.120.031893.

Srivastava, R., Mailo, J. & Dunbar, M. (2022, October). Perinatal stroke in fetuses, preterm and term infants. *Seminars in Pediatric Neurology*, 43, 100988. https://doi.org/10.1016/j.spen.2022.100988.

Section IV

Genetic and Chromosomal Disorders

16 Sickle Cell Disease (SCD)

Denise E. Maricle and Allante Lumas

Introduction

Sickle cell anemia (SCA) is one of a group of disorders known as sickle cell disease (SCD). SCD is an inherited blood disorder that affects the shape of the red blood cells responsible for transporting oxygen throughout the body. Although recognized for generations in Africa, SCA was first described in writing more than hundred years ago (1910) by James B. Herrick (Williams & Thein, 2018). Herrick was the first westerner to describe the elongated and sickle-shaped red blood cells endemic to SCD. In 1933, Lemuel Digs differentiated SCD from sickle cell trait. In 1949, Linus Pauling identified the contribution of abnormal hemoglobin, hemoglobin S (HbS), and E. A. Beet and James V. Neel identified that SCD was transmitted genetically. More recently it has been noted that SCD results from a single change in one gene that makes hemoglobin (Williams & Thein).

Red blood cells are usually round and flexible, but in SCD the red blood cells are shaped like crescents or sickles. The red blood cells become rigid and sticky, blocking or slowing blood flow to various areas of the body. Normal red blood cells can live for up to 120 days, but sickle cell red blood cells only live for 10–20 days. This can cause severe anemia due to the lack of healthy red blood cells circulating in the body. The severity of the changes to the red blood cells varies significantly between people resulting in variations in disease severity.

SCD is caused by a change in the gene that makes hemoglobin. The type of SCD manifested depends on the hemoglobin genes passed from parent to child. There are several types of SCD. The most common is sickle cell anemia (SCA) notated as HbSS. SCA is autosomal recessive requiring 2 affected genes, one from each parent; this results in two abnormal copies of B-Globin gene (HBB) on Chromosome 11 (the affected genes code for HbS). HbS has a variation in the beta-chain (β-chain) gene that causes a change in the properties of hemoglobin, resulting in the abnormal, rigid, sickling shape of red blood cells. Normal hemoglobin A contains two α chains and two β chains. Each α chain contains 141 amino acids and each β chain contains 146 amino acids. SCA results from the

DOI: 10.4324/9781032703923-20

single amino acid substitution of valine for glutamic acid in the beta-chain as a result of a nucleotide defect that causes the production of abnormal beta-chains in hemoglobin S. If both parents of a child carry the sickle cell trait, there is a one in four chance that their child will develop SCD.

Less common types of SCD include hemoglobin sickle cell disease (HbSC), which results from one abnormal HbS gene from one parent and one abnormal hemoglobin C (HbC) gene from the other parent. Sickle cell trait (HbAS) results from one HbS and one hemoglobin A (HbA) gene. Sickle beta thalassemia (HbS beta thalassemia) results from one HbS gene and one HbS beta thalassemia gene. There are two types of HbS beta thalassemia, zero (HbSbeta0) and plus (HbSbeta+). Other even rarer types of SCD include HbSD, HbSE, and HbSO. In these types, the individual has inherited a sickle cell gene from one parent and a gene for a defective form of hemoglobin, hemoglobin D, E, or O, from the other parent.

Epidemiology

SCD is common in African, Mediterranean, and Middle Eastern heritage groups. The highest sickle cell trait carrier rate is present in families who trace their ancestry to malaria endemic regions (Meier & Miller, 2012). In 1954, it was determined that the sickle cell trait conveys a protective factor against malaria, a common disease in Africa and other equatorial regions. Three-fourths of SCD occurs in Africa and 80% in sub-Saharan Africa. Worldwide approximately 43 million people are carriers of the sickle cell trait, and as of 2015, about 4.3 million are affected by SCD. In the United States about 100,000 individuals are affected by SCD (one out of every 365 African Americans, and one out of every 16,300 Latinos) with over 2 million who are carriers of sickle cell trait. SCD is more common in the United States than diseases such as cystic fibrosis, hemophilia, or phenylketonuria (PKU).

Diagnosis

Typically, a blood test that scans for the sickle cell form of hemoglobin is used to test for SCD. Most commonly this is hemoglobin electrophoresis, but other tests such as high-performance liquid chromatography (HPLC) or DNA testing may be used (Chernecky & Berger, 2013). In the USA, testing for SCD is part of newborn screenings, but this is not necessarily true in other countries.

Prenatal testing can also be used to identify SCD. Measures such as amniocentesis and chorionic villus sampling (CVS; testing a portion of the placenta) are commonly used (Sauntharaja & Vichinsky, 2018). CVS can be completed at 10–12 weeks of pregnancy, whereas amniocentesis does not reliably show results until 15–20 weeks of gestation. Most commonly ARMS-PRC (amplification refractory mutation system [ARMS] plus polymerase chain reaction [PCR]) along with CVS has been used in the prenatal diagnosis of SCD. ARMS-PCR uses an allele specific polymerase chain reaction to detect a single-base pair mutation, which in SCD is the mutation of the GAG sequence to GTG in the 6th position of the B globin gene, resulting in the encoding of valine instead of glutamine (Singh, Shrivastava, & Shrikhande, 2015).

Characteristic Symptoms and Medical Complications

Pain and anemia are characteristic symptoms of all SCD types (Meier & Miller, 2012), but pain is the major symptom seen in most individuals with SCA. Chronic pain results when the sickle-shaped red blood cells block blood flow in the tiny capillaries in the chest, abdomen, and joints.

The pain of SCD may be acute or chronic. Acute, severe pain often requires a hospital stay. Chronic pain is common. Chronic pain is defined as pain present most days and lasting for more than six months (Osunkwa, et al., 2020). These painful episodes can be immobilizing, making daily life uncomfortable and difficult. There are no obvious triggers for the pain, although cold, stress, illness, and dehydration can bring on a pain crisis. Chronic pain is also associated with depression, anxiety, fatigue, and sleep disruptions. Research on the neurobiology of SCD pain suggests that initial pain episodes start a cascade of physiological changes that are mediated by inflammation which ultimately alters the nervous system permanently (Nogrady, 2021). Ongoing research suggests that chronic SCD pain might result from overstimulation of the CNS, which causes hypersensitivity within the nerve fibers, resulting in even nonpainful stimuli being interpreted as painful (Nogrady, 2021; Okpala & Tawil, 2002).

Anemia (aplastic crisis) results from a shortage of red blood cells. Anemia is characterized by a lack of enough healthy red blood cells to carry adequate oxygen to body tissues. Having anemia can make the person feel tired and weak. In SCD anemia, red blood cells are not being replaced quickly enough. Children with SCD are vulnerable to iron deficiency anemia, where they lack iron in their blood. Without enough iron, the body can't produce enough hemoglobin in the red blood cells, which enables them to carry oxygen.

Anemia causes severe fatigue. Fatigue is one of the most common symptoms in SCD, but very little is known about its prevalence, frequency, severity or how it interferes in daily life for individuals with SCD (Ameringer et al., 2014). Fatigue can be either acute or chronic. When acute, the fatigue may be so debilitating and overwhelming that the person is unable to carry out daily activities. Fatigue may also be an indicator of an impending acute pain crisis. Very little is known about the relationship of fatigue and pain or fatigue and anemia in individuals with SCD (Ameringer et al.). More is known about the social costs of fatigue in that it results in increased healthcare use, reduced work or school productivity, loss of work or school days, and a very high reliance on the assistance of caregivers (Ameringer & Smith, 2011).

Swelling in the extremities may result when the sickle-shaped red blood cells block circulation in the feet and hands. Infections are also common when an individual has SCD. The sickle-shaped red blood cells damage the spleen, which increases the person's vulnerability to infection, particularly bacterial infections. Delayed growth in puberty is also a common feature which results from the shortage of red blood cells. Individuals with SCD may also experience vision difficulties that result when the tiny blood vessels that supply the eyes are plugged resulting in damage to the retina; this can cause blindness.

Medical complications associated with SCD are complex and life-altering. Medical complications resulting from SCD can start as early as 6 months of age and increase with frequency over time. Children with SCD are at higher risk for strokes as the sickle-shaped cells can block blood flow to the brain. About 10% of individuals with SCD experience a stroke, and up to 17% may have a silent cerebral infarct (SCI) before age 20 (Meier & Miller, 2012). Silent cerebral strokes are often only detectable with fMRI, while overt strokes show clear evidence of injury on other neuroimaging measures. Overt strokes commonly occur in the frontal and parietal lobes (Smith & Baker, 2011). Acute chest syndrome (ACS) and pulmonary hypertension are also common risks for SCD. ACS may result when the sickle-shaped cells block the vessels and capillaries in the lungs resulting in infection, whereas pulmonary hypertension is the result of high blood pressure in the lungs. At least one episode of ACS is seen in about 30% of individuals (Meier & Miller). Symptoms of ACS include fever, cough, chest pain, labored or rapid breathing, and shortness of breath. It is not uncommon for there to be organ damage in SCD. Chronically low blood-oxygen levels can damage organs, such as the kidneys, liver, and spleen. Splenic sequestration results when the sickle-shaped red blood cells get trapped in the spleen, resulting in enlargement of the spleen, circulatory collapse, and severe stomach pain. About 30% of children under the age of 6 with SCD experience splenic sequestration. Splenic sequestration results in a large amount of blood pooling in the spleen; treatment is a splenectomy or surgical removal of the spleen. Excess bilirubin caused by red blood cell destruction results in about a third of children with SCD having gallstones by the age of 7. The bilirubin collects in the gallbladder forming gallstones. As a result of complications, children with SCD may appear severely jaundiced (yellowing of the eyes) and ultimately will require surgery to remove the gallbladder. SCD can cause other vascular or circulatory problems such as leg ulcers, deep vein thrombosis (blood clots in veins of the leg or the lungs), priapism in males (prolonged, painful erections), or vascular necrosis (cellular death of bone components due to interrupted blood supply).

Treatment

SCD is a lifelong condition. Treating SCD includes managing acute and chronic complications and helping control the symptoms of the disease. For now, there is no cure for SCD, but blood transfusions are a common intervention. Although blood transfusions play a prominent role in the management of SCD complications, frequent transfusions can also lead to iron overload. Iron overload may increase the risk for damage to multiple organs, and as a result, medical providers may recommend iron chelation. Iron chelation involves the use of drugs such as Deferoxamine or Deferasirox, which work to bind to the iron and allow the body to excrete the bound particles. Recently stem cell transplants have been tried with some success (Khaddour et al., 2022). Red blood cells are created in bone marrow and hematopoietic stem cells (aka: blood stem cells) are found in the peripheral blood and bone marrow. A stem cell is an immature cell that can develop into all types of blood cells, including white blood cells, red blood cells, and platelets. However, blood stem cell transplants are incredibly risky as prior to the stem cell infusion, high doses of chemotherapy and/or total body irradiation are administered to kill off all the previous cells. Stem cell transplants in SCD involve allogenic transplantation, which requires a matched donor (Khaddour et al.). Chemotherapy and radiation have significant neuropsychological effects that might need to be considered for a child with SCD treated via a stem cell transplant. In 2023–2024 the FDA approved a powerful treatment for SCD; Casgevy (Vertex Pharmaceutical and CRISPR Therapeutics) uses gene editing to modify stem cells by editing the DNA found in the stem cells to remove the gene that causes SCD. These modified blood stem cells increase the production of fetal hemoglobin (HbF) which facilitates oxygen delivery and reduces or prevents the sickled cells. The treatment is lengthy and costs more than 2.2 million dollars per patient. This does not include costs associated with lengthy hospital stays or necessary treatments such as blood transfusions and chemotherapy. Although a ground-breaking treatment, it does not appear to be a cure for SCD. Rather, this treatment in combination with other treatments is designed to reduce the symptoms associated with SCD.

Children and adolescents with SCD are prescribed a variety of medications to treat their disease and its symptoms. Hydroxyurea, an oral medicine, is one of the most common. Approved in 2017 for children, it is useful in SCD as it helps the red blood cells stay round and flexible by increasing hemoglobin F; it is also thought to help reduce pain episodes and hospitalizations. L-glutamine oral powder is an amino acid used to reduce pain crises, prevent infection, and slow down damage to the blood vessels. Crizanlizumab is used in people with SCD to reduce how often certain episodes (vaso-occlusive crises) occur. It acts like an oil to prevent red blood cells from becoming sticky. It is often prescribed with hydroxyurea. Crizanlizumab is only supposed to be prescribed for individuals 16 and older. Voxelotor (aka: Oxybryta) is another medication used to treat SCD in children 12 years of age and older. Voxelotor is in a class of medications called hemoglobin S (HbS) polymerization inhibitors. It works by helping hemoglobin hold onto more oxygen and stop red blood cells from becoming misshapen. Finally, some analgesics (ibuprofen, acetaminophen), narcotics (tramadol, oxycodone, fentanyl), and penicillin are used prophylactically for pain relief and to reduce the chance of infection (Brandow et al., 2020).

Common home remedies utilized in SCD include folic acid supplements (folic acid helps make healthy bone marrow and new red blood cells), a healthy diet, hydration, and regular exercise. Individuals with SCD are discouraged from being at high altitudes (avoid flying), using tobacco or other smoking-related products, avoiding temperature extremes. They should be careful about vaccines and the use of some over-the-counter painkillers. Nonpharmacological therapies addressing pain management and fatigue might include hypnosis, imagery, mindfulness or relaxation techniques, acupressure or acupuncture, biofeedback, TENS stimulation, integrated physical therapy, therapeutic recreation, and art or music therapy.

Implications for the School

Qualification for Special Education Services

A child with SCD will likely qualify under the Other Health Impairment (OHI) classification of the IDEA or Section 504 of the Rehabilitation Act of 1973. This allows for modification of school schedules, alternative attendance requirements, provision of health-related services by medical staff (e.g., nurses), or therapies such as physical or occupational therapy or adaptive PE.

Regardless of whether the child is classified under IDEA and receives an Individualized Education Plan (IEP) or under Section 504 and has an Accommodation Plan (AP), an Education Health Care Plan (EHCP) or an Individualized Health Care Plan (IHP), and an Emergency Procedures Plan (EPP) should be developed and attached to the child's IEP or AP.

Assessment in the Schools

For most children with SCD screening for cognitive abilities and academic achievement will be sufficient except for a known or suspected stroke, or a change in cognitive status or academic progress. The type of cognitive or learning difficulty exhibited will depend on where in the brain the stroke(s) occurred. See Chapter 15 Pediatric Stroke/Cardiovascular Accident. Children with SCD are vulnerable to executive function deficits (e.g., memory, attention, and visual-motor processing) which may impact educational achievement and therefore should be monitored (Crosby et al., 2015). Additionally, children with SCD often exhibit psychological, psychiatric, and social-emotional difficulties, and it is necessary to evaluate social-emotional and behavioral functioning in addition to their health status. Research has shown that individuals with SCD may experience anxiety, depression, or issues related to low self-concept and embarrassment (Salih, 2019).

It is critical to assess the child's level of fatigue and pain. There are several measures available to assess fatigue (Ameringer et al., 2014), but most have been developed for adults and not validated with children or individuals with SCD. The Multidimensional Fatigue Symptom Inventory, Short Form (MFSI-SF: Stein et al., 1998) consists of 30 items assessing fatigue during the past month. The Brief Fatigue Inventory (BFI; University of Texas MD Anderson Cancer Center) consists of 10 items measuring fatigue over the past 24 hours. The Patient Reported Outcome Measurement Information Systems (PROMIS; Revicki et al., 2009) Fatigue Short Form (V1.0-fatigue-shortform 6a) uses 7 items to evaluate fatigue over the past week. Evaluation of fatigue should be part of the daily routine for a child with SCD and accommodations or adjustments made based on the child's self-report of fatigue levels.

Several measures of pain are also available. A commonly used measure is the Wong-Baker FACES Pain Rating Scale (www.wongbakerfaces.org). This self-report scale for children ages 3–18 years is available in multiple languages. The Adolescent Pediatric Pain Tool (APPT; Fernandes et al., 2014) is designed to measure the intensity, location, and quality dimensions of pain. The APPT is intended for use with children ages 8–17 and is available in English and Spanish. The Patient Reported Outcome Measurement Information System (PROMIS) Pediatric Pain Interference Scale (PPIS) is a screening tool for chronic pain (Revicki et al., 2009). The PPIS was initially developed for adults, but a specific pediatric pain item bank was later developed for use with children ages 8–17 years old (Varni et al., 2010). The PPIS assesses pain during daily activities over the previous seven days (interference on physical, psychological, and social functioning).

The Pain Coping Questionnaire (PCQ) is a screening tool designed to assess coping strategies for children experiencing pain (Reid et al., 1998). Developed with children aged 8–18 years, it has been used with individuals aged 5–20 years. This tool was developed with children with arthritis but has been used with children with other chronic pain conditions such as migraines, back pain, fibromyalgia, and non-cancer related pain. The Pediatric Pain Coping Inventory (PPCI) is used to assess pain coping strategies (Varni et al., 1996). It was developed with children aged 5–16 years. The PPCI was designed to provide standardized assessment of the mechanisms the child utilizes to cope with pain. The Coping Strategies Questionnaire (CSQ) is a screening tool designed to assess the use of cognitive and behavioral strategies to cope with pain (Rosenstiel & Keefe, 1983). Based on the SCQ, the Coping Strategies Questionnaire Revised for

SCD Children (CSQ-SCD) has seven scales about coping with pain: distraction, catastrophizing, ignoring pain sensations, reinterpreting pain sensations, praying, increasing activity level, and calming self-statements. Evaluation of pain should be part of the daily routine for a child with SCD and daily accommodations or adjustments made based on the child's self-report of pain levels. The child's report of pain needs to be taken seriously and validated.

Pain can be treated with rest, hydration, temperature adjustments, medications, learned coping strategies such as mindfulness, and/or notification of parent and excused absence. If mobility due to pain is an issue, consider modifying classroom locations to lessen the distance or time between classes. Provide the child with books and needed materials in each classroom to limit the need to carry a backpack. Alternative adaptive equipment (e.g., ergonomic desks, seating, computer tables) can also be used to support mobility and decrease pain or stress on the body.

School-Based Interventions and Accommodations to Consider

Most individuals with SCD can be fully included in regular education programming with some accommodations (Dyson, 2011). However, attendance and work completion policies may need to be adjusted based on the child's fatigue and pain levels, as well as the need for periodic medical treatment or hospitalization. Many children with SCD will miss school due to illness or treatment; 20–30 days of absenteeism a year is common (Crosby et al., 2015). The individual may have difficulty concentrating, trouble with forgetfulness, or irritability due to high levels of fatigue or pain. Hydration is critical and schools should ensure adequate hydration by allowing access to a water bottle at all times. Additionally, more frequent bathroom breaks may be needed as children with SCD produce more urine, even when more dehydrated than typical children, so provision of a special bathroom pass may be helpful. Children and adolescents with SCD may need accommodations for extreme temperature (e.g., heat or cold) with common sense accommodations consisting of seating away from vents for heating and air conditioning, allowing layered clothing choices, allowing the use of a blanket and/or providing permission to not exercise or participate in recess in extreme weather. School nurses need to keep this in mind when caring for injuries and avoid the use of cold packs or heating pads. Accommodations for physical education classes should be considered and based on the child's reported fatigue and pain levels. For example, a child with SCD may need more time to recover from vigorous activities than peers. If a child is having difficulty with fatigue, consider options for participating in activities that are less strenuous, such as being the PE teacher's "assistant" or "scorekeeper." If a child looks particularly pale or shows a low or decreased tolerance for physical activity, this may be a sign that their anemia has become worse. Adaptive PE should be considered with consultation from the adaptive PE coordinator. All school personnel should be responsive to complaints of pain and should not encourage the child to "bear" it. Rather, if permissible administer a pain reliever and/or attempt to assist the child in managing the pain (e.g., excusing them from the activity, or changing their seating location). In addition, all school personnel should be trained in monitoring for emotional well-being, watching for signs of stroke, and working at open communication with the family. An emergency plan should be in place to address medical emergencies such as a fever, stroke, or ACS. ACS is a medical emergency due to its rapid onset and severity; however, individuals unfamiliar with SCD's medical complications may mistake it for more common illnesses such as influenza, a cold, or SARS-CoV-2 (COVID-19) and delay critical treatment. Parents should be contacted immediately if their child has a temperature of 101 degrees, as this is a serious concern, and can lead to complications such as pneumonia or sepsis, which is a leading cause of death in children with SCD. A great resource is Tips for Supporting Students with Sickle Cell Disease (cdc.gov/ncbddd/sicklecell/documents/tipsheet).

Resources

American Sickle Cell Anemia Association: ascaa.org

Digital technology: iCanCope App: http://icancope.ca/

National Organization for Rare Disease: raredisease.org

Sickle Cell Consortium: sicklecellconsortium.org

Sickle Cell Disease Association of America: sicklecelldisease.org

Gray Johnson, J. & Williams, L. (2012) *Living with Sickle Cell Disease: The Struggle to Survive.*

Platt, A. F., Eckman, J., Hsu, L. & Vennemann, A. (2016). *Hope and Destiny: A Patient's and Parent's Guide to Sickle Cell Disease and Sickle Cell Trait*, 4th Edition.

References

Ameringer, S., ElswickJr, R. K., & Smith, W. (2014). Fatigue in adolescents and young adults with sickle cell disease: Biological and behavioral correlates and health-related quality of life. *Journal of Pediatric Oncology Nursing*, 31(1), 6–17. https://doi.org/10.1177/1043454213514632.

Ameringer, S. & Smith, W. R. (2011). Emerging biobehavioral factors of fatigue in sickle cell disease. *Journal of Nursing Scholarship*, 43(1), 22–29. https://doi.org/10.1111/j.1547-5069.2010.01376.x.

Brandow, A., Patrick-Carroll, C., Creary, S., Edwards-Elliot, R., Glassberg, J., Hurly, R., Kutlar, A., Seisa, M., Stinson, H., Strouse, J. J., Yusef, F., Zempskey, W. & Long, E. (2020). American Society of Hematology 2020 guidelines for

SCD: Management of acute and chronic pain. *Blood Advances* 4(12), 2656–2701 https://doi.org/10.1182/bloodadvances.2020001851.

Chernecky, C. C. & Berger, B. J. (2013). *Sickle cell test-blood.* In C. C. Chernecky & B. J. Berger (Eds) *Laboratory Tests and Diagnostic Procedures* (6th ed., p. 1014). MO: Elsevier.

Crosby, L. E., Joffe, N. E., Irwin, M. K., Strong, H., Peugh, J., Shook, L., Kalinyak, K. A. & Mitchell, M. J. (2015). School performance and disease interference in adolescents with sickle cell disease. *Physical Disabilities* 34(1), 14–30. doi:10.14434/pders.v34i1.13918.

Dyson, S. (2011). *Sickle cell and thalassemia health and safety: A guide to school policy.* Retrieved September 2, 2024 from sicklecelleducation.com.

Fernandes, A. M., De Campos, C., Batalha, L., Perdigao, A., & Jacob, E. (2014). Pain assessment using the Adolescent Pediatric Pain Tool: A systematic review. *Pain Research and Management*, 19, 212–218. https://doi.org/10.1155/2014/979416.

Khaddour, K., Hana, C., & Mewawalla, P. (2022). Hematopoietic stem cell transplantation. In *StatPearls* [Internet], Treasure Island, FL. StatPearls Publishing.

Meier, E. R. & Miller, J. L. (2012). Sickle cell disease in children. *Drugs*, 72, 895–906. https://doi.org/10.2165/11632890-000000000-00000.

Nogrady, B. (2021). Why severe sickle cell pain has been neglected. *Nature*, 596 (7873), 10–12. doi:10.1038/d41586-021-02142-0.

Okpala, I. & Tawil, A. (2002). Management of pain in sickle-cell disease. *Journal of the Royal Society of Medicine*, 95(9), 456–458. https://doi.org/10.1177/014107680209500909.

Osunkwa, J., O'Connor, H. & Saah, E., (2020). Optimizing the management of chronic pain in SCD. *Hematology*, 1, 562–569. DOI.org/10.1182/hematology.202000143.

Reid, G. J., Gilbert, C. A., & McGrath, P. J. (1998). The Pain Coping Questionnaire: Preliminary validation. *Pain*, 76(1–2),83–96. https://doi.org/10.1016/S0304-3959(98)29–23.

Revicki, D. A., Chen, W. H., Harnam, N., Cook, K. F., Amtmann, D., Callahan, L. F., Jensen, P. M., & Keefe, F. J. (2009). Development and psychometric analysis of the PROMIS pain behavior item bank. *Pain*, 146(1–2),158–169. https://doi.org/10.1016/j.pain.2009.07.029.

Rosenstiel, A.K., & Keefe, F.J. (1983). The use of coping strategies in chronic low back pain patients: Relationship to patient characteristics and current adjustment. *Pain*, 17(1), 33–44. https://doi.org/10.1016/0304-3959(83)90125–90122.

Salih, K. M. A. (2019). The impact of sickle cell anemia on the quality of life of sicklers at school age. *Journal of Family Medicine and Primary Care*, 8(2), 468–471. https://doi.org/10.1016/0304-3959(83)90125–90122.

Saunthararajah, Y., & Vichinsky, E. P. (2018). Sickle cell disease: clinical features and management. In *Hematology* (pp. 584–607). Elsevier.

Singh, P.J., Shrivastava, A.C., & Shrikhande, A.V. (2015). Prenatal diagnosis of SCD by technique of PCR. *Indian Journal of Hematology and Blood Transfusions*, 31(2), 233–241.

Smith, J. T. & Baker, D. A. (2011). Sickle cell disease. In *Handbook of Neurodevelopmental and Genetic Disorders in Children* (2nd ed., pp. 338–361). Guilford Press.

Stein, K. D., Martin, S. C., Hann, D. M., & Jacobsen, P. B. (1998). A multidimensional measure of fatigue for use with cancer patients. *Cancer Practice*, 6, 143–152. https://doi.org/10.1046/j.1523-5394.1998.006003143.x.

Varni, J. W., Stucky, B. D., Thissen, D., Dewitt, E. M., Irwin, D. E., Lai, J. S., Yeatts, K., & Dewalt, D.A. (2010). PROMIS Pediatric Pain Interference Scale: An item response theory analysis of the pediatric pain item bank. *Journal of Pain*, 11(11), 1109–1119. https://doi.org/10.1016/j.jpain.2010.02.005.

Varni, J. W., Waldron, S. A., Gragg, R. A., Rapoff, M. A., Bernstein, B. H., Lindsley, C. B., & Newcomb, M. D. (1996). Development of the Waldron/Varni Pediatric Pain Coping Inventory. *Pain*, 67, 10. https://doi.org/10.1016/0304-3959(96)03077–03071.

Williams, T. N. & Thein, S. L. (2018). Sickle cell anemia and its phenotypes. *Annual Review Of Genomics And Human Genetics*, 19, 113–147. https://doi.org/10.1146/annurev-genom-083117-021320.

17 Cystic Fibrosis (CF)

Andrea Wierzchowski

Introduction

Cystic fibrosis (CF) is an inherited, chronic, genetic condition that arises when both parents are carriers, and both pass on a mutated cystic fibrosis transmembrane conductance regulator (CFTR) gene to their offspring (Chalmers, 2021). This mutation causes dysfunction to the CFTR protein where chloride cannot properly move the surface of the cells. Chloride is a component of salt. Without chlorine transitioning properly, it cannot attract water, thus causing mucus, sweat, and digestive fluids to become thick and sticky instead of thin and slippery. Bacteria is trapped, particularly within the lungs, liver, pancreas, digestive, and reproductive systems, causing significant blockage in the airways and infection.

The progressive nature of the disease can be slow and punishing, requiring urgent and frequent medical attention, and at times surgical intervention, such as lung or liver transplants. Over the last several decades, clinical advancements and greater exploration into the molecular nature of the CFTR gene have provided therapeutic improvements to better mitigate the disease (Scotet et al., 2020). This has modified the epidemiology of CF. Historically, individuals born with CF died within 18 months, and now they are living in to their 50s and 60s with self-reports of a decent quality of life (Farrell et al., 2020).

Identification and Diagnosis

CF was recognized apart from celiac disease and termed cystic fibrosis of the pancreas in 1938 (Davis, 2006). The breakdown of the disease was originally thought to be within the mucus glands until a critical discovery was made in 1948. It was observed that individuals with CF had heat prostration and their sweat produced five times the excess amount of sodium and chloride. The identification of CF through sweat tests became more accurate than blood samples, and the utilization of two positive sweat tests is still the most reliable way of diagnosing CF today (Davis). In 1983, it was confirmed via use of sweat ducts that chloride transport and

DOI: 10.4324/9781032703923-21

sodium reabsorption was the basic defect in CF. Through positional cloning, the CFTR gene was discovered in 1989, and now more than 2000 mutations have been identified (Farrell et al. 2020). This discovery has paved the way for the development of specific pharmacological therapies.

If genetic testing is accessible, the diagnosis can be given while the baby is still in utero. With a positive diagnosis, genetic counseling provides psychoeducation, expectations, and a treatment plan (U.S. Department of Health and Human Services | National Heart Lung and Blood Institute, n.d.). However, if genetic testing does not occur, more than half of CF diagnoses come from newborn screenings. As of 2010, every newborn in the United States has a blood test to screen for the CFTR protein (U.S. Department of Health and Human Services | National Heart Lung and Blood Institute). If the test is positive, then a sweat test is performed. High chloride content of between 30–59 mmol/L indicates that additional testing may be required, and greater than or equal to 60 mmol/L points to a diagnosis of CF (North Carolina Newborn Screening Program, 2023). If the diagnosis is missed at birth, most children are eventually diagnosed by the age of 2 based on additional symptoms.

Epidemiology and Prognosis

Globally, 162,428 people are estimated to be living with CF across 94 countries (Scotet et al., 2020). Patient registries are available in approximately 45 countries and used to identify 90% of the estimated diagnosed population. Little is known about lower-income countries due to their lack of registries. It is estimated that 57,076 patients worldwide are undiagnosed.

CF occurs across all races and ethnicities; however, white individuals of north European descent have the highest prevalence. In Europe, the incidence rates average 1/4500 in Western Europe and 1/6000 in Northern and Central Europe (Scotet et al., 2020). Incidence rates are 1/3300 in Canada and 1/4000 in the United States. In larger, more developed countries in South and Central America, such as Argentina and Costa Rica, the average incidence is 1/6100 and 1/15,000 respectively. In Asian and Middle Eastern populations, the incidence rates are widely variable. In Jordan rates are 1/2560, in India 1/10,000–1/100,000, and 1/350,000 in Japan. Minimal data is available for African populations.

In 1938, nearly every individual diagnosed with CF died within the first year of life (McBennett et al., 2022). Since then, therapeutic remedies have become more refined allowing most pediatric patients to be able to transition to adulthood (Farrell et al. 2020). With successful therapeutic advancements being able to specifically target the root genetic makeup of CF, fewer and fewer individuals will be carriers of the gene, moving toward elimination of the disease.

Additionally, an individual's life expectancy can be increased by transplant. The average survival rate of lung transplantation is approximately six years, with a range of between five and ten years (Bos et al., 2020). The survival rate with a liver transplant typically ranges from 5 to 20 years (Mayo Clinic, 2024).

Characteristics, Symptoms, and Treatment

The severity of CF can differ from child to child, even within the same family. Broad characteristics in infants (birth to one year) may include delayed growth and failure to gain weight, meconium causing severe constipation, no bowel movement in the first 24–48 hours following birth, and "salty" skin (Children's Health, n.d.). Children who are one year and older may experience low bone density, male and female infertility, clubbed toes and fingers, and/or pancreatitis.

Symptoms are generally broken down into two categories, respiratory and digestive (Chalmers, 2021). Respiratory symptoms may include thick mucus, persistent cough, reoccurring colds, wheezing, shortness of breath, exercise intolerance, repeated lung infections, bronchitis, pneumonia, inflamed nasal passages, stuffy nose, and chronic sinusitis (Children's Health, n.d.). Digestive symptoms may consist of pale or clay-colored stools that are foul-smelling or greasy, stools that have mucus or float, diarrhea, intestinal gas and blockage, chronic and severe constipation, swollen belly from constipation, rectal prolapse, nausea, loss of appetite, poor weight gain, inflamed pancreas, gallstones, diabetes, and liver disease.

Treatment Team

CF requires specialists who work as part of a multidisciplinary team to give optimal care within their area of expertise. This may consist of a genetic counselor, general physician, pulmonologist, gastroenterologist, cardiothoracic surgeon, abdominal surgeon, registered dietitians, medical assistants, nurses (inpatient/outpatient), nurse practitioners, physical, speech, occupational, and respiratory therapists, psychologists/neuropsychologists, social workers, research coordinators, school administrators, school nurses, and school psychologists.

Medical Course and Procedures

Depending on the timing of diagnosis, treatment planning can begin with genetic counseling (Children's Health, n.d.). When diagnosed as a newborn, monthly progress monitoring takes place until 6 months old. Visits are then extended to every two months until the child is 1 year old. After that, children typically have quarterly visits. Medical procedures may consist of airway clearance therapies, inhalants to relax airways, enzyme therapy, antibiotics and anti-inflammatory drugs, stool softeners, acid-reducing drugs, chest physical therapy (CPT), and surgery.

Due to the progressive nature of this disease, hospital admissions are frequent. An analysis of nationwide admission trends for CF patients from 2003 to 2013 showed an increase from 8328 discharges in 2003 to 12,590 discharges in 2013 (Agrawal et al., 2017). While this trend demonstrates that the pediatric population is transitioning into adulthood and living longer, they are still experiencing significant illnesses that warrant admission throughout the course of the disease (Dickinson & Collaco, 2021).

Pharmacology

The sequencing of the CFTR gene has led to the development of small molecule combination pharmacological therapies targeting the root cause of CF, such as Trikafta, Symdeko/Symkevi, Orkambi, and Kalydeco (Guo et al., 2022). Headaches are the most common side effect of CFTR modulators that school personnel need to consider when designing an intervention program. Children and adolescents may also be prescribed bronchodilators (e.g., albuterol), mucus thinners (i.e., mucolytics) and antibiotics. Access to these medications and treatments during school hours may require accommodation through an Individual Education Plan (IEP).

Psychiatric and Neuropsychological Implications

Psychiatry

Individuals with CF and their family members may need help identifying and learning how to cope with their thoughts and feelings. Flexibility and frequent adjustments have to occur in living with CF. It is important that activities do not revolve around the disease (Cystic Fibrosis Foundation, n. d.). Factors that have been shown to cause a decline in mental health are decreased lung function, lower body mass index, poorer adherence to medical care, worsening health-related quality of life, more frequent hospitalizations, increased healthcare costs, and the required isolation from others with CF (Goldbeck et al., 2014). Rates of depression in children and adolescents averaged 18.7% and 27.2% for adults (Lord et al., 2022). Anxiety prevalence in children and adolescents ages 12–19 was 26% and 28.4% in adults. Caregiver depression rates were 32.8% and 38.4% for anxiety.

Neuropsychology

Pediatric

Information on pediatric populations with CF is scant, with the majority of the literature focusing on neuropsychological testing post-lung transplant. In one study, 11 children with a mean age of 11.5 participated in pre- and post-testing showing improvements for verbal learning, aspects of mood, behavior, and adaptive functioning after transplant. The majority of cognitive domains suggested age-appropriate abilities, with a relative weakness in executive functioning (Gold et al., 2020). Emotional or behavioral difficulties were not endorsed by caregivers.

Adult

The research is limited with adults as well. One study documented 31 CF patients over the age of 17 demonstrating cognitive impairment, as defined by scores being one or more standard deviations from the mean, in areas of attentional deficits (23%), verbal immediate and delayed memory (32%), working memory (61%), and executive functioning (19%) (Maddrey et al., 1998).

These results align with deficits within fronto-striatal circuitry and could be consistent with neurodevelopmental disorders such as attention-deficit/hyperactivity disorder (ADHD). In later years, individuals with CF should be monitored for mild to major neurocognitive disorder (i.e., dementia). Overall, these gaps in the literature warrant further neuropsychological research across the lifespan.

Academic Considerations and Accommodations

What can be difficult about CF is that internally the individual is suffering, but externally, their presentation may appear neurotypical. Students and their families are encouraged to meet with special education staff and school administrators early on to request a 504 Accommodation Plan or the initiation of an IEP under the classification of Other Health Impairment (OHI).

The following accommodations could be considered in an IEP or 504 Plan.

- Alternate education plan to account for frequent absences for medical treatments.
- Reduced requirements and extra time on assignments.
- Homebound services with consistent teachers, Zoom virtual instruction.
- Extra time to eat during lunch, snack throughout the school day, and transition between classes.
- Provide nursing support and a sterile environment for treatments, medications, oxygen, nutritional supplements, and enzymes.
- Drink 6–12 ounces of fluid every 20–30 minutes.
    - Consider sports drinks with carbohydrates and electrolytes.
- Frequent access to the bathroom to account for abdominal pain, foul-smelling gas, or diarrhea, as well as increased fluid intake.

- Ask the class not to draw attention to the student if they pass gas frequently.
- Easy access to water, trashcan, and tissue for coughing.
- Allow the student to clean their hands with alcohol-based hand gel.
- Allow the student to place their head on their desk if fatigued.
- Encourage exercise and mobility to loosen the mucus that clogs the lungs and strengthen the muscles used to breathe.
- To help determine the appropriate level of physical activity, physical therapy, and adaptive PE evaluations may be appropriate.
- Practice the 6-foot distance (2 meters) from others with a cold, flu, or an infection in all settings, especially indoors.
- Encourage everyone to wash their hands by making soap and water and/or alcohol-based hand gel readily available in the classroom.
- Clean all supplies (e.g., pencil sharpener, lab equipment, etc.).
- Avoid sharing personal items, such as straws or eating utensils.
- Encourage students to cover their cough or sneeze. Throw the tissue away immediately, then wash or clean hands. If a tissue is not available, encourage students to cough or sneeze into their inner elbow and away from the individual with CF.
- Allow full-time mask usage.
- Allowance to remain indoors during orange and red ozone days.
- Provide counseling support to aid with coping with CF in the academic setting.
- Provide a peer buddy or social support group to offset isolation.

First-Hand Account of Living with CF

As a healthcare provider, sometimes there is no better way to learn about an issue than to try to immerse yourself in another's lived experience, especially when you cannot fully relate to certain aspects (e.g., race, gender, orientation, etc.). Dr. Wierzchowski invited Ms. Victoria Lopez, a client of four years, and her family to share their personal insights on living with CF.

The Journey of a CF Fighter and their Parents

Victoria was born as a healthy eight-pound baby in 2001, prior to standardized CF diagnostic screening. She had difficulty with weight gain and was treated both inpatient and outpatient for failure to thrive. At approximately eight months old, Victoria weighed 13 pounds and contracted pneumonia during the summer. Victoria's mother was finally referred to a gastroenterologist who immediately brought in a pulmonologist who asked two specific questions: "When you kiss her is she salty?" and "When she poops is she smelly?" The providers conducted a sweat test, and upon positive results, Victoria was admitted and kept in the hospital for six weeks. The original pediatrician had missed the diagnosis because of race. The family identifies as Mexican American, and the predominant race diagnosed with CF is White. The family would eventually meet another Latino family who had a child with CF, but not until Victoria was four years old. This parent would help connect Victoria's mother to a CF community of parents who stayed up to date with information.

All the information that existed on CF around 2002 was handed to Victoria's parents in a blue binder. They were also provided with two phone numbers for parents whose children had been diagnosed with CF. Victoria's mother reported feeling overwhelmed because neither she nor Mr. Lopez had heard of CF. They did not understand any of the diagnostic information being given to them. Victoria's life expectancy in 2002 was five years. The pulmonologist told Victoria's parents to go home, grieve, and feel all the emotions they needed to, because when they returned to the hospital it would be time to be full-time caregivers to a child with CF. Upon discharge, Victoria's mother recounted being terrified to bring her home because she had to learn an extensive medical treatment plan including antibiotic administration, CPT, and enzyme therapy. The only medication that Victoria's mother recalled being prescribed during that time was Xopenex, which was an inhaler to open up the airways.

Within five years, pulmozyme and hypertonic saline had been released and helped with excretion. Victoria was administered several inhalant respiratory medications every two to four hours depending on her breathing. Victoria was one of the first people to trial a CPT vest at a local hospital in Dallas, Texas. The vest inflates like a life jacket and shakes to loosen the mucus in the lungs. She used this device 3–4 times a day. Clinic visits were maintained every two months.

Day care was strongly discouraged so Victoria's mother turned to extended family for support to maintain employment. When Victoria started kindergarten, a 504 Plan was created and consisted of nursing support for enzyme treatments, and prevention from going outside in orange or red ozone layers.

At eight, Victoria was formally diagnosed with asthma, and at nine, with CF-related diabetes (CFRD). At 11, pharmacotherapy moved to intravenous (IV) antibiotic medication because of the increased quantities she had to take. Victoria's mother had to learn how to administer IV treatments so that Victoria could remain an outpatient and attempt to continue school. For a brief period, Victoria was able to do IV antibiotics in the morning prior to school and in the evening when she got home from school. Victoria recalled teachers not accommodating her need to lay her head down due to fatigue. Her lung capacity was at 70%, and she utilized an oxygen concentrator full-time. At age 12 (middle school), Victoria started home bound services where two consistent teachers would provide instruction (e.g., two days/week). Her workload was reduced, and grades were based on a percentage of what she was able to complete. Victoria's mother strongly emphasized consistent communication with the school and always kept them informed of absences. Victoria was in the hospital continuously for either bronchoscopy treatments or chronic staph infections in her lungs that led to respiratory syncytial virus (RSV). Physicians began to discuss future lung transplantation.

At this time, Victoria had her first major surgery for Mediport placement. During surgery, Victoria experienced an asthma attack and was placed on a ventilator for one week. This was a traumatic experience for the family. When Victoria awoke, she did not remember what happened. She had to participate in physical and speech therapy to learn how to walk and talk again. She was discharged after two weeks with instructions to continue in-home physical therapy.

For the next four years, Victoria was in the hospital every two weeks for three to four days at a time. She was participating in treatments to try to salvage her lungs. Victoria's mother would be with her full-time, while continuing to work remotely. Mr. Lopez maintained full-time employment and would care for their other daughter when not at work. They also relied heavily on extended family to help. The family stressed that every evening, including extended family, they would meet to have dinner together at the hospital. In addition, every holiday was spent in the hospital for four years.

At age 15, Victoria met with an advanced pulmonologist and was evaluated for a bilateral lung transplant. Her lung capacity was now 40%. There are a host of criteria that have to be met to qualify for a lung transplant, and while it is ironic, a recipient has to be "sick enough" to be officially listed in the national registry. On Victoria's 16th birthday, she was admitted into the hospital and officially listed for transplant. It was anticipated that she would be in the hospital until she had the transplant; however, she recovered enough to be discharged home on oxygen. Victoria's mother felt helpless and conflicted. With a lung transplant, there is not a living donor, and Victoria's mother wrestled daily with the fact that someone would have to die for her child to live. She reported relying on her faith throughout Victoria's medical journey, even more so during this period that led up to transplant.

After waiting approximately four months, Victoria received a call for the transplant. The family accepted the offer, and after approximately eight hours in surgery, Victoria had a new set of lungs. Victoria was placed on extracorporeal membrane oxygenation (ECMO) for one day because her body was so weak. Despite surgery going well, Victoria reported severe pain upon waking, to the degree that she thought dying would have been less painful. Inpatient recovery was four weeks and she then transitioned to a rehabilitation hospital to enhance breathing, talking, and walking again. In hindsight, Victoria wished that she had been given more preparation and insight as to how painful waking up and learning how to breathe would be.

Victoria is now prescribed 24 medications, and while her inhalants for CF have stopped, they have been replaced with antirejection medications. There can be a misconception that a transplant will cure everything, and the individual will feel brand new, but it is more realistic to conceptualize the process as trading one condition for another. Victoria acknowledged that she underwent transplant for her family. She was able to graduate from high school, has attended some college, and now maintains employment. Victoria started Trikafta in 2022, and that is the only CF medication she is on now besides creon24 for her pancreas, which aids in food digestion. CF is no longer concentrated in her lungs but remains in her pancreas.

Psychological Interventions

Victoria began psychotherapy at age 16 after her transplant. Her treatment plan was multimodal, consisting of psychotherapy and psychotherapeutic medication managed by a psychiatrist. She would attend therapy two times per week after school and psychotherapeutic medication consisted of an anxiolytic, antidepressant, and a mood stabilizer. Victoria shared that her mental health declined substantially after her lung transplant, particularly because of the grueling adjustment to her new lungs.

She transitioned to seeing Dr. Wierzchowski in 2020. Treatment consisted of using an existential/humanistic approach for individual therapy and family systems for family therapy. Dyadic work has included sibling and parent–child sessions at different points over the years. Individual sessions have been maintained consistently once a week for four years. Treatment has focused on concepts such as anxiety, depression, medical traumas, processing death and dying, grief, self-efficacy, self-concept, validation of experience, resilience and overcoming challenges, understanding healthy friendships and social connectedness, healthy coping strategies, communication skills, adaptive functioning, executive functioning strategies, and initiating and maintaining employment. Victoria has also participated in a 12-week intensive outpatient program (4 hours/day), which aided in working through the traumatic nature of living with CF from childhood into adulthood, including transplantation.

From a developmental perspective, Erik Erikson's stages and book *Identity, Youth, and Crisis* (1968), have been helpful in aiding Victoria to move through important developmental milestones at a later chronological age. The psychosocial delays are accounted for by being in "survival mode" and being on the brink of death from CF. The "normal" aspects of childhood and teenage life were simply nonexistent. In a sense, Victoria is healing and picking up where she left off before her health substantially declined.

For many years, Victoria did not enjoy being alive. With the assistance of psychotherapeutic medication and intensive psychotherapy, she is beginning to explore and identify what she finally wants from life. Victoria is allowing herself to assume the confidence to set goals and enjoy life without having to live in fear of being ill all the time. Indeed, she is a fighter.

The Importance of Multidisciplinary Interaction

Victoria's current multidisciplinary team consists of psychiatry, pulmonology, gastroenterology, otolaryngology (ENT), endocrinology, nephrology, urology, neurology, psychology, and chiropractic. Her psychologist is in close contact with psychiatry and pulmonology as she sees Victoria on a weekly basis and can pick up on nuances in physical and psychological health that may be time sensitive. For example, Victoria was in session and fatigued to the point where she could not keep her eyes open. Precautionary COVID-19 testing was recommended. Victoria tested positive and was able to be admitted into the hospital immediately to receive a three-day course of Remdesivir.

Additional Words of Wisdom

Victoria's mother attested to making the most out of every moment because anyone in that situation can go to a dark place (e.g. depression and suicidal). She shared that they would make posters, decorate the room, dress up when possible, use dark humor to cope, and bring a crock pot and cook her favorite food in the hospital room. Victoria added that she is grateful for the resources that exist now to process all the emotions and stressors associated with CF.

Conclusion

Nearing 100 years since CF's identification, the advancements in the treatment of CF have been radical. Currently, those with CF, such as Victoria, have endured a challenging medical and psychological course. These individuals provide us with gratitude and teach us grit and resilience. With the ability to increase the amount of CFTR protein through pharmaco-modulated treatment, carriers of the CF gene will eventually diminish, reducing the progression of the disease all together. Until then, providers are encouraged to play an active role in understanding and accommodating the individual's needs.

Resources

- Cystic Fibrosis Foundation: https://www.cff.org
- Healthcare Professionals: https://www.cfsourcehcp.com
- Everyday CF: https://www.everyday-cf.com/cystic-fibrosis-health
- Empowering families living with CF: https://bluecaboose.org/
- Helping children with life-threatening medical conditions: https://hopekids.org/

References

Agrawal, A., Agarwal, A., Mehta, D., Sikachi, R. R., Du, D., & Wang, J. (2017). Nationwide trends of hospitalizations for cystic fibrosis in the United States from 2003 to 2013. *Intractable & Rare Diseases Research*, 6(3), 191–198. https://doi.org/10.5582/irdr.2017.01043.

Bos, S., Vos, R., Van Raemdonck, D. E., & Verleden, G. M. (2020). Survival in adult lung transplantation: Where are we in 2020? *Current Opinion in Organ Transplantation*, 25(3), 268–273. https://doi: 10.1097/MOT.0000000000000753.

Chalmers, S. (2021). What is cystic fibrosis? A Mayo Clinic expert explains. Retrieved January 30, 2024 from https://www.mayoclinic.org/diseases-conditions/cystic-fibrosis/symptoms-causes/.

Children's Health (n.d.). *Cystic fibrosis (CF) program*. Retrieved February 12, 2024 from https://www.childrens.com/specialties-services/specialty-centers-and-programs/pulmonology/programs-and-services/cystic-fibrosis-program.

Cystic Fibrosis Foundation (n.d.). Therapeutics development network. Retrieved February 8, 2024 from https://www.cff.org/researchers/therapeutics-development-network.

Davis, P. B. (2006). Cystic fibrosis since 1938. *American Journal of Respiratory and Critical Care Medicine*, 173(5), 475–482. https://doi.org/10.1164/rccm.200505-840oe.

Dickinson, K. M. & Collaco, J. M. (2021). Cystic fibrosis. *Pediatrics in Review*, 42 (2), 55–67. https://doi.org/10.1542/pir.2019-0212.

Farrell, P. M., Rock, M. J., & Baker, M. W. (2020). The impact of the CFTR gene discovery on cystic fibrosis diagnosis, counseling, and preventive therapy. *Genes*, 11(4), 401. https://doi.org/10.3390/genes11040401.

Gold, A., Young, J. M., Solomon, M., & Grasemann, H. (2020). Neuropsychological outcomes following pediatric lung transplantation. *Pediatric Pulmonology*, 55(9), 2427–2436. https://doi.org/10.1002/ppul.24915.

Goldbeck, L., Fidika, A., Herle, M., & Quittner, A. (2014). Psychological interventions for individuals with cystic fibrosis and their families. *The Cochrane Database of Systematic Reviews*, 6. https://doi.org/10.1002/14651858.CD003148.pub3.

Guo, J., Garratt, A., & Hill, A. (2022). Worldwide rates of diagnosis and effective treatment for cystic fibrosis. *Journal of Cystic Fibrosis*, 21(3), 456–462. https://doi.org/10.1016/j.jcf.2022.01.009.

Lord, L., McKernon, D., Grzeskowiak, L., Kirsa, S., & Ilomäki, J. (2022). Depression and anxiety prevalence in people with cystic fibrosis and their caregivers: A systematic review and meta-analysis. *Social Psychiatry and Psychiatric Epidemiology*, 58(2), 287–298. https://doi.org/10.1007/s00127-022-02307-w.

Maddrey, M. A., Cullum, C. M., & Prestidge, C. (1998). Neuropsychological dysfunction in adults with cystic fibrosis. *Archives of Clinical Neuropsychology*, 13 (1), 118–119. https://doi.org/10.1093/arclin/13.1.118a.

Mayo Clinic (2024, January 19). *Liver transplant*. Retrieved February 12, 2024 from https://www.mayoclinic.org/tests-procedures/liver-transplant/about/pac-20384842.

McBennett, K. A., Davis, P. B., & Konstan, M. W. (2022). Increasing life expectancy in cystic fibrosis: Advances and challenges. *Pediatric Pulmonology*, 57, S5–S12. https://doi.org/10.1002/ppul.25733.

North Carolina Newborn Screening Program (2023). *Cystic fibrosis (CF) sweat test fact sheet for parents.* Retrieved February 8, 2024 from https://www.ncdhhs.gov/sweattest-handoutpdf.

Scotet, V., L'Hostis, C., & Férec, C. (2020). The changing epidemiology of cystic fibrosis: Incidence, survival and impact of the CFTR gene discovery. *Genes*, 11 (6), 589. https://doi.org/10.3390/genes11060589.

U.S. Department of Health and Human Services | National Heart Lung and Blood Institute (n.d.). *Cystic fibrosis.* Retrieved January 30, 2024 from https://www.nhlbi.nih.gov/health/cystic-fibrosis/diagnosis.

18 Genetic Disorders Impacting Cognition

Grace A. Mucci, Elizabeth Pearce and Shania Hao

Introduction

Approximately 1 in 2000 people are affected by a genetic disorder (Lopes et al., 2018). This translates to about 2% to 5% of all live births. It is estimated that there are over 6000 known genetic disorders, and new ones are being identified every day (OMIM, 2024). Genetic disorders can be caused by a single-gene mutation (inherited or *de Novo*), an autosomal dominant or autosomal recessive inheritance, or can occur through environmental causes. Several of the most common genetic disorders described within this chapter are known to impact cognition.

Down Syndrome/Trisomy 21

Down syndrome (DS) is the most common chromosomal abnormality affecting 1:600 live births with a ratio of 1.3:1 male to females (Centers for Disease Control and Prevention, 2023). DS occurs when a human has a full or partial extra copy of chromosome 21 (Antonarakis et al., 2020). There are several types, with the most common being Trisomy 21 (94% of all DS), where there is a third chromosome 21 in addition to the usual two. The cause of the extra copy of the chromosome is still unknown. Medical comorbidities include congenital heart defects, hematological disorders (primarily leukemia), dermatological conditions, gastrointestinal disorders, respiratory difficulties, hearing and visual disturbances, immune dysfunction, impaired fertility, and obstructive sleep apnea (Ivan & Cromwell, 2014). Psychiatric and behavioral comorbidities include autism spectrum disorder, depression, attention-deficit/hyperactivity disorder, oppositional-defiant behavior, and aggression (Wajuihian, 2016).

Prenatal screenings can estimate the likelihood of a fetus having DS. Screening tests usually involve a blood test and an ultrasound, providing a diagnosis with almost 100% certainty. Diagnostic procedures include chorionic villus sampling (CVS) and amniocentesis. Diagnosis at birth is made using identification of the common physical traits associated with DS. In addition to evaluating physical features, a chromosomal analysis

DOI: 10.4324/9781032703923-22

called a karyotype is done to confirm the diagnosis (Centers for Disease Control and Prevention, 2023.

Common physical features of DS include a flattened face and almond-shaped eyes that slant upwards. Additionally, children with DS may have a short neck, small ears, poor muscle tone, and loose joints. Children may also exhibit tiny white spots on the iris of the eye, as well as a single line across the palm of the hand, referred to as the palmar crease (Centers for Disease Control and Prevention). Neuropsychological correlates of DS include cognitive impairment (mild, moderate, severe, or profound) and early developmental delay (Pulsifer, 2021). Many of the cognitive deficits are expressed over the individual's life, and include language and communication deficits, executive dysfunction, adaptive skill delays, social skills deficits, motor skill delays, and academic difficulties (Grieco et al., 2015; Daunhauer et al., 2020; Krell et al., 2021). In addition to progressive intellectual impairment, individuals with DS also show difficulties with higher order cognitive functions such as verbal working memory, executive dysfunction, and learning (Loveall et al., 2017). Language skills tend to be acquired more slowly and are frequently related to the severity of cognitive functioning deficits, as well as physical characteristics impacting oral motor functioning (Yamauchi et al., 2019).

Turner Syndrome

Turner syndrome (TS) is a sex chromosome aneuploidy characterized by the partial or complete absence of one of the X chromosomes in females. TS can be divided into three types: Monosomy X (45%), Mosaic (44%), and Ring Turner (rarest, de Novo causation). TS is not typically inherited, rather it most often results from a random error during early fetal development. TS is prevalent in 1:2500 live female births. Individuals with TS who still possess some genetic material from the second X chromosome exhibit less of a deficit than those missing the chromosome in its entirety (Norman, 2022).

TS results in a variety of symptoms and individuals can be differentially affected. Physical manifestations include short stature, delayed puberty, ovarian failure, infertility, webbed neck, gonadal dysgenesis (abnormalities of ovaries, testes, and gonads), and lymphatic clearance defects, as well as cardiac conditions (Viuff & Gravholt, 2022). Specific physical traits, such as short stature and ovarian failure, were correlated with the region Xp11.2-p22.1 on the X chromosome (Luo et al., 2022). Individuals with TS are at an increased risk for hearing loss, diabetes, hypertension, aortic abnormalities, dyslipidemia (a metabolic disorder with abnormal lipids or lipoproteins in the blood), higher rates of liver disease, and elevated liver enzymes (Mitsch et al., 2023; Singh et al., 2021).

Although verbal processing appears to be intact, individuals with TS may experience deficits in arithmetic, visuospatial processing, visual memory, visual constructional skills, and visuospatial working memory, similar to a non-verbal learning disorder profile (Park et al., 2023). This may result from reduced functional connectivity during working memory tasks (Zhao et al., 2019). Lower levels of educational success may result from social isolation and poor self-concept (Culen et al., 2017). TS is associated with social-cognitive processing and executive functioning impairments, resulting in difficulties in social competence, social cognition, and self-esteem (Wolstencroft & Skuse, 2019). Thus, individuals with TS are at risk of social skill deficits. Since many with TS are not diagnosed until near the end of adolescence after failure to sexually mature, early diagnosis is crucial to maximize growth, address learning needs, and improve social functioning (Swauger et al., 2021).

Treatment for TS typically includes routine pediatric care with continued monitoring of blood pressure and the cardiovascular systems, as well as growth hormone treatment (Gravholt et al., 2018). Sex steroid treatment, such as daily growth hormone injections and estrogen therapy beginning around age 11–12, is also common (Mitsch et al., 2023). In school, individuals with TS may be eligible under the classification of Other Health Impairment, and will likely be eligible for OT, APE, speech and potentially learning disability support (SLD most commonly in math) services as well as social skills support.

Fragile X Syndrome

Fragile X syndrome (FXS) is an X-linked dominant disorder and is caused by the mutation of the fragile X messenger ribonucleoprotein 1 (FMR1) gene on the X chromosome. The prevalence of Fragile X is 1:4000–5000 males and 1:6000–8000 females. Fragile X is a broad-spectrum disorder, meaning it involves learning disabilities, emotional problems, and intellectual deficits. About 12% of those diagnosed have at least one seizure, with a higher rate of seizures in males (13.7%) than females (6.2%) (Berry-Kravis et al., 2021).

Males with FXS have a higher incidence of ID compared to females. The majority of males with FXS exhibit ASD features, including hand biting, hand flapping, perseverative speech, and self-stimulating behaviors (Bartholomay et al., 2019). Other symptoms include speech delays, anxiety, and hyperactive behavior (Ezell et al., 2019). Males tend to get diagnosed earlier with FXS because females with FXS usually exhibit less severe cognitive impairment and milder phenotypes leading to later diagnoses. Females tend to be less affected by FXS because they have two X chromosomes (Bartholomay et al.).

Those with FXS tend to have strengths in verbal memory, including verbal ability and long-term memory for verbal information (Huddleston et al., 2014). Females with average IQ, but with the full mutation usually demonstrate learning disabilities, attentional and organizational problems, executive dysfunction, and math problems (Bartholomay et al., 2019).

Additional neuropsychological implications include a short attention span, impulsivity, hyperactivity, and sensory sensitivities (Razak et al., 2020). Those with FXS are easily hyper-aroused and often demonstrate tantrums, aggressiveness, difficulties with transitions, and perseverations (Crawford et al., 2020). Individuals with FXS also show delayed development of nonverbal communication and use of gestures, body language, and facial expressions (Fielding-Gebhardt et al., 2020).

Noonan Syndrome

Noonan syndrome (NS) is an autosomal dominant disorder. Although several genes have been linked to NS, more than half of NS cases are caused by a mutation in the PTPN11 gene. Symptoms of NS include multiple congenital anomalies with variable expressivity across individuals, as well as heterogenous phenotypic manifestations that can change with age. NS is the most common genetic disorder in children with congenital heart disease. With a prevalence of 1:100–1:2500 births, those diagnosed with NS show highly variable neurocognitive and behavioral outcomes (Pierpont, 2016).

Physical characteristics include short stature, craniofacial anomalies, a broad, high forehead, and hypertelorism (increased distance between two body parts, in NS it is often seen in the distance between eyes). In addition, characteristics may be evidenced such as low-set posteriorly rotated ears with a thick helix, high-arched eyebrows, short neck with excess nuchal skin, epicanthal folds, downward-slanting palpebral fissures, deeply grooved philtrum, ptosis (drooping of the upper eyelid), low posterior hairline, high arched palate, and an abnormally small jaw (micrognathia) (Pierpont, 2016). NS is also associated with congenital heart defects, including pulmonary valve stenosis, hypertrophic obstructive cardiomyopathy, atrial and ventricular septal defects, and persistent ductus arteriosus (Pierpont & Digilio, 2018).

Research has demonstrated that neurocognitive functioning varies depending upon the genetic phenotype (Pierpont, 2016). Intellectual functioning tends to range from mild intellectual deficiency to superior abilities, however the majority display average to mildly below average intelligence. Attention and related functions are the most common neuropsychological finding, which suggests possible frontal lobe-subcortical circuitry problems (Pierpont). Additional neuropsychological implications include visuo-constructional, motor, visual perceptual and sensory deficits. Delays in language acquisition and articulation are common. Individuals with NS are also often described as "clumsy," poor in sports, and as having motor development delays.

Treatment for NS is usually patient specific since complications are specific to each individual. In individuals with congenital heart defects, patients can be treated with certain medications or surgical interventions.

Early interventions such as speech therapy, physical therapy, and other social and medical services have also been used to treat NS.

Klinefelter Syndrome

Klinefelter syndrome (KS) (47, XXY) is a non-inherited genetic disorder and occurs when one extra X chromosome is present, resulting in an XXY presentation affecting 1:500–1:1000 males. Many males with KS go undiagnosed. Common features of KS include tall height, long legs, and short torso. Many men with KS are infertile and may exhibit smaller testes (hypogonadism) and penis, breast growth, less facial and body hair, reduced muscle tone, narrower shoulders and wider hips, weaker bones, decreased sexual interest, and lower energy. Those with KS are at an increased risk of metabolic syndrome and osteoporosis (Gravholt et al., 2018).

Klinefelter syndrome can result in a wide range of intellectual abilities, with individuals demonstrating on average IQ 10–15 points lower than controls. Language development is often delayed, with verbal deficits most common, and mixed results can be seen with executive functions (Gravholt et al., 2018). Psychiatric comorbidities, such as depression, anxiety, ASD, ADHD, and schizophrenia, and social skill deficits are common and often untreated. Early identification and hormonal therapy may help offset these difficulties (Ballegeer et al., 2018). Lifelong testosterone replacement therapy (TRT) initiated at the onset of puberty can help with the development of normal pubertal growth. Mastectomies have been performed on males with enlarged breasts. Fertility treatment, speech and physical therapy, counseling, and educational support are often employed (Gravholt et al.).

Stickler Syndrome

Stickler syndrome (SS) refers to a group of disorders of connective tissue, which can affect multiple organ systems. Mutations in SS appear to be associated with the genes responsible for collagen formation needed for connective tissues throughout the body (Boothe et al., 2020). There are several types:

- Type I: mutations over the entire COL2A1 gene on chromosome 12q13.11; accounts for about 80% of all cases; autosomal dominant inheritance.
- Type II: mutations of the COL11A1 gene on chromosome 1p21; autosomal dominant inheritance.
- Type III: mutations of the COL11A2 gene on chromosome 6p21.3; affects the joints and hearing without involving the eyes; autosomal dominant inheritance.
- Types IV, V, and VI are increasingly rare: autosomal recessive inheritance.

The clinical features of SS are typically variable, even among those affected within the same family, but may include abnormal facial features (i.e., flattened facial structure and nasal bridge; small jaw, cleft palate); eye abnormalities, myopia, and cataracts; sensorineural hearing loss; joint problems; and cardiac conditions (50% experience mitral valve prolapse). While intelligence is often average, some may develop learning difficulties. Early identification of SS is important to allow for prompt surveillance and treatment of abnormalities such as skeletal malformations and retinal detachment.

Angelman Syndrome

Angelman syndrome (AS) primarily affects the nervous system and causes severe developmental delay and learning disabilities. The prevalence rate is equal among males and females, with 1:12,000–20,000 live births. Angelman syndrome results from the loss of function of the UBe3A gene in the 15th maternal chromosome, which provides instructions for making a protein that is vital for how the nervous system develops and functions. Infants with AS appear normal at birth, but often have feeding problems in the first months of life and show significant speech impairment and developmental delays before the age of 3 (Margolis et al., 2015).

Seizures are a primary feature of AS with >80% developing seizures within the first three years. Physically, infants may exhibit microcephaly (abnormally small head), flatness in the back of the head, as well as tongue thrusting. Physical characteristics also include light hair, skin and eye color, and scoliosis. Those with AS may also exhibit hand flapping and arms uplifted while walking, hypotonia, ataxia, hyperactivity, and sleep problems (Margolis et al., 2015).

Neuropsychological implications of AS include developmental delay, ID, and severe speech impairment. Another common characteristic includes having a happy demeanor with frequent laughter, which resulted in AS historically being referred to as "happy puppet" syndrome. Treatment of AS revolves around appropriate therapies for physical and neurological problems. Patients may require treatment with physiotherapy or bracing to resolve scoliosis. Many problem behaviors of AS can be improved with consistency of treatment, with help from a behavioral therapist if necessary (Margolis et al., 2015).

CHARGE Syndrome

CHARGE syndrome is a rare disorder that affects multiple organ systems during early fetal development, occurring in 1:10,000–15,000 live births (de Geus et al., 2017) and affects males and females equally. The most common features include coloboma (abnormality of eye), cranial nerve and heart defects, blocked nasal passages, retardation of growth and development, hypogonadotropic hypogonadism, ear abnormalities, and sensory hearing loss. Many cases are initially misdiagnosed or undiagnosed, especially in children with less obvious symptoms or fewer problems. The cause of CHARGE is usually a change in the CHD7 gene, or in more rare cases, changes in the region of chromosome 8q12.2 where the CHD7 gene is located.

Diagnosis of CHARGE syndrome is usually made by a geneticist based on four criteria: coloboma, cranial nerve abnormalities, choanal atresia (nasal formation abnormalities), and CHARGE ears (unusual external ears) (Usman & Sur, 2023). Characteristic facial features include asymmetric facial nerve palsy, cleft lip or palate, esophageal atresia, or tracheoesophageal fistula. Many children with CHARGE also develop scoliosis. Symptoms can vary significantly from one child to another.

Many of the structural abnormalities prevalent in CHARGE patients can be corrected through surgery. Interventions may be required for factors such as feeding problems and speech–language deficits. For treatment of sleep disturbances, usual treatments for obstructive sleep apnea can reduce symptoms. Cochlear implants may be used to treat hearing deficits. Most children with CHARGE are developmentally delayed. This is primarily due to sensory deficits or frequent illnesses and hospitalizations during development (Dijk et al., 2019). However, children with CHARGE have been shown to be able to catch up later in childhood if they present with average intellectual abilities. Common behaviors of the disorder include autistic-like behaviors such as hand waving or head banging (Hartshorne et al., 2017). Given the complexities of CHARGE syndrome, careful management and coordinated care among specialists provides the best chance for better outcomes (Usman & Sur, 2023).

Williams Syndrome

Williams syndrome (WS) occurs through a deletion of a portion of the long arm of Chromosome 7 that contains the elastin gene (ELN). The prevalence of WS is 1:7500–20,000 live births and can be maternal or paternal in origin. There are many medical complications in WS, including ocular/visual and ear/auditory deficits. Additional problems encompass respiratory, cardiovascular, gastrointestinal, renal, growth, metabolism, hypercalcemia, hernias, hypotonia, early puberty, hoarse voice, and musculoskeletal complications. It is common to experience a delay in meeting developmental milestones, such as speech, language, and communication; delays in fine and gross motor skills; as well as excessive worrying and severe anxiety (Morris & Mervis, 2021).

Neuropsychological correlates of WS include language difficulties, but usually with strengths in auditory rote memory. Those with WS often exhibit better performance on verbal than visuospatial construction measures. Patients may demonstrate deficits with attention, social, and thought problems. They may also resemble the non-verbal learning disorder phenotype, and many have intellectual disability. Treatment for WS typically involves managing specific symptoms, such as hypertension and anxiety, with medications and other therapies (Kozel et al., 2021).

Implications for Assessment and Intervention

Pediatric psychologists are unlikely to be assessing and diagnosing the genetic disorder itself, as that is typically the purview of physicians and geneticists. However, practitioners do commonly assess children and adolescents with genetic disorders for difficulties in cognition/intellectual functioning, academic skills, behavior or pathology, social-emotional skills, and adaptive functioning. It is for this reason pediatric practitioners need to be familiar with various genetic disorders.

Assessments with individuals presenting with a genetic disorder should be comprehensive, may be more elaborate than a typical psychoeducational assessment, and likely to require neuropsychological assessment. These children might need significant assessment for differential diagnosis (i.e., intellectual disorder [ID] vs. autism, or some other combination). They may be recommended for restrictive educational placements (e.g., functional life skills classrooms) and frequently require justifications for a variety of supports and services (e.g., OT, PT, APE, SL therapy, guardianship, job placement, supervised living, etc.). Therefore, when conducting assessment with these children, first gather information regarding the disorder to determine what areas of functioning are likely to be impacted and complete a comprehensive background and developmental history to gain information for each specific child. The chosen testing battery should include tests that evaluate typical or known areas of dysfunction for that genetic disorder and the constellation of symptoms and behaviors being expressed by the individual. For example, when evaluating a child with TS, it will be important to evaluate visuospatial processing and mathematics abilities. It is also important to collect data from a variety of sources and perspectives, such as parents, caregivers, teachers, and when possible, the child themselves. Gathering information from medical professionals and previous psychoeducational assessment would also be beneficial.

When selecting measures, ensure that they have good psychometric properties and if possible, have normative data that is applicable to the disorder. The clinician may need to use intellectual and language tasks that have lower floors and tasks that do not require a motor response. For example, using a test such as the Stanford-Binet (SB-5) (Roid, 2003) that has extended floors and ceilings may provide a more accurate measure of significantly below average cognitive functioning than a more commonly utilized measure such as the Wechsler Scales (Sansone et al., 2014; Wechsler, 2014). Behavioral ratings and emotional measures may or may not be applicable to the child as they may not yield appropriate findings and reflect the phenotype of the disorder rather than the child's true experiences.

Children with genetic disorders impacting intellectual functioning, academic functioning, language, and adaptive functioning are typically eligible for early intervention services (birth to 3) and special education services (pre-K to age 21) under IDEIA. Those not meeting criteria for IDEIA are eligible for all of the same services under Section 504 of the Rehabilitation Act of 1973. Educational interventions often focus on basic academic skills and functional life skills such as attempting to improve daily-life skills, dressing, sleep hygiene, and acquiring the skills needed for independence (Krell et al., 2021). Children with these genetic conditions frequently require services for speech fluency and language development. The associations between difficulties with speech fluency and the level of language functioning should be taken into consideration when planning both assessment and treatment (Næss et al., 2021). Vision and hearing challenges are also common with this population and will need to be addressed in the assessment and academic settings as well as considered in intervention planning (Wajuihian, 2016). Health and wellness are a critical component when addressing the needs of children with these genetic disorders and it may be necessary to consider developing an Education Health Care Plan (EHCP), Individualized Health Care Plan (IHP), or an Emergency Procedures Plan (EPP) into the IEP. For instance, for children with DS, structured plans for physical activity during early childhood may decrease the risk of cardiovascular disease, heart problems, and obesity (Donaldson & Gault, 2021). Additionally, many of these children and adolescents take a variety of medications and those side effects should be considered in both assessment and intervention. Transition to adult services is often also a necessary component for children living with these genetic conditions. Assessment and intervention may need to consider job training and support services, independent and supervised living options, genetic and sexual health counseling, as well as legal guardianship.

Conclusion

Genetic disorders are caused by inherited and random mutations on genes, affecting growth and development. It should be emphasized that genetic disorders may manifest or "express" themselves in diverse ways, ranging from minor to major impact on a child's developmental trajectory. While it is not possible to cover all genetic disorders, particularly since some are quite rare, this chapter briefly reviewed those disorders that are more commonly known to affect cognition. Given the heterogeneity of these disorders, it is incumbent upon those who work with these youth to identify each individual's cognitive strengths and weaknesses, vulnerabilities, and need for ongoing intervention and surveillance in order to help those affected live their best lives possible.

Resources

Genetic and Rare Diseases Information Center: https://rarediseases.info.nih.gov

OMIM: https://omim.org/

Orphanet: https://www.orpha.net/consor/cgi-bin/index.php

GeneReviews: https://www.ncbi.nlm.nih.gov/books/NBK1116/

Clinical Genomic Database: https://research.nhgri.nih.gov/CGD/search/

UpToDate: https://www.uptodate.com/contents/search

ClinGen Actionability Knowledge Repository: https://actionability.clinicalgenome.org/ac/

References

Antonarakis, S. E., Skotko, B. G., Rafii, M. S., Strydom, A., Pape, S. E., Bianchi, D. W., Sherman, S. L., & Reeves, R. H. (2020). Down syndrome. *Nature Reviews Disease Primers*, 6(1), 9. https://www.nature.com/articles/s41572-019-0143-7.

Bartholomay, K. L., Lee, C. H., Bruno, J. L., Lightbody, A. A., & Reiss, A. L. (2019). Closing the gender gap in Fragile X syndrome: Review on females with FXS and preliminary research findings. *Brain Sciences*, 9(1), 11. https://doi.org/10.3390/brainsci9010011.

Ballegeer, R., Demyttenaere, K., & Simons, W. (2018). The Klinefelter syndrome: A systematic review of secondary psychiatric comorbidities. *Tijdschrift Voor Psychiatrie*, 60(9), 606–618. https://europepmc.org/article/med/30215449.

Berry-Kravis, E., Filipink, R. A., Frye, R. E., Golla, S., Morris, S. M., Andrews, H., Choo, T. H., Kaufmann, W. E., & FORWARD Consortium (2021). Seizures in Fragile X syndrome: Associations and longitudinal analysis of a large clinic-based cohort. *Frontiers in Pediatrics*, 9, 736255. https://doi.org/10.3389/fped.2021.736255.

Boothe, M., Morris, R., & Robin, N. (2020). Stickler syndrome: a review of clinical manifestations and the genetics evaluation. *Journal of Personalized Medicine*, 10 (3), 105. https://doi.org/10.3390/jpm10030105.

Centers for Disease Control and Prevention (2023). *Down syndrome*. Retrieved February 16, 2024, from https://www.cdc.gov/ncbddd/birthdefects/downsyndrome.htm.

Crawford, H., Abbeduto, L., Hall, S. S., Hardiman, R., Hessl, D., Roberts, J. E., Scerif, G., Stanfield, A, C, Turkm J., & Oliver, C. (2020). Fragile X syndrome: An overview of cause, characteristics, assessment, and management. *Paediatrics and Child Health*, 30(11), 400–403. https://doi.org/10.1016/j.paed.2020.08.007.

Culen, C., Ertl, D. A., Schubert, K., Bartha-Doering, L., & Haeusler, G. (2017). Care of girls and women with Turner syndrome: Beyond growth and hormones. *Endocrine Connections*, 6(4), R39–R51. https://doi.org/10.1530/EC-17-0036.

Daunhauer, L. A., Will, E., Schworer, E., & Fidler, D. J. (2020). Young students with Down syndrome: Early longitudinal academic achievement and neuropsychological predictors. *Journal of Intellectual & Developmental Disability*, 45 (3), 211–221. https://doi.org/10.3109/13668250.2020.1726016.

de Geus, C. M., Free, R. H., Verbist, B. M., Sival, D. A., Blake, K. D., Meiners, L. C., & van Ravenswaaij-Arts, C. M. A. (2017). Guidelines in CHARGE syndrome and the missing link: Cranial imaging. *American Journal of Medical Genetics. Part C, Seminars in Medical Genetics*, 175(4), 450–464. https://doi.org/10.1002/ajmg.c.31593.

Dijk, D. R., Bocca, G., & van Ravenswaaij-Arts, C. M. (2019). Growth in CHARGE syndrome: Optimizing care with a multidisciplinary approach. *Journal of Multidisciplinary Healthcare*, 12, 607–620. https://doi.org/10.2147/JMDH.S175713.

Donaldson, M., & Gault, E. J. (2021). Promoting healthy behavior in Turner syndrome—the challenge begins in childhood. *Acta Paediatrica*, 110(8), 2298–2300. https://doi.org/10.1111/apa.15906.

Ezell, J., Hogan, A., Fairchild, A., Hills, K., Klusek, J., Abbeduto, L., & Roberts, J. (2019). Prevalence and predictors of anxiety disorders in adolescent and adult males with autism spectrum disorder and fragile X syndrome. *Journal of Autism and Developmental Disorders*, 49(3), 1131–1141. https://doi.org/10.1007/s10803-018-3804-6.

Fielding-Gebhardt, H., Warren, S. F., & Brady, N. C. (2020). Developmental trajectory of communication repair in children with fragile X syndrome. *Autism & Developmental Language Impairments*, 5, 2396941520909014. https://doi.org/10.1177/2396941520909090.

Gravholt, C. H., Chang, S., Wallentin, M., Fedder, J., Moore, P., & Skakkebæk, A. (2018). Klinefelter syndrome: Integrating genetics, neuropsychology, and endocrinology. *Endocrine Reviews*, 39(4), 389–423. https://doi.org/10.1210/er.2017-00212.

Grieco, J., Pulsifer, M., Seligsohn, K., Skotko, B., & Schwartz, A. (2015). Down syndrome: Cognitive and behavioral functioning across the lifespan. *American Journal of Medical Genetics Part C: Seminars in Medical Genetics*, 169(2), 135–149. https://doi.org/10.1002/ajmg.c.31439.

Hartshorne, T. S., Stratton, K. K., Brown, D., Madhavan-Brown, S., & Schmittel, M. C. (2017). Behavior in CHARGE syndrome. *American Journal of Medical Genetics. Part C, Seminars in Medical Genetics*, 175(4), 431–438. https://doi.org/10.1002/ajmg.c.31588.

Huddleston, L. B., Visootsak, J., & Sherman, S. L. (2014). Cognitive aspects of fragile X syndrome. Wiley interdisciplinary reviews. *Cognitive Science*, 5(4), 501–508. https://doi.org/10.1002/wcs.1296.

Ivan, D. L. & Cromwell, P. (2014). Clinical practice guidelines for management of children with Down syndrome: Part II. *Journal of Pediatric Health Care, 28*(3), 280–284. doi:10.1016/j.pedhc.2013.05.003.

Kozel, B. A., Barak, B., Kim, C. A., Mervis, C. B., Osborne, L. R., Porter, M., & Pober, B. R. (2021). Williams syndrome. *Nature Reviews Disease Primers*, 7(1), 42. https://www.nature.com/articles/s41572-021-00276-z.

Krell, K., Haugen, K., Torres, A., & Santoro, S. L. (2021). Description of daily living skills and independence: A cohort from a multidisciplinary Down syndrome clinic. *Brain Sciences*, 11(8), 1012. DOI: https://doi.org/10.3390/brainsci11081012.

Lopes, M. T., Koch, V. H., Sarrubbi-Junior, V., Gallo, P. R., & Carneiro-Sampaio, M. (2018). Difficulties in the diagnosis and treatment of rare diseases according to the perceptions of patients, relatives, and health care professionals. *Clinics*, 73, e68. https://doi.org/10.6061/clinics/2018/e68.

Loveall, S. J., Conners, F. A., Tungate, A. S., Hahn, L. J., & Osso, T. D. (2017). A cross-sectional analysis of executive function in Down syndrome from 2 to 35 years. *Journal of Intellectual Disability Research*, 61(9), 877–887. https://doi.org/10.1111/jir.12396.

Luo, H., Ni, L., Yang, Y. Q., Zhang, X. M., Huang, H., Tan, S., Ling, C., Liang, L., Wang, L., Dan, T., Zhou, S. X., & Yang, C. (2022). Characterization of a rare mosaic X-ring chromosome in a patient with Turner syndrome. *Molecular Cytogenetics*, 15(1), 15. https://link.springer.com/article/10.1186/s13039-022-00593-2.

Margolis, S. S., Sell, G. L., Zbinden, M. A., & Bird, L. M. (2015). Angelman syndrome. *Neurotherapeutics*, 12(3), 641–650. https://doi.org/10.1007/s13311-015-0361-y.

Mitsch, C., Alexandrou, E., Norris, A. W., & Pinnaro, C. T. (2023). Hyperglycemia in Turner syndrome: Impact, mechanisms, and areas for future research. *Frontiers in Endocrinology*, 14, 1116889. https://doi.org/10.3389/fendo.2023.1116889.

Morris, C. A. & Mervis, C. B. (2021). Williams syndrome. *Cassidy and Allanson's Management of Genetic Syndromes*, 1021–1038. https://doi.org/10.1002/9781119432692.ch63.

Næss, K. B., Nygaard, E., Hofslundsengen, H., & Yaruss, J. S. (2021). The association between difficulties with speech fluency and language skills in a national age cohort of children with down syndrome. *Brain Sciences*, 11(6), 704. https://doi.org/10.3390/brainsci11060704.

Norman, M. Z. (2022). Turner syndrome: What school psychologists should know. *Communique*, 51(3), 4–6.

OMIM (2024). *Gene Map Statistics*. Retrieved February 16, 2024, from www.omim.org.

Park, S. Y., Kim, S. J., Lee, M., Lee, H. I., Kwon, A., Suh, J., Song, K., Chae, H. W., Joo, B., & Kim, H. S. (2023). Neurocognitive and psychosocial profiles of children with Turner syndrome. *Annals of Pediatric Endocrinology & Metabolism*, 28(4), 258–266. doi:10.6065/apem.2244222.111.

Pierpont, E. I. (2016). Neuropsychological functioning in individuals with Noonan syndrome: A systematic literature review with educational and treatment recommendations. *Journal of Pediatric Neuropsychology*, 2, 14–33. https://doi.org/10.1007/s40817-015-0005-5.

Pierpont, M. E. & Digilio, M. C. (2018). Cardiovascular disease in Noonan syndrome. *Current Opinion in Pediatrics*, 30(5), 601–608. doi:10.1097/MOP.0000000000000669.

Pulsifer M. (2021). Down syndrome: Neuropsychological phenotype across the lifespan. *Brain Sciences*, 11(11), 1380. https://doi.org/10.3390/brainsci11111380.

Razak, K. A., Dominick, K. C., & Erickson, C. A. (2020). Developmental studies in fragile X syndrome. *Journal of Neurodevelopmental Disorders*, 12, 1–15. https://doi.org/10.1186/s11689-020-09310-9.

Roid, G. H. (2003). *Stanford-Binet Intelligence Scales* (5th ed., SB:V). Itasca, IL: Riverside Publishing.

Sansone, S. M., Schneider, A., Bickel, E., Berry-Kravis, E., Prescott, C., & Hessl, D. (2014). Improving IQ measurement in intellectual disabilities using true deviation from population norms. *Journal of Neurodevelopmental Disorders*, 6 (1), 16. DOI: https://link.springer.com/article/10.1186/1866-1955-6-16.

Singh, I., Noel, G., Barker, J. M., Chatfield, K. C., Khanna, A. D., Nokoff, N., & Davis, S. M. (2021). Hepatic abnormalities in youth with Turner Syndrome. *Journal of the Endocrine Society*, 5(Supplement_1), A798–A799. https://doi.org/10.1111/liv.15358.

Swauger, S., Backeljauw, P., Hornung, L., Shafer, J., Casnellie, L., & Gutmark-Little, I. (2021). Age at, and indication for diagnosis of Turner syndrome in the pediatric population. *American Journal of Medical Genetics. Part A*, 185(11), 3411–3417. https://doi.org/10.1002/ajmg.a.62459.

Usman, N., & Sur, M. (2023). CHARGE syndrome. In *StatPearls* [Internet]. StatPearls Publishing. doi: https://www.ncbi.nlm.nih.gov/books/NBK559199/.

Viuff, M. & Gravholt, C. H. (2022). Turner syndrome and fertility. *Annales d'endocrinologie*, 83(4), 244–249. https://doi.org/10.1016/j.ando.2022.06.001.

Wajuihian, S. O. (2016). Down syndrome: An overview. *African Vision and Eye Health*, 75(1), 1–6. https://hdl.handle.net/10520/EJC194996.

Wechsler, D. (2014). *Wechsler Intelligence Scale for Children*, (5th ed., WISC-V). Pearson.

Wolstencroft, J. & Skuse, D. (2019). Social skills and relationships in Turner syndrome. *Current Opinion in Psychiatry*, 32(2), 85–91. doi:10.1097/YCO.0000000000000472.

Yamauchi, Y., Aoki, S., Koike, J., Hanzawa, N., & Hashimoto, K. (2019). Motor and cognitive development of children with Down syndrome: The effect of acquisition of walking skills on their cognitive and language abilities. *Brain and Development*, 41(4), 320–326. https://doi.org/10.1016/j.braindev.2018.11.008.

Zhao, C., Yang, L., Xie, S., Zhang, Z., Pan, H., & Gong, G. (2019). Hemispheric module-specific influence of the X chromosome on white matter connectivity: Evidence from girls with Turner syndrome. *Cerebral Cortex*, 29(11), 4580–4594. https://doi.org/10.1093/cercor/bhy335.

19 Deletion Disorders

Destiny Orantes, Ashley Schiros and Kevin M. Antshel

Introduction

Deletion disorders are syndromes that result from deletion of genetic material on part of a chromosome. These syndromes often include congenital anomalies, distinctive facial dysmorphisms, physical and/or intellectual disability, and other associated symptoms that are often specific to the deleted genetic material. This chapter provides an overview of five more common deletion disorders and discusses methods of diagnosing and treating deletion disorders.

Cri-Du-Chat Syndrome

Cri-du-chat syndrome (CdCS) was identified in 1963 by Lejeune and colleagues. CdCS was named in reference to the characteristic high-pitch cry, which was likened to the sound of a meowing cat (Rodríguez-Caballero et al., 2010). This characteristic "cat-like" cry is thought to result from a small, narrow, diamond-shaped larynx and small, hypotonic epiglottis. CdCS incidence ranges from 1:15,000 to 1:50,000 infants (Cerruti Mainardi, 2006) and occurs more frequently in boys (3:1). The main clinical features of CdCS include a high-pitched monochromatic cry, severe psychomotor and intellectual delays, broad nasal bridge, microcephaly (small head), monolid eyes (one eye fold instead of two), micrognathia (underdeveloped lower jaw), and abnormal dermatoglyphics (ridge patterns on the skin, as with fingerprints). Low birth weight, round face, hypertelorism (wider than typical distance between the eyes), and down-turned corners of the mouth occur in over 80% of children with CdCS. Co-occurring health conditions include myopia, cataracts, scoliosis, flat foot, bone deformity wherein the distal tibia is turned inward toward the body, hernia, and abdominal separation.

CdCS is a genetic disorder that results from a deletion on the short arm (p) of chromosome 5. Most often CdCS results from *de novo* deletion. Larger deletions are associated with a more severe presentation and cognitive impairments. Approximately 10% of CdCS cases occur from an

DOI: 10.4324/9781032703923-23

inherited chromosomal translocation, wherein a balance translocation becomes unbalanced in the next generation, resulting in genetic material loss (Cerruti Mainardi). CdCS from an unbalanced translocation results in a more severe clinical profile.

Neonatal presentation of CdCS includes asphyxia, impaired suction, cyanotic cries, and hypotonia. During the first year of life, psychomotor delays become evident. Growth and development delays during the first two years of life are often due to feeding difficulties (e.g., impaired ability to swallow, reflux, weak suction). As the child ages, hypotonia is replaced with hypertonia, and microcephaly becomes more apparent. Orofacial abnormalities are common with 50% of children with CdCS having a high palate and 75% presenting with a small mandible, teeth misalignment, enamel hypoplasia, and poor oral hygiene (Rodríguez-Caballero et al., 2010).

Children with CdCS experience significant speech delays and often have stronger receptive language and comprehension skills with more impaired expressive language abilities. Approximately 50% of children with CdCS experience hyperactivity (Cerruti Mainardi, 2006). Inattention, aggression, stereotyped movement disorder, and self-injurious behaviors are also common in children with CdCS (Sigafoos, O'Reilly, & Lancioni, 2009) Self-injurious behavior in CdCS often consists of hitting the head against objects or body parts and self-biting.

Wolf-Hirschhorn Syndrome

Wolf-Hirschhorn syndrome was first identified in the 1960s. HL (1961) and Hirschhorn et al. (1965) were the first to describe WHS in cases of infants with low birth weight, seizures, delayed physical development, and a distinctive craniofacial structure. This craniofacial structure is characterized by microcephaly, prominent forehead, wide nose bridge, and hypertelorism—historically referred to as a "Greek warrior helmet." Several hundred cases of WHS have been extensively detailed in medical and scientific literature; however, the current prevalence estimate of WHS in the United Stated is fewer than 1:50,000 (Shannon et al., 2001).

The presentation of WHS is variable with features ranging in frequency and severity. Many of the most common features of WHS are related to craniofacial characteristics: short philtrum, distinctive downturned corners of mouth, microcephaly, hypodontia (missing adult teeth), micrognathia, high hairline and prominent forehead, hypertelorism and a wide nasal bridge (Paradowska-Stolarz, 2014). Pervasive delays in growth are frequent in WHS and include fetal weight below the tenth percentile, low birth weight, and continued delays in physical development, growth, and hypotonia throughout childhood. Infants and children with WHS frequently exhibit global delays in meeting physical, academic, and social-emotional milestones. Severe intellectual disability, cerebellar ataxia (e.g., lack of coordination, difficulty judging distances), and epilepsy also occur with high frequency in WHS. Congenital heart defects, renal issues, scoliosis, and skeletal growth delays are features of WHS that occur with moderate frequency.

Symptoms of WHS first occur prenatally. Prenatal growth deficiencies are the most common concern leading to early identification of WHS, with facial dysmorphism and central nervous system anomalies regularly identified in utero (Tang et al., 2023). Epilepsy is a foremost concern, occurring in over 90% of WHS cases. The peak incidence of epilepsy in WHS is 6–12 months of age, with tonic-clonic seizures occurring in 70% of individuals and 50% of infants experiencing status epilepticus in the first years of life (Paprocka et al., 2022). Symptoms, such as status epilepticus and severe growth deficits can be fatal, and approximately 35% of individuals who have WHS die within the first two years of life (Shannon et al., 2001). Individuals with less severe clinical presentations often live into adulthood; however, the course of WHS is chronic with persistent adaptive and cognitive deficits.

WHS is caused by a heterozygous deletion occurring in the terminal section of chromosome 4p. Specifically the 4p16.3 region known as the Wolf-Hirschhorn region, and deletion size in this region can range from less than 2Mb up to 30Mb. Many genes are found in this region, although the *WHSC1* is the only gene that is deleted in every known case of WHS (Bergemann, Cole, & Hirschhorn, 2005). Although WHS is usually due to a partial deletion in 4p16.3, translocations have also been linked to the disorder. Genetic deletions or translocations that result in WHS can be either *de novo* or inherited. The size of deletion in 4p is related to WHS phenotype (Nevado et al., 2020). A deletion of less than 3.5Mb is considered small and associated with a milder phenotype (e.g., facial characteristics, growth delay, mild intellectual disability, seizures). Large deletions occur more frequently and are defined as a deletion of 5–18Mb. A large deletion is associated with more extensive structural malformations of facial, skeletal, and organ structure, severe growth delay, low muscle tone, and more significant neurodevelopmental impairment. The most severe phenotype occurs from a very large deletion, which exceeds 22–25 Mb.

22q11.2 Deletion Syndrome

The syndrome resulting from the deletion of chromosome 22q11.2, known as 22q11.2 deletion syndrome (22q11.2 DS), DiGeorge syndrome (DGS), or velocardiofacial syndrome (VCFS), is associated with hypoparathyroidism, hypocalcemia, thymic hypoplasia, heart defects associated with malformation of the outflow tract of the heart, facial dysmorphisms, and cleft palate. The syndrome exhibits a complex phenotype with considerable variability, encompassing craniofacial, neurological, cognitive, behavioral, ocular, speech and hearing, musculoskeletal, and internal organ manifestations, as well as airway, gastrointestinal, or renal abnormalities

(Kobrynski & Sullivan, 2007). The estimated incidence of 22q11.2 DS ranges from 1:3000 to 1:6000 live births (McDonald, Codrea, & Gavin, 2015), making it one of the most common syndromic conditions.

This syndrome happens when there is missing genetic material from a specific part of chromosome 22. This results in only one copy of certain genes instead of the usual two. The deletion types and sizes in 22q11.2 DS exhibit significant variability due to low-copy-number repeat sequences flanking the deleted region. Approximately 90% of individuals with 22q11.2 DS display a 2.54 Mb heterozygous deletion involving four low copy number repeats in around 40 genes. Notable genes in this region include *TBX1, PRODH, COMT* and *SNAP29*. 22q11.2 DS occurs *de novo* in approximately 90% to 95% of affected individuals with less than 10% of all cases being transmitted genetically from parent to child (Du, de la Morena, & van Oers, 2020).

22q11.2 DS is the most common cause of syndromic palatal anomalies and velopharyngeal dysfunction (Jackson et al., 2019). It is a significant risk factor for schizophrenia/psychosis (up to 1 in 4 individuals with 22q11.2 DS will develop psychosis in adulthood; Cleynen et al., 2021), and is the second most common cause of developmental delay and congenital heart disease after Down syndrome. Craniofacial dysmorphism in 22q11.2 DS is characterized by a diverse array of facial phenotypic features including an elongated face, hypertelorism, a broad nasal bridge, hooded eyelids, up slanted palpebral fissures, a long nose with a bulbous tip, a short philtrum, a small mouth, micrognathia, and low-set, posteriorly rotated, small ears. Cleft palate, velopharyngeal insufficiency, and hypotonia, accompanied by hypernasal speech, have been estimated to occur in as many as 30%–80% of children with 22q11.2 DS. Velopharyngeal operations are quite common during childhood to improve speech quality (Cárdenas-Nieto et al., 2020). Congenital heart disease is identified in approximately 60% to 80% of children affected by 22q11.2 DS (Goldmuntz, 2020). Endocrine anomalies including hypoparathyroidism, hypocalcemia, thyroid dysfunction, and growth retardation are also commonly reported in 22q11.2 DS impacting up to 65% of children with the genetic condition.

The intellectual abilities of most individuals with 22q11.2 DS fall within the borderline range (IQ 70–85), with at least 30% exhibiting mild intellectual disability. In addition to schizophrenia, anxiety disorders, attention-deficit/hyperactivity disorder (ADHD), and autism spectrum disorder are also prevalent in individuals with 22q11.2 DS (Schneider et al., 2014). Males are more likely to exhibit symptoms of ADHD, and younger individuals (below 12 years) tend to show both ADHD and anxiety symptoms. Notably, the psychiatric phenotype in 22q11.2 DS evolves over time, with a higher prevalence of ADHD and anxiety disorders in childhood shifting to increased rates of psychosis and mood disorders during adolescence and young adulthood (Swillen & McDonald-McGinn, 2015). An ADHD diagnosis during childhood is associated with an increased risk for developing a psychotic disorder and experiencing psychotic symptoms during adolescence and young adulthood (Jhawar et al., 2021).

Written expression, attention, and cognitive flexibility each improve over time with 22q11.2 DS, yet youth with 22q11.2 DS never "close the gap" with their typically developing same-age peers. This means that despite growth, developmental delays in these domains persist over time. Reading comprehension, math, verbal fluency, and working memory all exhibit a developmental lag trajectory in 22q11.2 DS. Finally, social functioning as reported by parents and teachers remains consistently poor compared to typically developing peers. Individuals with 22q11.2 DS experience increasing social impairments and peer rejection (Jhawar et al., 2021).

Prader-Willi Syndrome

Prader-Willi syndrome (PWS) is a neurodevelopmental genomic imprinting disorder with a lack of gene expression on chromosome 15. PWS was first identified by Andrea Prader and Heinrich Willi in 1956, when they described a syndrome with the phenotypic characteristics of abnormal growth, short stature, small hands and feet, hypotonia, early onset of childhood obesity, insatiable hunger, intellectual disability, and cryptorchidism (undescended testicles) in males. PWS occurs in approximately 1:15,000 individuals and is more frequent among Caucasian individuals (Butler et al., 2019). Children with PWS have mild craniofacial dysmorphisms, with a disproportionately long and narrow head, strabismus, and a small, upturned nose with a thin upper lip and down-turned corners of the mouth. Enamel hypoplasia, sticky saliva, and dry mouth are also commonly seen among children with PWS.

There are two clinical stages to PWS. The first consists of failure to thrive, and the second of hyperphagia and onset of obesity. Prenatal signs of PWS include reduced fetal activity, low birthweight, increased head-abdomen circumference ratio, polyhydramnios (amniotic fluid build-up), breech presentation, and pre- and post-term delivery complications. At birth, features of PWS include hypotonia, hypopigmentation, feeding problems, and hypogonadism. In infancy, feeding problems and hypotonia persist, as well as developmental delays, temperature instability, orthopedic problems, and growth hormone deficiency present. Children with PWS develop behavioral difficulties, including temper tantrums, excessive food-seeking behavior, intellectual delays, learning problems, repetitive asking, compulsive behavior, disruptive behavior, and cognitive rigidity. Over 60% of children with PWS experience skin excoriation. Complications associated with PWS include diabetes mellitus, osteoporosis, fatty liver, right-sided heart failure, obstructive sleep apnea, hypoventilation, gastrointestinal dysmotility, stasis ulcers, and water intoxication (Butler et al., 2019).

The most common cause of PWS is a *de novo* deletion of the paternal 15q11-q13 region, which accounts for approximately 60% of PWS cases (Butler et al., 2019). This *de novo* deletion can be described as a type I or type II deletion. The type I deletion is larger, whereas the type II deletion is smaller, but both involve the proximal breakpoint and the distal breakpoint of chromosome 15q. Five percent of individuals with PWS have an atypical deletion, which is smaller than those with type I or type II deletions. The second cause of PWS is maternal disomy 15, in which there are two maternal chromosome 15s. Autism spectrum disorder (ASD) is common among individuals with maternal disomy 15. The risk of psychosis is increased among all subtypes, but the risk of bipolar disorder and cyclic psychosis is elevated in PWS with the maternal disomy subtype. The third genetic cause is exceedingly rare and occurs when the father contributes a microdeletion of the imprinting center received from his mother.

Clinical diagnostic thresholds for PWS are based on age and major and minor diagnostic features. For children under 3 years old, five clinical diagnostic points are required, three of which must come from the major criteria to meet the criteria for PWS. For children over 3 years old, eight clinical diagnostic points are required, four of which must come from the major features to meet the criteria for PWS. Major clinical diagnostic criteria include: (1) hyperphagia; (2) hypogonadism; (3) characteristic facial features; (4) global developmental delay and mild to moderate intellectual disability; (5) neonatal and infantile hypotonia; (6) feeding problems and failure to thrive in infancy; (7) excessive or rapid weight gain with onset between 12 months and 6 years of age. Minor clinical diagnostic criteria include: (1) decreased fetal movement; (2) short stature; (3) sleep disturbance/sleep apnea; (4) behavioral difficulties; (5) hypopigmentation; (6) small hands and feet; (7) eye abnormalities; (8) narrow hands with straight ulnar border; (9) speech articulation defects and skin-picking; (10) thick viscous saliva.

Management for PWS requires a multidisciplinary approach in which geneticists, dieticians, mental health practitioners, primary care physicians, and orthopedic specialists work together to manage the comorbid conditions, behavioral problems, weight gain, and hormone deficiencies (Butler et al., 2019). To manage hyperphagia and obesity, there must be rigorous control of diet, securing food in the environment, and regimented exercise plans. Growth hormone replacement, sex steroids, thyroid hormone, and glucocorticoids are indicated if deficiencies are present.

Smith Magenis Syndrome

Smith Magenis syndrome (SMS) was first identified in the 1980s (Smith, 1982; Smith et al., 1986) where nine unrelated patients were identified having a genotypic deletion at chromosome 17p11.2 and a shared phenotype of brachycephaly (short head or lower than normal ratio of skull length to width), a protruding lower jaw, hoarse voice, speech delay, psychomotor and growth retardation, and behavioral concerns. The birth incidence of SMS is estimated to be between 1:15,000 to 1:25,000 births (Smith et al., 2001). SMS is often identified by the distinctive facial dimorphism coupled with speech delay and behavioral concerns.

The phenotypes of SMS range in symptom presentation and severity, although sleep disturbances and behavioral dysregulation are often the most impairing features of the syndrome. The sleep disturbances associated with SMS affect 65% to 100% of individuals and include early sleep onset/offset and repeated or prolonged nighttime waking, resulting in poor sleep quality and reduced sleep duration (De Leersnyder, 2013). These sleep difficulties stem from atypical circadian rhythms and abnormal secretion of melatonin, likely because of loss of genetic material in 17p11.2 that is responsible for circadian regulation of melatonin. Notably, sleep disturbances can affect daytime behaviors, such that reduced sleep quality is correlated with increased maladaptive behaviors in individuals with SMS. The maladaptive behaviors in SMS occur in upwards of 80% of individuals and range from oppositional behaviors and distractibility to frequent temper tantrums, aggression, and self-injurious behaviors (Elsea & Girirajan, 2008). Head banging, skin picking, and wrist biting are the most frequent self-injurious behaviors seen in SMS and typically start by age two (Bouras, Dykens, & Smith, 1998). Self-injurious behaviors unique to SMS include pulling out fingernails and toenails and inserting objects into bodily orifices (Dykens, 1997). The behavioral phenotype of SMS also includes ADHD comorbidity and stereotypical behaviors, such as a spasmodic upper body squeeze (Finucane et al., 1994). Although the onset of the behavioral phenotype is typically in childhood, an exacerbation of maladaptive behavior commonly occurs during puberty.

The genetic cause of SMS is ascribed to deletion in chromosome 17p, specifically 17p11.2 (Smith et al., 2001). The majority of individuals with SMS exhibit deletion in 17p11.2, but approximately 10% of cases are caused by pathogenic variants in the *RAI1* gene resulting in lack of allele functioning. Although multiple genes are located in 17p11.2, *RAI1* is the gene primarily associated with SMS. *RAI1* codes for a protein that regulates transcription and is involved in a variety of behavioral, neurodevelopment, and circadian rhythms functioning, and its function loss is responsible for most symptoms seen in SMS.

Deletion Disorder Diagnosis

Clinical suspicion for deletion disorders requires specialized genetic imaging techniques for diagnosis. Fluorescence in situ hybridization (FISH) is the most common technique used to identify genetic deletions (Halder et al., 2013). Chromosomal microarray analysis may be performed to identify deletion size more precisely.

Implications for Assessment and Intervention

These five genetic syndromes involve many similar assessment and intervention considerations.

Assessment

CdCS, WHS, 22q11.2 DS, PWS, and SMS are all characterized by cognitive, academic, and social developmental delays or deficits and are therefore very likely to qualify for special education services under the Individuals with Disabilities Education Act (IDEA). An Individualized Education Plan (IEP) which includes speech/language, occupational and/or physical therapy within the formal school setting is nearly universal for these five conditions. The genetic syndrome itself is often the qualifying condition (Other Health Impairment) although intellectual disability, speech/language impairment, orthopedic impairment, autism, ADHD, specific learning disability, or multiple disabilities can serve as the qualifying condition for receipt of special education and related services.

In the educational environment, frequent evaluations over time are imperative to align educational expectations with the ability level of children with these conditions. Assessing academic performance and making curricular adjustments, especially during transition junctures (e.g., transition from elementary school to middle school) is crucial.

General assessment recommendations for working with youth with intellectual disabilities and/or developmental delays should be followed. In addition, all five conditions are characterized to varying degrees by inattention, hyperactivity, and anxiety symptoms. Thus, assessment should consider the extent to which these symptoms are impairing functioning above and beyond what is expected given the child's developmental delays. Finally, general assessment considerations for all conditions should focus on better understanding caregiver stress, coping, and mental health. It is our experience that the impacts of raising a child with a deletion disorder on parental stress, coping and mental health is underappreciated by providers and school personnel. All conditions can be chronically stressful for caregivers as each condition is associated with a range of medical, developmental, and mental health conditions. More specific assessment considerations for each individual deletion disorder are detailed in Table 19.1.

Intervention

Regarding interventions, specialized educational settings, social comfort, experiential schoolwork, and modified expectations matching competency levels can be beneficial to consider. Transition plans for adult work and living are essential. Traditional transition programs for the intellectual disability population will likely work well for CdCS, WHS, PWS, and

Table 19.1 Deletion Disorders: Unique Assessment and Intervention Components

Disorder	*Assessment*	*Intervention*
Cri-du-chat Syndrome (CdCS)	Expressive language is often more significantly impacted than receptive language • Psychological tests which place a large emphasis on verbal responding may underestimate true, innate abilities Self-injurious behaviors (e.g., biting, scratching, head banging; SIBs) are common	Speech/language therapy is likely to be integral and necessary throughout K-12 education Complete functional behavioral assessment (FBA) to develop a custom treatment program focused on changing specific aspects of the environment that may be contributing to SIBs Consider referral to psychiatry if SIBs persist or worsen
Wolf-Hirschhorn Syndrome	The very high prevalence of seizures (90+%) and motor ataxia should be carefully assessed for	Consult with neurology and physical/occupational therapy
22q11.2 DS Prader-Willi Syndrome (PWS)	The most significant specific assessment consideration in 22q11.2 DS is the risk for psychosis • The presentation of psychosis in the 22q11.2 DS population is like that of the non-22q11.2 DS population. • Thus, standard assessment considerations for psychosis, including the use of structured interviews such as the Structured Interview for Prodromal Symptoms (SIPS) should be considered with youth with 22q11.2 DS and their parents. Assessment should consider the extent to which common PWS phenomena such as skin excoriation, obstructive sleep apnea, and compulsive food-seeking/hyperphagic behaviors are present.	Consult with psychiatry Psychoeducation, family-based interventions, cognitive remediation and cognitive behavioral strategies can be helpful Complete functional behavioral assessment (FBA) to develop a custom treatment program focused on changing specific aspects of the environment that may be contributing to excoriation and compulsive food-seeking/hyperphagic behaviors Consult with neurology for treatment of sleep apnea For hyperphagia, consult with a nutritionist regarding dietary interventions For hyperphagia, a key intervention is making sure that individuals with PWS do not have unrestricted access to food

Disorder	*Assessment*	*Intervention*
Smith-Magenis Syndrome (SMS)	Sleep disturbances are very common in SMS and should be continually assessed, especially since total sleep is negatively associated with disruptive behaviors (e.g., oppositionality, temper tantrums, aggression) Self-injurious behaviors are also common in SMS and should be assessed	Sleep hygiene interventions such as limiting daytime napping and caffeine intake, avoiding screen time 2 hours before bed, removing electronics from the bedroom, white noise machines, etc. can be helpful Complete functional behavioral assessment (FBA) to develop a custom treatment program focused on changing specific aspects of the environment that may be contributing to SIBs

SMS yet may not adequately meet the needs of individuals with 22q11.2 DS who are relatively higher functioning. For youth with 22q11.2 DS, designing programming to maximize adaptive, social, and functional skills is essential towards promoting functional independence in adulthood.

Outside of the school setting, caregivers of youth with any of these conditions could routinely practice functional and social skills within home and community environments. Caregivers can use strategies like modeling, talking out loud, and direct instruction to provide explicit practice in using money, organizing belongings, and planning activities. Structured social opportunities outside of school-based interventions, such as therapy-based programs, non-profit organizations, and specialty camps, can be valuable to consider. More specific to 22q11.2 DS, early intensive treatment addressing anxiety and pragmatic language deficits can contribute to the development of confidence and peer engagement skills. More specific intervention considerations for each deletion disorder are detailed in Table 19.1.

Resources

Websites

https://fivepminus.org/resources/ Tool for parents, families, and professionals to learn more about Cri-du-chat syndrome as well as a source for resources.

http://wolfhirschhorn.org/ Compilation of information, discussions, stories, events, and pictures of people with WHS.

https://22q.org/ Tool for parents, families, and professionals to learn more about 22q11.2 DS as well as a source for resources.

www.pwsausa.org Prader-Willi Syndrome Association (USA) is an organization of families and professionals working together to raise awareness, offer support, provide education and advocacy and promote research to enhance the quality of life of those affected by PWS.

https://smith-magenis.org Resources for families that live with the syndrome as well as professionals who treat, educate, and care for people with SMS.

Books

Educating Children with the 22q11.2 Deletion Syndrome, Velo Cardio Facial Syndrome and DiGeorge, Third Edition (2020) by Donna Cutler-Landsman, Plural Publishing.

Neurobehavioral Manifestations of Prader-Willi Syndrome (2022) edited by Deepan Singh, Cambridge University Press

On the Road to Success with SMS: A Smith-Magenis Guidebook for Schools (2014) by Brenda Finucane and Barbara Hass-Givler, Amazon Kindle edition.

References

Bergemann, A. D., Cole, F., & Hirschhorn, K. (2005). The etiology of Wolf-Hirschhorn syndrome. *Trends in Genetics*, 21(3), 188–195. doi:10.1016/j.tig.2005.01.00.

Bouras, N., Dykens, E. M., & Smith, A. C. M. (1998). Distinctiveness and correlates of maladaptive behaviour in children and adolescents with Smith-Magenis syndrome. *Journal of Intellectual Disability Research*, 42(6), 481–489. doi:10.1046/j.1365-2788.1998.4260481.x.

Butler, M. G., Miller, J. L., & Forster, J. L. (2019). Prader-Willi syndrome-clinical genetics, diagnosis and treatment approaches: An update. *Current Pediatric Reviews*, 15(4), 207–244. doi:10.2174/1573396315666190716120925.

Cárdenas-Nieto, D., Forero-Castro, M., Esteban-Pérez, C., Martínez-Lozano, J., & Briceño-Balcázar, I. (2020). The 22q11.2 microdeletion in pediatric patients with cleft lip, palate, or both and congenital heart disease: A systematic review. *Journal of Pediatric Genetics*, 9(1), 1–8. doi:10.1055/s-0039-1698804.

Cerruti Mainardi, P. (2006). Cri du chat syndrome. *Orphanet Journal of Rare Diseases*, 1, 1–9. doi:10.1186/1750-1172-1-33.

Cleynen, I., Engchuan, W., Hestand, M. S., Heung, T., Holleman, A. M., Johnston, H. R., Monfeuga, T., McDonald-McGinn, D. M., Gur, R. E., Morrow, B. E., Swillen, A., Vorstman, J. A. S., Bearden, C. E., Chow, E. W. C., van den Bree, M., Emanuel, B. S., Vermeesch, J. R., Warren, S. T., Owen, M. J., … & Bassett, A. S. (2021). Genetic contributors to risk of schizophrenia in the presence of a 22q11.2 deletion. *Molecular Psychiatry*, 26(8), 4496–4510. doi:10.1038/s41380-020-0654-3.

De Leersnyder, H. (2013). Pediatric neurology part I: Chapter 34. *Smith-Magenis syndrome*, (Vol. 111, pp. 295–296). Elsevier Inc. doi:10.1016/B978-0-444-52891-9.00034-8.

Du, Q., de la Morena, M. T., & van Oers, N. S. (2020). The genetics and epigenetics of 22q11. 2 deletion syndrome. *Frontiers in Genetics*, 10, 486538. doi:10.3389/fgene.2019.01365.

Dykens, E. M. (1997). Brief report: Cognitive and behavioral profiles in persons with Smith-Magenis syndrome. *Journal of Autism and Developmental Disorders*, 27(2), 203–211. doi:10.1023/A:1025800126086.

Elsea, S. H. & Girirajan, S. (2008). Smith-Magenis syndrome. *European Journal of Human Genetics*, 16(4), 412–421. doi:10.1038/sj.ejhg.5202009.

Finucane, B. M., Konar, D., Givler, B. H., Kurtt, M. B., & ScottJr, C. I. (1994). The spasmodic upper-body squeeze: A characteristic behavior in Smith-Magenis syndrome. *Developmental Medicine & Child Neurology*, 36(1), 78–83. doi:10.1111/j.1469-8749.1994.tb11770.x.

Goldmuntz, E. (2020, March). 22q11.2 deletion syndrome and congenital heart disease. *American Journal of Medical Genetics Part C: Seminars in Medical Genetics*, 184(1), 64–72. doi:10.1002/ajmg.c.31774.

Halder, A., Jain, M., Chaudhary, I., Gupta, N., & Kabra, M. (2013). Fluorescence in situ hybridization (FISH) using non-commercial probes in the diagnosis of clinically suspected microdeletion syndromes. *Indian Journal of Medical Research*, 138(1), 135–142.

Hirschhorn, K., Cooper, H. L., & Firschein, I. L. (1965). Deletion of short arms of chromosome 4–5 in a child with defects of midline fusion. *Humangenetik*, 1(5), 479–482. doi:10.1007/BF00279124.

HL, C. (1961). Apparent deletion of short arms I chromosome (4 or 5) in a child with defects of midline fusion. *Mammology Chrom. Newsletter*, 4, 14–16.

Jackson, O., Crowley, T. B., Sharkus, R., Smith, R., Jeong, S., Solot, C., & McDonald-Mcginn, D. (2019). Palatal evaluation and treatment in 22q11. 2 deletion syndrome. *American Journal of Medical Genetics Part A*, 179(7), 1184–1195. doi:10.1002/ajmg.a.61152.

Jhawar, N., Brown, M. J., Cutler-Landsman, D., Kates, W. R., Angkustsiri, K., & Antshel, K. M. (2021). Longitudinal psychiatric and developmental outcomes in 22q11.2 deletion syndrome: A systematic review. *Journal of Developmental & Behavioral Pediatrics*, 42(5), 415–427. doi:10.1097/DBP.0000000000000927.

Kobrynski, L. J. & Sullivan, K. E. (2007). Velocardiofacial syndrome, DiGeorge syndrome: The chromosome 22q11.2 deletion syndromes. *The Lancet*, 370 (9596), 1443–1452. doi:10.1016/S0140-6736(07)61601-8.

Lejeune, J. (1963). Trois cas de délétion partielle du bras court d'un chromosome 5. *Comptes rendus de l'Académie des Sciences*, 257, 3098–3102.

McDonald, J., Codrea, A., & Gavin, B. (2015). A pilot music group for young people attending a community child and adolescent mental health service. *Irish Journal of Psychological Medicine*, 32(3), 259–264.

Nevado, J., Ho, K. S., Zollino, M., Blanco, R., Cobaleda, C., Golzio, C., Beaudry-Bellefeuille, I., Berrocoso, S., Limeras, J., Barrúz, P., Serrano-Martín, C., Cafiero, C., Málaga, I., Campos-Sánchez, E., Moriyón-Iglesias, T., Márquez, S, Markham, L., Twede, H., Lortz, A., … & Lapunzina, P. (2020). International meeting on Wolf-Hirschhorn syndrome: Update on the nosology and new insights on the pathogenic mechanisms for seizures and growth delay. *American Journal of Medical Genetics Part A*, 182(1), 257–267. doi:10.1002/ajmg.a.61406.

Paprocka, J., Kaminiów, K., Yetkin, O., Tekturk, P., Baykan, B., Leiz, S., Kluger, G., & Striano, P. (2022). Clinical and epilepsy characteristics in Wolf-Hirschhorn syndrome (4p-): A review. *Seizure*. doi:10.1016/j.seizure.2022.12.001.

Paradowska-Stolarz, A. M. (2014). Wolf-Hirschhorn syndrome (WHS)-literature review on the features of the syndrome. *Advances in Clinical and Experimental Medicine*, 23(3), 485–489. doi:10.17219/acem/24111.

Rodríguez-Caballero, Á., Torres-Lagares, D., Rodríguez-Pérez, A., Serrera Figallo, M. D. L. Á., Hernández Guisado, J. M., & Machuca-Portillo, G. (2010). Cri du chat syndrome: A critical review. *Medicina Oral, Patología oral y Cirugía bucal*, 15(3), e473–e478. doi:10.4317/medoral.15.e473.

Schneider, M., Debbané, M., Bassett, A. S., Chow, E. W., Fung, W. L. A., Van Den Bree, M. B. M., Owen, M., Murphy, K. C., Niarchou. M., Kates, W. R., Antshel, K. M., Fremont, W., McDonald-McGinn, D. M., Gur, R. E., Zackai, E. H., Vorstman, J., Duijff, S. N., Klaassen, P. W. J., Swillen, A., ... & International Consortium on Brain and Behavior in 22q11.2 Deletion Syndrome (2014). Psychiatric disorders from childhood to adulthood in 22q11.2 deletion syndrome: Results from the International Consortium on Brain and Behavior in 22q11.2 Deletion Syndrome. *American Journal of Psychiatry*, 171(6), 627–639. doi:10.1176/appi.ajp.2013.13070864.

Shannon, N. L., Maltby, E. L., Rigby, A. S., & Quarrell, O. W. J. (2001). An epidemiological study of Wolf-Hirschhorn syndrome: Life expectancy and cause of mortality. *Journal of Medical Genetics*, 38(10), 674–679. doi:10.1136/jmg.38.10.674.

Sigafoos, J., O'Reilly, M. F., & Lancioni, G. E. (2009). Cri-du-chat. *Developmental Neurorehabilitation*, 12(3), 119–121. doi:10.1080/17518420902975720.

Smith, A. C. M. (1982). Deletion of the 17 short arm in 2 patients with facial clefts. *American Journal of Human Genetics*, 34, 146A.

Smith, A. C., McGavran, L., Robinson, J., Waldstein, G., Macfarlane, J., Zonona, J., Reiss, J., Lahr, M., Allen, L., Magenis, E., Opitz, J. M., & Reynolds, J. F. (1986). Interstitial deletion of (17)(p11. 2p11. 2) in nine patients. *American Journal of Medical Genetics*, 24(3), 393–414. doi:10.1002/ajmg.1320240303.

Smith, A. C. M., Boyd, K. E., Brennan, C., Charles, J., Elsea, S. H., Finucane, B. M., Foster, R., Gropman, A., Girirajan, S., & Haas-Givler, B. (2001). Smith-Magenis syndrome. In M.P. Adam et. al. (Eds), *GeneReviews®*. University of Washington, Seattle.

Swillen, A. & McDonald-McGinn, D. (2015, June). Developmental trajectories in 22q11.2 deletion syndrome. In *American Journal of Medical Genetics Part C: Seminars in Medical Genetics*, 169(2), 172–181. doi:10.1002/ajmg.c.31435.

Tang, F., Zeng, Y., Wang, L., Yin, D., Chen, L., Xie, D., & Wang, J. (2023). Prenatal phenotype of Wolf-Hirschhorn syndrome: A case series and literature review. *Molecular Genetics & Genomic Medicine*, 11(6), e2155. doi:10.1002/mgg3.2155.

20 Neurofibromatosis Type 1 and Neurofibromatosis Type 2-Related Schwannomatosis

Angela Canas and Natalie Escalante

Introduction

Neurofibromatosis (NF) has historically referred to a group of three distinct genetic disorders including neurofibromatosis type 1 (NF1), neurofibromatosis type 2 (NF2), and schwannomatosis. This nomenclature recently changed to align with current research and clinical findings. NF2 was renamed and now represents one of the various types of schwannomatosis. Both NF1 and *NF2*-related schwannomatosis (formerly NF2; hereinafter referred to as *NF2*-SWN) are multisystemic, single-gene disorders caused by pathogenic variants that affect tumor suppressor proteins and result in uncontrolled neural cell proliferation involving the nerves, skin, and/or eyes. Both disorders are inherited in an autosomal dominant fashion and are diagnosed using specific clinical criteria, although molecular testing can be used to confirm the presence of a pathogenic variant. Despite sharing core features, these disorders have distinct genetic etiologies, phenotypic expressions, disease courses, and clinical management.

There are three forms of NF1. Constitutional NF1 results from a germline pathogenic variant in the NF1 gene. Germline variants affect reproductive cells, which contain the genetic material transmitted to offspring. Mosaic NF1 (MNF1) is caused by a postzygotic change in the NF1 gene, resulting in some cells having two functional NF1 genes and other cells having a pathogenic variant in one copy of the NF1 gene (Ejerskov et al., 2021). Individuals with MNF1 present with clinical features localized to one or more segments of the body or with generalized features of the disorder. Individuals with MNF1 typically develop more benign presentations than those with constitutional NF1, although Ejerskov and colleagues reported a higher frequency of plexiform neurofibromas and cognitive impairment than previously documented. Watson syndrome is characterized by café au lait macules, pulmonary stenosis, reduced intelligence (IQ), and short stature (Allanson et al., 1991). Most affected individuals also have relative macrocephaly and Lisch nodules, and about a third have neurofibromas.

DOI: 10.4324/9781032703923-24

Historically, two forms of NF2 have been referenced in the literature. The Wishart phenotype represents a more aggressive form involving multiple neoplasms with rapid progression that emerge under the age of 20 years, whereas patients with the Gardner phenotype exhibit a milder disease course characterized by fewer, slow-growing tumors that typically arise later in life (Coy et al., 2019). Current *NF2*-SWN phenotypes represent either constitutional/germline or mosaic/segmental pathogenic variants. The latter presentation is associated with more localized findings and a milder disease course. Constitutional/germline forms of NF1 and *NF2*-SWN will be the focus of this chapter.

Genetic Contributions

Both NF1 and *NF2*-SWN result from pathogenic variants that disrupt the production of specific tumor suppressor proteins leading to the uncontrolled proliferation of neural cells. NF1 and *NF2*-SWN are caused by pathogenic variants on chromosomes 17 and 22, respectively (Kresak & Walsh, 2016). The NF1 gene is responsible for producing neurofibromin, while the NF2 gene is responsible for producing merlin or schwannomin. Both proteins play a role in tumor suppression through their interaction with pathways involved in the cellular division cycle. Pathogenic variants involving these genes result in the partial or complete loss of protein function, which leads to rapid cellular proliferation and the various tumors characteristic of these conditions.

Approximately half of individuals with NF1 and *NF2*-SWN inherit the disorder from a parent in an autosomal dominant fashion (Kotch et al., 2023). The remaining half acquire the disorder from *de novo* or spontaneous pathogenic variants. If inherited, only a single copy (i.e., from one parent) of the affected gene is needed to acquire the disorder. For individuals with NF1 or *NF2*-SWN, there is a 50% chance, with each pregnancy, that their offspring will inherit the condition. Thus, a child with an affected parent has a 50% chance of inheriting the affected gene and subsequently presenting with the disorder.

Epidemiology

With an incidence rate of 1:2500 to 1:4000 births, NF1 is the most common tumor predisposition syndrome worldwide (Tabata et al., 2020). NF1 has been identified across all racial and ethnic groups and affects males and females equally (Anderson & Gutmann, 2015). Relative to the general population, the life expectancy of individuals with NF1 is reduced by up to 26 years, with malignancy representing the primary reason for death before 30 years of age (Uusitalo et al., 2015).

NF2-SWN has a much smaller incidence, with yearly birth rate estimates ranging between 1:25,000 (Children's Tumor Foundation, 2024) and

1:33,000 (National Organization for Rare Disorders, 2023) worldwide. No sex, racial, or ethnic differences have been found in *NF2*-SWN. Mortality is correlated with the age of diagnosis and the varying expression of the tumors associated with *NF2*-SWN (Forde et al., 2020). Early age of symptom onset, a constitutional presentation, and the presence of intracranial meningiomas are considered negative prognostic indicators.

Diagnosis

Previously, NF diagnoses were based on 1988 National Institutes of Health clinical consensus criteria. In 2020, the criteria for NF1 and NF2 were revised (see Legius et al., 2021 and Plotkin et al., 2022 for updated criteria). Genetic testing is not necessary to confirm clinical diagnoses. In NF1, molecular confirmation is typically reserved for individuals who do not meet clinical criteria but are suspected of presenting with the condition and to distinguish NF1 from other conditions with overlapping features (Legius et al.). In *NF2*-SWN, genetic testing is recommended for individuals with more than a 1% chance of presenting with the condition (Halliday et al., 2023).

Characteristics and Symptoms

Medical and Neurological Implications

There is notable variability in the phenotypic expression of NF1 and *NF2*-SWN (Messina & Signorelli, 2020). This variability is likely related to the underlying genotype. In NF1, for example, large or complete 1.4-Mb gene deletions have been associated with a higher tumor burden, an increased risk of malignancy, and more frequent and severe neurocognitive difficulties (Friedman, 2022). In *NF2*-SWN, truncating variants have been associated with the greatest disease-related morbidity and mortality (Evans, 2023). For a review of the various genotypic-phenotype correlations evidenced in NF1 and *NF2*-SWN, refer to Friedman (2022) and Evans (2023).

NF1 is characterized by multiple café au lait macules, skinfold freckling, peripheral and central nervous system (CNS) tumors, ocular hamartomas, and bone lesions (Legius et al., 2021). Cutaneous pigmentary features are the most common finding. Café au lait macules are flat areas of hyperpigmentation that are typically ovoid-shaped, well-defined, and several millimeters in size (Friedman, 2022). They are usually the first clinical sign of NF1, appearing between birth and early childhood. Once established, they remain stable in size and number. Individuals with NF1 can also present with freckling in the inguinal and/or axillary regions, and in other skinfold areas not typically exposed to sunlight (Miller et al., 2019). Skinfold freckles typically emerge between 3 and 5 years of age.

Neurofibromas are benign peripheral nerve sheath tumors (PNSTs) presenting as discrete nodular growths or as diffuse plexiform lesions (Ferner et al., 2006). Cutaneous/subcutaneous neurofibromas are relatively small, well-circumscribed nodules that typically develop in adolescence to early adulthood but can also appear during childhood. They grow slowly but can increase in size and quantity during periods of hormonal change (Well et al., 2020). Although they do not carry a high potential for malignant transformation, they can result in discomfort (e.g., stinging, itching, bleeding, or pain) and cosmetic burden (Ferner et al.). Cutaneous neurofibromas are the most common NF1-related tumor, presenting in up to 99% of adults with NF1 (Friedman, 2022). Plexiform neurofibromas are complex, diffuse lesions involving several nerve fascicles that present superficially or infiltrate muscle, bone, and viscera (Jack et al., 2020). Unlike cutaneous neurofibromas, plexiform neurofibromas emerge during early childhood to adolescence (Miller et al., 2019). They can be disfiguring, disabling, painful, and/or life-threatening. Plexiform neurofibromas are seen in up to 50% of individuals with NF1 and carry an increased risk for malignant transformation.

Malignant PNSTs (MPNSTs) are aggressive sarcomas that typically arise from pre-existing plexiform neurofibromas (Jack et al., 2020). They can be deep and difficult to detect, metastasize quickly, affect crucial life functions (e.g., mobility, sight, swallowing), and carry a poor prognosis. Individuals with NF1 have an 8% to 13% lifetime risk of developing a MPNST (Evans et al., 2002). MPNSTs are the most common malignancy and the most common cause of death in individuals with NF1 (Staedtke et al., 2017).

Optic pathway gliomas (OPG) are grade I pilocytic astrocytomas that typically involve the anterior visual pathway (Listernick et al., 1997). Although often asymptomatic, they can result in reduced visual acuity, visual field defects, optic nerve atrophy, pupillary defects, strabismus, proptosis, and other symptoms. OPGs can also cause precocious puberty due to infiltration into the hypothalamus, which regulates growth hormone. The risk for developing a symptomatic OPG is greatest in children under 7 years old. OPGs are the most common CNS tumor in individuals with NF1. Fifteen to 30% of children with NF1 develop an OPG; of these, 30% to 50% will be symptomatic, and about 30% will require treatment (Fisher et al., 2012).

Lisch nodules are elevated, pigmented hamartomas on the iris (Alkatan et al., 2020), and choroidal abnormalities are bright, patchy nodules representing proliferating Schwann cells (Vagge et al., 2015). Both ocular manifestations are purely morphological and do not result in visual disturbances (Mallone et al., 2022). Lisch nodules are seen in >95% of adults with NF1 (Friedman, 2022). Prevalence rates for choroidal abnormalities range between 70% and 100% (Vagge).

NF1 is also associated with some distinctive and relatively uncommon skeletal abnormalities (Friedman, 2022; Miller et al., 2019). Sphenoid wing dysplasia (abnormal development of the sphenoid bone of the skull) is usually congenital, unilateral, and static but can be progressive and lead to facial and orbital disfiguration. Long bone dysplasia typically emerges in infancy or toddlerhood and involves the tibia or fibula, resulting in anterior and lateral bowing. Long bone dysplasia can progress to a fracture with permanently delayed or improper healing (pseudoarthrosis) and a "false joint" appearance. Lastly, dystrophic scoliosis is characterized by the acute angulation of a short spine segment, with underlying vertebral-body and rib abnormalities. This condition typically emerges in early childhood and progresses rapidly.

Additional NF1-related clinical manifestations include, but are not limited to: (a) cardiovascular conditions and vasculopathies (e.g., vascular stenoses, aneurysms, stroke, hypertension); (b) neurological complications (e.g., migraines, seizures, aqueductal stenosis/hydrocephalus, macrocephaly, various brain tumors); (c) endocrine issues (e.g., growth hormone deficiency, precocious puberty); (d) gastrointestinal issues (e.g., constipation, gastric abdominal pain); and (e) other skeletal abnormalities (e.g., osteopenia/osteoporosis, chest wall deformities, limb length discrepancies). For a review of these and other manifestations in NF1, refer to Friedman (2022) and Miller and colleagues (2019).

Areas of hyperintensity on T2-weighted magnetic resonance imaging (MRI) are present in over half of children with NF1 (Miller et al., 2019). T2 hyperintensities are most often seen in the basal ganglia, thalamus, cerebellum, and brainstem. They typically emerge between 2 and 10 years of age and regress by the second decade of life. The nature and significance of these lesions remain undetermined (Di Stasi et al., 2023). Additional brain abnormalities, including increased white and grey matter volumes in specific brain regions, increased size of subcortical structures (e.g., corpus collosum), atypical symmetry of the planum temporale, and microstructural integrity alterations, have been documented in this population (Baudou et al., 2020).

NF2-SWN is primarily characterized by bilateral vestibular schwannomas (VS; formerly acoustic neuromas). These benign tumors develop on the vestibulocochlear nerve and can result in tinnitus, sensorineural hearing loss, and balance dysfunction (Evans, 2023). They can also expand medially, resulting in brainstem compression and hydrocephalus. Age of onset is typically between 18 and 24 years, although approximately 10% of people develop symptoms during childhood (Children's Tumor Foundation, 2024). By 30 years of age, nearly every affected individual will have developed bilateral VS (Deep et al., 2020). Some individuals will also develop other cranial and peripheral nerve schwannomas (60%), meningiomas (50%–80%), and intramedullary tumors (5%–33%; Gregory et al., 2023). Depending on tumor location, facial weakness, speaking/swallowing difficulties, seizures, and vision impairment may be present (Children's Tumor Foundation; CTF, 2024). Pediatric onset *NF2*-SWN is associated with a more severe disease course but is often under-identified given its differing symptom presentation (Evans, 2023). Children with *NF2*-SWN often present with skin and eye problems initially, as well as mononeuropathy, weakness, and/or an isolated meningioma or schwannoma.

Neuropsychological Implications

Individuals with NF1 are at increased risk for cognitive, academic, and psychosocial impairments. Neuropsychological difficulties present across the lifespan and adversely affect quality of life (QOL), academic functioning, and vocational attainment. NF1-related medical complications and associated treatments can result in or compound neuropsychological deficits (Potter & Mendoza, 2019). Structural and morphological brain alterations have also been associated with neuropsychological outcomes and functional impairment (Baudou et al., 2020).

Studies investigating the neuropsychological sequela of NF1 have revealed wide-ranging outcomes. However, there is a consensus that a large majority of individuals with NF1 experience significant impairment in at least one area of cognitive functioning, with a recent meta-analysis revealing differences in IQ, visuospatial processing, and academic achievement (Crow et al., 2022). Globally, individuals with NF1 typically exhibit low average-to-average IQ, with a distinct downward shift on the bell curve (i.e., 10–15 standard points below the normative mean; Lehtonen et al., 2012). The prevalence rate of intellectual disability (ID) is notably higher than in the general population (Crow et al., 2022) but significantly lower than in other CNS-related genetic disorders.

Academic difficulties are among the most commonly reported concerns in this population. The presence of specific learning disorders (SLD) is reported to range between 20% and 70%, with the broad range due largely to how *learning disability* has been operationalized and applied across time and studies (Hyman et al., 2005). Historically, NF1 was associated with nonverbal learning disability (NVLD), which encompasses deficits in nonverbal reasoning, visual-spatial processing, fine motor functioning, and mathematics within the context of intact verbal functions. This profile has not been consistently evidenced in NF1, and current research suggests more variable phenotypic presentations. Studies have consistently revealed significantly higher rates of SLD in children with NF1 when compared to normative samples and unaffected sibling controls. Specifically, difficulties in reading (i.e., phonological processing, decoding, reading fluency, reading comprehension), mathematics (i.e., computation, applied problem solving), and written expression (i.e., spelling, handwriting) have been documented (Chaix et al., 2017; Lehtonen et al., 2012).

Language delays have been evidenced in children with NF1 as young as 10 months of age (Kolesnik et al., 2017). Problems with speech articulation, vocabulary knowledge, and phonological processing can persist throughout childhood and are correlated with reduced literacy skills. Additionally, weaknesses in verbal reasoning/verbal concept formation (Lehtonen et al., 2012) and difficulties in aspects of complex nonliteral language, including sarcasm and metaphor comprehension (Haebich et al., 2023), have been documented.

Impairments in nonverbal functions, including fluid reasoning, visuospatial perception and organization, and visual-motor integration, remain among the most common and well-documented in children with NF1 (Crow et al., 2022). Although nonverbal deficits have been consistently replicated across studies, many tasks intending to assess nonverbal functions also tap other cognitive domains, particularly attention, executive functioning (EF), and IQ. Van Eylen and colleagues (2017) found that nonverbal performance remained intact when EF and IQ were controlled.

Findings related to verbal and visual explicit memory in individuals with NF1 are variable. Some studies have failed to produce significant differences in memory performance between children with NF1 and controls, while other studies have documented explicit memory weaknesses (Bulgheroni et al., 2019). Although memory tends to be preserved (Janusz, 2020), attention, EF, visuospatial, and language difficulties, and their effects on adequate encoding (and subsequent recall) of information should be considered.

Problems with attention are frequently evidenced in children with NF1. Research documents difficulties with selective, sustained, and divided attention, as well as response inhibition – across visual and auditory tasks. Attention-deficit/hyperactivity disorder (AD/HD) is one of the most common cognitive phenotypes in this population. Up to 60% of individuals with NF1 meet diagnostic criteria for AD/HD (Lidzba et al., 2012). Children with NF1 and comorbid AD/HD tend to experience more severe cognitive problems (e.g., sustained attention, verbal processing, learning), as well as an increased risk for social, emotional, and behavioral difficulties (McNeill et al., 2019; Pride et al., 2012).

Difficulties in EF are frequently cited in studies of children with NF1. In a meta-analytic study, Beaussart and colleagues (2018) found significant impairments in working memory, planning/organization, cognitive flexibility, and inhibition, even after controlling for IQ and AD/HD. Unlike explicit memory, visual and verbal working memory are among the most frequently documented EF impairments in this population (Schwetye & Gutmann, 2014).

Gross and fine motor difficulties, including manual dexterity, coordination, balance, gait, and psychomotor speed, are commonly seen in children with NF1 (Acosta et al., 2006). Rietman and colleagues (2017) found motor problems across a broad range of domains, noting AD/HD and ASD as significant predictors of motor outcomes. Research also suggests a correlation between lower IQ and increased difficulties in balance, gait, running speed, and agility (Champion et al., 2014).

Difficulties in social awareness, motivation, cognition, and communication are common in NF1 (Walsh et al., 2013). Children with NF1 report fewer friendships and reduced self-esteem, possess underdeveloped social skills, and engage in fewer prosocial behaviors (Domon-Archambault et al., 2018; Payne et al., 2020). Symptoms of autism are frequent, with up to 30% of children with NF1 meeting diagnostic criteria for ASD. An increased risk for mood, anxiety, and conduct disorders has also been documented (McNeill et al., 2019; Schwetye & Gutmann, 2014). Impairments in adaptive functioning have been reported, with a recent cross-sectional study of 104 children with NF1 revealing conceptual, social, and/or practical adaptive difficulties in nearly half of the sample (Eby et al., 2019).

Given its rarity and reduced brain involvement in comparison to NF1, there is limited research on the neuropsychological implications of *NF2*-SWN. Nonetheless, it can be assumed that the symptoms of *NF2*-SWN are apt to impact an individual's cognition and overall QOL. Individuals with *NF2*-SWN can have progressive hearing loss due to VS and its associated treatment (Potter & Mendoza, 2019). Pediatric hearing loss is a risk factor for delayed speech and language development, as well as problems with working memory and EF (Lieu et al., 2020). Severe hearing loss can also adversely impact phonological processing, reading, and processing speed (Olivier et al., 2019). Consequently, these problems can impact academic performance, occupational attainment, and QOL. Halliday and colleagues (2019) also reported the presence of internalizing symptoms in 29% of their sample, as well as features of AD/HD and ASD in a small proportion (3.5%) of individuals. More research is needed to identify a neuropsychological profile associated with *NF2*-SWN.

Treatment

Medical

Given the congenital and incurable nature of NF1 and *NF2*-SWN, disease management primarily involves routine surveillance, as well as symptom prevention and intervention, with palliative care recommended for terminal manifestations. Although surveillance standards exist for all patients with NF1 and *NF2*-SWN, treatment regimens vary based on particular clinical presentations.

Although most cutaneous neurofibromas do not warrant treatment, in extreme cases, they can be surgically removed. Surgical resection is the mainstay of treatment for plexiform neurofibromas, although successful removal may be complicated by extensive encroachment on surrounding structures and nerves, rapid tumor recurrence, and an increased risk of malignant transformation. Chemotherapy is not effective, and radiotherapy is contraindicated due to the risk for malignant transformation. MEK inhibitors are a treatment option for inoperable plexiform neurofibromas (Gross et al., 2020). Recently, Solumetinib (Koselugo) was approved to treat NF1-related symptomatic plexiform neurofibromas in children.

Surgical excision with tumor-free margins is the usual treatment for MPNSTs. Chemotherapy can be used to reduce the tumor size with the aim of making it amenable to surgery or as palliative therapy in those with metastatic disease. Unfortunately, the prognosis is poor (i.e., 5-year overall survival rate; Staedtke et al., 2017) with life expectancy likely dependent on the size and location of the tumor, time of diagnosis, and presence of recurrence or metastasis.

Yearly ophthalmological examinations are recommended for all individuals with NF1 under 8 years of age, and then every two years until 18 years of age (Listernick et al., 2007). OPGs can wax/wane, stabilize, or spontaneously resolve. The first line of treatment for progressive or infiltrative OPGs is chemotherapy (Packer et al., 1997). Radiotherapy is not indicated in children because of potential secondary malignancy, as well as neuropsychological, vascular, and endocrine consequences (Sievert & Fisher, 2009). Severe proptosis and extensive gliomas may be treated surgically (Avery et al., 2011).

Children with NF1 require yearly spine assessment to monitor for scoliosis. (Ferner et al., 2006). Because of its rapidly progressive nature and associated deformities, dystrophic scoliosis warrants early surgical intervention. Likewise, early detection and surgical intervention of sphenoid wing dysplasia may help prevent facial disfigurement (Rijken et al., 2023). Imaging of the tibia and fibula is recommended in children who exhibit bowing, with the aim of preventing fractures through bracing (Ofluoglu et al., 2008). Pseudoarthrosis treatment typically involves multiple surgeries and/or amputation of the affected limb (Wientroub & Grill, 2000).

Treatment for *NF2*-SWN-associated tumors includes surgical resection, radiation, and/or chemotherapy, although intervention may be deferred if the tumors are stable (Kotch et al., 2023). There is no consensus or clear guidelines for surgery, as the presence of a tumor and associated symptoms (e.g., hearing loss) do not always correlate with tumor burden. Further, there are considerable surgery risks including worsening of symptoms or facial nerve damage. Surgery may be indicated if there is brainstem compression/dysfunction or obstructive hydrocephalus, despite tumor size (Blakeley et al., 2011). The use of radiation on *NF2*-SWN-associated tumors may result in secondary malignancies, vascular complications, and ipsilateral hearing loss (Kotch et al.). Effective, systematic chemotherapies to treat VS are limited, and surgery remains the primary treatment approach.

Cochlear implants may be an effective treatment for hearing loss due to *NF2*-SWN but requires the cochlear nerve to be intact (Deep et al., 2020). If the tumor progresses, resection may be required, limiting the utility of the implants. In that case, an auditory brainstem implant (ABI) may be considered. An ABI can help with speech perception and hearing environmental sounds, but results are mixed.

Neuropsychological and Psychiatric

Approaches to treating the array of cognitive and psychiatric difficulties experienced by individuals with NF1 and *NF2*-SWN are akin to those used in the general population. The variability in the phenotypic expression of NF1 and *NF2*-SWN, the comorbidities experienced by individuals with these conditions, and individual resources should be considered in treatment planning. In addition to educational support, community-based treatments include (a) applied behavior analysis therapy and social skills training for ASD; (b) concomitant psychopharmacological and psychotherapeutic interventions for anxiety and depression; (c) outpatient speech, occupational, and physical therapies; (d) EF coaching and academic tutoring for learning difficulties; and (e) medication for AD/HD symptoms.

Implications for the School

Qualification for Special Education Services

Students with NF1 and *NF2*-SWN should be considered for educational support under IDEA or the Rehabilitation Act of 1973 (Section 504), depending on the nature and severity of their physical and neurocognitive impairments and the presence of neurological/medical comorbidities. For example, a student with NF1 who does not present with intellectual, academic, language, or visual impairments but has been diagnosed with AD/HD could be supported through Section 504. In contrast, a child who requires academic or therapeutic intervention would be best served under the special education umbrella. A child with NF1 is most likely to qualify under the Other Health Impairment (OHI) classification, although additional classifications of SLD, Speech Impairment (SI), Autism (AU), and Visual Impairment (VI) may be necessary. In rarer cases, children with NF1 could qualify under ID in addition to OHI and other relevant classifications. Students with *NF2*-SWN will likely qualify under the OHI and/or Deaf or Hard of Hearing (DHH) classifications, depending on the presence and severity of hearing loss.

Assessment

Children with NF1 and *NF2*-SWN should be routinely assessed. More frequent evaluation may be warranted when there are suspected changes in cognitive status, and in cases involving surgery, tumor progression, stroke, epilepsy, etc. When assessing these populations, certain precautions should be taken to ensure adequate assessment of skills and abilities, including consideration of hearing and vision impairments. The examiner will also need to consider the impact of neuropathy, headache/pain, AD/HD-related behaviors, and internalizing symptomatology.

Disease-related visual impairments and blindness (VI/B) is critical to consider during assessment. Although some common measures may appear to be suitable for assessing children with VI/B, utilizing general population norms may not be appropriate (Joyce et al., 2022). The degree of VI, age of onset, and level of educational attainment prior to the onset of vision loss should be considered, as individuals with a later onset may have poorer immediate and working memory abilities and greater difficulty discriminating shapes and textures compared to individuals who have been visually impaired longer. While some well-known assessments (e.g., WRAT-5, WJ IV ACH) have Braille adaptations, they do not have VI/B norms, and performance should be interpreted cautiously. Other less common measures that utilize VI/B norms include the Cognitive Test for the Blind, Intelligence Test for Visually Impaired Children, Test of Gross Motor Development, Third Edition, and McCarron Assessment of Neuromuscular Development, Sixth Edition, VI/B Version. For a comprehensive review of VI/B assessment, refer to Joyce and colleagues (2022).

For children with *NF2*-SWN assessment of hearing is important (Grenon & Whitaker, 2022). Examiners should consult with speech and language pathologists and other colleagues who have experience with DHH individuals and utilize sign interpreters with expertise in psychological/psychoeducational evaluations when possible. Non-verbal communication such as eye gaze, facial expressions, and head tilts should be observed and considered. Although using non-verbal measures may be beneficial in some cases, these measures are not language-free, often containing both verbal directions and requiring some form of internal dialogue for successful completion. Over relying on nonverbal measures may lead to misrepresentation of strengths and weaknesses.

Fatigue, pain, and neuropathy are common in pediatric NF1 and *NF2*-SWN and should be considered during testing. Frequent rest and positioning breaks, strategic scheduling, brief testing sessions, adjustments to overhead lighting, and various seating options are recommended to optimize performance. In cases of weakness or neuropathy, the examiner may want to abbreviate the number of fine motor tasks, provide oral administration of self-report measures, and/or avoid motor-based speeded tests.

The presence of internalizing and externalizing disorders may impact or impede the assessment process, including performances on measures of attention, EF, memory, and IQ (Barisa, 2020; Kirk & Boada, 2020). Children with behavioral dysregulation may need frequent breaks or multiple test sessions. Lastly, children with NF1 or *NF2*-SWN may exhibit non-credible performance. Research indicates that even experienced evaluators cannot reliably discriminate between test scores indicating simulated impairment from those indicating actual impairment (Larrabee & Kirkwood, 2020). Basing conclusions on non-credible performance may lead to inappropriate classifications or services, thus evaluators should include performance validity tests during assessments.

Interventions and Accommodations

Interventions and accommodations should be designed in consultation with vision, audiology, speech/language, and orientation/mobility specialists. Support for individuals who are DHH include hearing aids, amplification systems, augmentative communication devices, and speech/language services (Pingale & Fletcher, 2022). Accommodations for VI include corrective lenses, special lighting, preferential seating, use of audiobooks, oral administration, and speech-to-text technology. Additional supports may include extended time on tasks/tests, scheduled breaks for eye fatigue, multisensory/multimodal teaching, reduced workload, maintaining a consistent environment (e.g., avoid re-arranging tables, desk, chairs, supplies), and possibly Braille instruction. Adapted physical education, ensuring safety during transitions, and adult assistance during drills and emergency situations should be considered. Additional academic supports may be needed based on the child's cognitive profile. School personnel should work collaboratively with each child's family to ensure appropriate supports and resources.

Resources

Children's Tumor Foundation: ctf.org

Neurofibromatosis Network: nfnetwork.org

References

Acosta, M. T., Gioia, G. A., & Silva, A. J. (2006). Neurofibromatosis type 1: New insights into neurocognitive issues. *Current Neurology and Neuroscience Reports*, 6(2), 136–143. https://doi.org/10.1007/s11910-996-0036-5.

Alkatan, H. M., Bakry, S. S., Alabduljabbar, A. (2020). Ocular findings in neurofibromatosis. In F. Signorelli & R. Messina (Eds), *Neurofibromatosis: Current trends and future directions* (pp. 73–82). IntechOpen.

Allanson, J. E., Upadhyaya, M., Watson, G. H., Partington, M., MacKenzie, A., Lahey, D., MacLeod, H., Sarfarazi, M., Broadhead, W., & Harper, P. S. (1991). Watson syndrome: Is it a subtype of type 1 neurofibromatosis? *Journal of Medical Genetics*, 28(11), 752–756. https://doi.org/10.1136/jmg.28.11.752.

Anderson, J. L., & Gutmann, D. H. (2015). Neurofibromatosis type I. In M. P. Islam & E. S. Roach (Eds), *Handbook of clinical neurology (Vol. 132): Neurocutaneous syndromes* (1st ed., pp. 75–86). Elsevier. https://doi.org/10.1016/B978-0-444-62702-5.00004-4.

Avery, R. A., Fisher, M. J., & Liu, G. T. (2011). Optic pathway gliomas. *Journal of Neuro-ophthalmology*, 31(3), 269–278. doi:10.1097/WNO.0b013e31822aef82.

Barisa, M. T. (2020). Mood disorders: Depression, mania, and anxiety. In K. J. Stucky, M. W. Kirkwood, & J. Donders (Eds), *Clinical neuropsychology dtudy guide and board review* (pp. 639–667). Oxford University Press.

Baudou, E., Nemmi, F., Biotteau, M., Maziero, S., Peran, P., & Chaix, Y. (2020). Can the cognitive phenotype in neurofibromatosis type 1 (NF1) be explained by neuroimaging? A review. *Frontiers in Neurology*, 10, 1373. https://doi.org/10.3389/fneur.2019.01373.

Beaussart, M., Barbarot, S., Mauger, C., & Roy, A. (2018). Systematic review and meta-analysis of executive functions in preschool and school-age children with neurofibromatosis type 1. *Journal of the International Neuropsychological Society*, 24(9), 977–994. https://doi.org/10.1017/S1355617718000383.

Blakeley, J. O., Evans, D. G., Adler, J., Brackmann, D. E., Chen, R., Ferner, R. E., Hanemann, C. O., Harris, G., Huson, S. M., Jacob, A., Kalamaridès, M., Karajannis, M. A., Korf, B. R., Mautner, V., McClatchey, A. I., Miao, H., Plotkin, S. R., Slattery, W. H., Stemmer-Rachamimov, A., … Giovannini, M. (2011). Consensus recommendations for current treatments and accelerating clinical trials for patients with neurofibromatosis type 2. *American Journal of Medical Genetics: Part A*, 158(1), 24–41. https://doi.org/10.1002/ajmg.a.34359.

Bulgheroni, S., Taddei, M., Saletti, V., Esposito, S., Micheli, R., & Riva, D. (2019). Visuoperceptual impairment in children with NF1: From early visual processing to procedural strategies. *Behavioural Neurology, 2019*, 1–10. https://doi.org/10.1155/2019/7146168.

Chaix, Y., Lauwers-Cancès, V., Faure-Marie, N., Gentil, C., Lelong, S., Schweitzer, E., Rodriguez, D., Iannuzzi, S., Kemlin, I., Dorison, N., Rivier, F., Carniero, M., Preclaire, E., Barbarot, S., Lion-François, L., & Castelnau, P. (2017). Deficit in phonological processes: A characteristic of the neuropsychological profile of children with NF1. *Child Neuropsychology*, 24(4), 558–574. https://doi.org/10.1080/09297049.2017.1313970.

Champion, J. A., Rose, K. J., Payne, J. M., Burns, J., & North, K. N. (2014). Relationship between cognitive dysfunction, gait, and motor impairment in children and adolescents with neurofibromatosis type 1. *Developmental Medicine and Child Neurology*, 56(5), 468–474. https://doi.org/10.1111/dmcn.12361.

Children's Tumor Foundation (2024). *NF2-related schwannomatosis.* Retrieved October 4, 2024 from https://www.ctf.org/understanding-nf/nf2/.

Coy, S., Rashid, R., Stemmer-Rachamimov, A., & Santagata, S. (2019). An update on the CNS manifestations of neurofibromatosis type 2. *Acta Neuropathologica*, 139(4), 643–665.

Crow, A. J. D., Janssen, J. M., Marshall, C., Moffit, A., Brennan, L., Kohler, C. G., Roalf, D. R., & Moberg, P. J. (2022). A systematic review and meta-analysis of intellectual, neuropsychological, and psychoeducational functioning in neurofibromatosis type 1. *American Journal of Medical Genetics. Part A*, 188(8), 2277–2292. https://doi.org/10.1002/ajmg.a.62773.

Deep, N. L., Patel, E. J., Shapiro, W. H., Waltzman, S. B., Jethanamest, D., McMenomey, S. O., Roland, J. T., & Friedmann, D. R. (2020). Cochlear implant outcomes in neurofibromatosis Type 2: Implications for management. *Otology & Neurotology*, 42(4), 540–548. doi:10.1097/MAO.0000000000002994.

Di Stasi, M., Cocozza, S., Buccino, S., Paolella, C., Di Napoli, L., D'Amico, A., Melis, D., Ugga, L., Villano, G., Ruocco, M., Scala, I., Brunetti, A., & Elefante, A. (2023). The role of unidentified bright objects in the neurocognitive profile of neurofibromatosis type 1 children: A volumetric MRI analysis. *Acta Neurologica Belgica*, 124(1), 223–230. https://doi.org/10.1007/s13760-023-02381-0.

Domon-Archambault, V., Gagnon, L., Benoît, A., & Perreault, S. (2018). Psychosocial features of neurofibromatosis type 1 in children and adolescents. *Journal of Child Neurology*, 33(3), 225–232. https://doi.org/10.1177/0883073817749367.

Eby, N. S., Griffith, J. L., Gutmann, D. H., & Morris, S. M. (2019). Adaptive functioning in children with neurofibromatosis type 1: Relationship to cognition, behavior, and magnetic resonance imaging. *Developmental Medicine and Child Neurology*, 61(8), 972–978. https://doi.org/10.1111/dmcn.14144.

Ejerskov, C., Raundahl, M., Gregersen, P. A., & Handrup, M. M. (2021). Clinical features and disease severity in patients with mosaic neurofibromatosis type 1: A single-center study and literature review. *Orphanet Journal of Rare Diseases*, 16(1), 1–9.

Evans, D. G. R. (2023). *NF2-related schwannomatosis*. GeneReviews. NCBI Bookshelf. https://www.ncbi.nlm.nih.gov/books/NBK1201/.

Evans, D. G. R., Baser, M. E., McGaughran, J., Sharif, S., Howard, E., & Moran, A. (2002). Malignant peripheral nerve sheath tumors in neurofibromatosis 1. *Journal of Medical Genetics*, 39(5), 311–314. https://doi.org/10.1136/jmg.39.5.311.

Ferner, R. E., Huson, S. M., Thomas, N., Moss, C., Willshaw, H., Evans, D. G., Upadhyaya, M., Towers, R., Gleeson, M., Steiger, C., & Kirby, A. (2006). Guidelines for the diagnosis and management of individuals with neurofibromatosis 1. *Journal of Medical Genetics*, 44(2), 81–88. https://doi.org/10.1136/jmg.2006.045906.

Fisher, M. J., Loguidice, M., Gutmann, D. H., Listernick, R., Ferner, R. E., Ullrich, N. J., Packer, R. J., Tabori, U., Hoffman, R. O., Ardern-Holmes, S. L., Hummel, T. R., Hargrave, D. R., Bouffet, E., Charrow, J., Bilaniuk, L. T., Balcer, L. J., & Liu, G. T. (2012). Visual outcomes in children with neurofibromatosis type 1-associated optic pathway glioma following chemotherapy: A multicenter retrospective analysis. *Neuro-oncology*, 14(6), 790–797. https://doi.org/10.1093/neuonc/nos076.

Forde, C., King, A. T., Rutherford, S. A., Hammerbeck-Ward, C., Lloyd, S. K., Freeman, S. R., Pathmanaban, O. N., Stapleton, E., Thomas, O. M., Laitt, R. D., Stivaros, S., Kilday, J. P., Vassallo, G., McBain, C., Kerrigan, S., Smith, M. J., McCabe, M. G., Harkness, E. F., & Evans, D. G. (2020). Disease course of neurofibromatosis type 2: A 30-year follow-up study of 353 patients seen at a single institution. *Neuro-oncology*, 23(7), 1113–1124. https://doi.org/10.1093/neuonc/noaa284.

Friedman, J. M. (2022). *Neurofibromatosis 1*. GeneReviews. NCBI Bookshelf. https://www.ncbi.nlm.nih.gov/books/.

Gregory, G. E., Islim, A. I., Hannan, C. J., Jones, A. P.., Hammerbeck-Ward, C., Rutherford, S. A., Freeman, S. R., Lloyd, S., Kalamaridès, M., Smith, M. J., Couper, K., McBain, C. A., Jenkinson, M. D., Brough, D., King, A. T., Evans, D. G., & Pathmanaban, O. N. (2023). The clinical, genetic, and immune landscape of meningioma in patients with NF2-schwannomatosis. *Neuro-oncology Advances*, 5(Supplement_1), i94–i104. https://doi.org/10.1093/noajnl/vdac127.

Grenon, G. & Whitaker, R. (2022). Assessing and intervening with children who are deaf and hard of hearing. In D. C. Miller, D. E. Maricle, C. L. Bedford, & J. A. Gettman (Eds), *Best practices in school neuropsychology* (pp. 285–300). John Wiley & Sons.

Gross, A. M., Wolters, P. L., Dombi, E., Baldwin, A., Whitcomb, P., Fisher, M. J., Weiss, B., Kim, A., Bornhorst, M., Shah, A. C., Martin, S., Roderick, M. C., Pichard, D. C., Carbonell, A., Paul, S. M., Therrien, J., Kapustina, O., Heisey,

K., Clapp, D. W., … Widemann, B. C. (2020). Selumetinib in children with inoperable plexiform neurofibromas. *New England Journal of Medicine*, 382(15), 1430–1442. doi:10.1056/NEJMoa1912735.

Haebich, K. M., Pride, N. A., Collins, A., Porter, M., Anderson, V., Maier, A., Darke, H., North, K. N., & Payne, J. M. (2023). Understanding nonliteral language abilities in children with neurofibromatosis type 1. *Neuropsychology*, 37 (8), 872–882. https://doi.org/10.1037/neu0000916.

Halliday, D., Emmanouil, B., & Evans, D. G. R. (2023). Updated protocol for genetic testing, screening, and clinical management of individuals at risk of NF2-related schwannomatosis. *Clinical Genetics*, 103(5), 540–552. https://doi.org/10.1111/cge.14310.

Halliday, D., Emmanouil, B., Vassallo, G., Lascelles, K., Nicholson, J. C., Chandratre, S., Anand, G., Wasik, M., Pretorius, P., Evans, D. G., & Parry, A. (2019). Trends in phenotype in the English paediatric neurofibromatosis type 2 cohort stratified by genetic severity. *Clinical Genetics*, 96(2), 151–162. https://doi.org/10.1111/cge.13551.

Hyman, S. L., Shores, A., & North, K. N. (2005). The nature and frequency of cognitive deficits in children with neurofibromatosis type 1. *Neurology*, 65(7), 1037–1044. https://doi.org/10.1212/01.wnl.0000179303.72345.ce.

Jack, A. S., Durcanova, B., Wright, Z. G., Shah, V., & Jacques, L. (2020). Peripheral nerve tumors in neurofibromatosis 1, neurofibromatosis 2, and schwannomatosis. In F. Signorelli & R. Messina (Eds), *Neurofibromatosis: Current trends and future directions* (pp. 9–30). IntechOpen.

Janusz, J. (2020). Chromosomal and genetic syndromes. In K. J. Stucky, M. W. Kirkwood, & J. Donders (Eds), *Clinical neuropsychology study guide and board review* (pp. 315–344). Oxford University Press.

Joyce, A. W., Dial, J. G., & Dial, C. L. (2022). Assessing and intervening with children who are visually impaired. In D. C. Miller, D. E. Maricle, C. L. Bedford, & J. A. Gettman (Eds), *Best practices in school neuropsychology* (pp. 301–312). John Wiley & Sons.

Kirk, J. W. & Boada, R. (2020). Attention-deficit/hyperactivity disorder. In K. J. Stucky, M. W. Kirkwood, & J. Donders (Eds), *Clinical neuropsychology study guide and board review* (pp. 281–296). Oxford University Press.

Kolesnik, A. M., Jones, E. J. H., Garg, S., Green, J., Charman, T., & Johnson, M. H. (2017). Early development of infants with neurofibromatosis type 1: A case series. *Molecular Autism, 8(1)*, 1–13. https://doi.org/10.1186/s13229-017-0178-0.

Kotch, C., Brosius, S., De Raedt, T., & Fisher, M. J. (2023). Updates in the management of central and peripheral nervous system tumors among patients with neurofibromatosis type 1 and neurofibromatosis type 2. *Pediatric Neurosurgery*, 58(5), 267–280. https://doi.org/10.1159/000529507.

Kresak, J. & Walsh, M. (2016). Neurofibromatosis: A review of NF1, NF2, and schwannomatosis. *Journal of Pediatric Genetics*, 5(2), 98–104. doi:10.1055/s-0036-1579766.

Larrabee, G. J., & Kirkwood, M. (2020). Symptom and performance validity testing. In K. Stucky, M. Kirkwood, & J. Donders (Eds.), *Clinical neuropsychology study guide and board review* (pp. 214–227). Oxford University Press, USA.

Legius, E., Messiaen, L., Wolkenstein, P., Pancza, P., Avery, R. A., Berman, Y., Blakeley, J. O., Babovic-Vuksanovic, D., Cunha, K., Ferner, R. E., Fisher, M., Friedman, J. M., Gutmann, D., Kehrer-Sawatzki, H., Korf, B., Vf, M.,

Peltonen, S., Rauen, K., Riccardi, V., ... Plotkin, S. R. (2021). Revised diagnostic criteria for neurofibromatosis type 1 and Legius syndrome: An international consensus recommendation. *Genetics in Medicine*, 23(8), 1506–1513. https://doi.org/10.1038/s41436-021-01170-5.

Lehtonen, A., Howie, E., Trump, D., & Huson, S. M. (2012). Behaviour in children with neurofibromatosis type 1: Cognition, executive function, attention, emotion, and social competence. *Developmental Medicine and Child Neurology*, 55(2), 111–125. https://doi.org/10.1111/j.1469-8749.2012.04399.x.

Lidzba, K., Granström, S., Lindenau, J., & Mautner, V. (2012). The adverse influence of attention-deficit disorder with or without hyperactivity on cognition in neurofibromatosis type 1. *Developmental Medicine and Child Neurology*, 54(10), 892–897. https://doi.org/10.1111/j.1469-8749.2012.04377.x.

Lieu, J. E. C., Kenna, M., Anne, S., & Davidson, L. (2020). Hearing loss in children: A review. *JAMA*, 324(21), 2195. doi:10.1001/jama.2020.17647.

Listernick, R., Ferner, R. E., Liu, G. T., & Gutmann, D. H. (2007). Optic pathway gliomas in neurofibromatosis 1: Controversies and recommendations. *Annals of Neurology*, 61(3), 189–198. https://doi.org/10.1002/ana.21107.

Listernick, R., Louis, D. N., Packer, R. J., & Gutmann, D. H. (1997). Optic pathway gliomas in children with neurofibromatosis 1: Consensus statement from the NF1 optic pathway glioma task force. *Annals of Neurology*, 41(2), 143–149. https://doi.org/10.1002/ana.410410204.

Mallone, F., Lucchino, L., Giustini, S., Lambiase, A., & Moramarco, A. (2022). An update on choroidal abnormalities and retinal microvascular changes in neurofibromatosis type 1. *Orphanet Journal of Rare Diseases, 17*(1), 223. https://doi.org/10.1186/s13023-022-02369-8.

McNeill, A. M., Hudock, R. L., Foy, A. M. H., Shanley, R., Semrud-Clikeman, M., Pierpont, M. E., Berry, S. A., Sommer, K., Moertel, C. L., & Pierpont, E. I. (2019). Emotional functioning among children with neurofibromatosis type 1 or Noonan syndrome. *American Journal of Medical Genetics. Part A*, 179(12), 2433–2446. https://doi.org/10.1002/ajmg.a.61361.

Messina, R. & Signorelli, F. (2020). Introductory chapter: Neurofibromatosis: Current trends and future directions. In F. Signorelli & R. Messina (Eds), *Neurofibromatosis: Current trends and future directions* (pp. 3–6). IntechOpen.

Miller, D. T., Freedenberg, D., Schorry, E., Ullrich, N. J., Viskochil, D., Korf, B. R., Chen, E., Trotter, T. L., Berry, S. A., Burke, L. W., Geleske, T. A., Hamid, R., Hopkin, R. J., Introne, W. J., Lyons, M. J., Scheuerle, A. E., & Stoler, J. M. (2019). Health supervision for children with neurofibromatosis type 1. *Pediatrics*, 143(5), e20190660. https://doi.org/10.1542/peds.2019-0660.

National Organization for Rare Disorders. (2023, July 31). *NF2-related schwannomatosis: Symptoms, causes, treatment | NORD*. Retrieved October 2, 2024 from https://rarediseases.org/rare-diseases/neurofibromatosis-2/#affected.

Ofluoglu, O., Davidson, R. S., & Dormans, J. P. (2008). Prophylactic bypass grafting and long-term bracing in the management of anterolateral bowing of the tibia and neurofibromatosis 1. *The Journal of Bone and Joint Surgery*, 90 (10), 2126–2134. doi:10.2106/JBJS.G.00272.

Olivier, T. W., Bass, J. K., Ashford, J. M., Beaulieu, R., Scott, S. M., Schreiber, J. E., Palmer, S., Mabbott, D. J., Swain, M. A., Bonner, M., Boyle, R., Chapeiski, M. L., Evankovich, K. D., Armstrong, C. L., Knight, S. J., Wu, S., Onar-Thomas, A., Gajjar, A., & Conklin, H. M. (2019). Cognitive implications of ototoxicity in pediatric patients with embryonal brain tumors. *Journal of Clinical Oncology*, 37(18), 1566–1575. https://doi.org/10.1200/JCO.18.01358.

Packer, R. J., Ater, J., Allen, J., Phillips, P., Geyer, R., Nicholson, H. S., Jakacki, R., Kurczynski, E., Needle, M., Finlay, J., Reaman, G., & Boyett, J. M. (1997). Carboplatin and vincristine chemotherapy for children with newly diagnosed progressive low-grade gliomas. *Journal of Neurosurgery*, 86(5), 747–754. https://doi.org/10.3171/jns.1997.86.5.0747.

Payne, J. M., Walsh, K. S., Pride, N. A., Haebich, K. M., Maier, A., Chisholm, A., Glad, D. M., Casnar, C. L., Rouel, M., Lorenzo, J., Del Castillo, A., North, K. N., & Klein-Tasman, B. (2020). Social skills and autism spectrum disorder symptoms in children with neurofibromatosis type 1: Evidence for clinical trial outcomes. *Developmental Medicine and Child Neurology*, 62(7), 813–819. https://doi.org/10.1111/dmcn.14517.

Pingale, V. & Fletcher, T. (2022). Assessing and intervening with children with sensorimotor impairment. In D. C. Miller, D. E. Maricle, C. L. Bedford, & J. A. Gettman (Eds), *Best practices in school neuropsychology* (pp. 527–540). John Wiley & Sons.

Plotkin, S. R., Messiaen, L., Legius, E., Pancza, P., Avery, R. A., Blakeley, J. O., Babovic-Vuksanovic, D., Ferner, R., Fisher, M. J., Friedman, J. M., Giovannini, M., Gutmann, D. H., Hanemann, C. O., Kalamarides, M., Kehrer-Sawatzki, H., Korf, B. R., Mautner, V-F., MacCollin, M., Papi, L., … Evans, D. G. (2022). Updated diagnostic criteria and nomenclature for neurofibromatosis type 2 and schwannomatosis: An international consensus recommendation. *Genetics in Medicine*, 24(9), 1967–1977. https://doi.org/10.1016/j.gim.2022.05.007.

Potter, B. S. & Mendoza, L. (2019). Cognitive issues experienced by individuals living with neurofibromatosis. In F. Signorelli & R. Messina (Eds), *Neurofibromatosis: Current trends and future directions* (pp. 53–69). IntechOpen.

Pride, N. A., Payne, J. M., & North, K. N. (2012). The impact of ADHD on the cognitive and academic functioning of children with NF1. *Developmental Neuropsychology*, 37(7), 590–600. https://doi.org/10.1080/87565641.2012.695831.

Rietman, A. B., Oostenbrink, R., Bongers, S., Gaukema, E., Van Abeelen, S., Hendriksen, J. G., Looman, C. W. N., De Nijs, P. F. A., & De Wit, M. (2017). Motor problems in children with neurofibromatosis type 1. *Journal of Neurodevelopmental Disorders*, 9(1), 1–10. https://doi.org/10.1186/s11689-017-9198-5.

Rijken, B. F. M., Van Veelen-Vincent, M. L. C., & Mathijssen, I. M. J. (2023). Sphenoid dysplasia in patients with neurofibromatosis type 1: Clinical features and imaging findings including cerebrospinal fluid alterations. *European Journal of Paediatric Neurology*, 42, 28–33. https://doi.org/10.1016/j.ejpn.2022.11.006.

Schwetye, K. E. & Gutmann, D. H. (2014). Cognitive and behavioral problems in children with neurofibromatosis type 1: Challenges and future directions. *Expert Review of Neurotherapeutics*, 14(10), 1139–1152. https://doi.org/10.1586/14737175.2014.953931.

Sievert, A. J. & Fisher, M. J. (2009). Pediatric low-grade gliomas. *Journal of Child Neurology*, 24(11), 1397–1408. https://doi.org/10.1177/0883073809342005.

Staedtke, V., Bai, R., & Blakeley, J. O. (2017). Cancer of the peripheral nerve in neurofibromatosis type 1. *Neurotherapeutics*, 14(2), 298–306. https://doi.org/10.1007/s13311-017-0518-y.

Tabata, M. M., Li, S., Knight, P., Bakker, A., & Sarin, K. Y. (2020). Phenotypic heterogeneity of neurofibromatosis type 1 in a large international registry. *JCI Insight*, 5(16), e136262. doi:10.1172/jci.insight.136262.

Uusitalo, E., Leppävirta, J., Koffert, A., Suominen, S., Vahtera, J., Vahlberg, T., Pöyhönen, M., Peltonen, J., & Peltonen, S. (2015). Incidence and mortality of neurofibromatosis: A total population study in Finland. *Journal of Investigative Dermatology*, 135(3), 904–906. doi:10.1038/jid.2014.465.

Vagge, A., Camicione, P., Capris, C., Sburlati, C., Panarello, S., Calevo, M. G., Traverso, C. E., & Capris, P. (2015). Choroidal abnormalities in neurofibromatosis type 1 detected by near-infrared reflectance imaging in paediatric population. *Acta Ophthalmologica*, 93(8), e667–e671. https://doi.org/10.1111/aos.12750.

Van Eylen, L., Plasschaert, E., Wagemans, J., Boets, B., Legius, E., Steyaert, J., & Noens, I. (2017). Visuoperceptual processing in children with neurofibromatosis type 1: True deficit or artefact? *American Journal of Medical Genetics. Part B, Neuropsychiatric Genetics*, 174(4), 342–358. https://doi.org/10.1002/ajmg.b.32522.

Walsh, K. S., Vélez, J. I., Kardel, P. G., Imas, D. M., Muenke, M., Packer, R. J., Castellanos, F. X., & Acosta, M. T. (2013). Symptomatology of autism spectrum disorder in a population with neurofibromatosis type 1. *Developmental Medicine and Child Neurology*, 55(2), 131–138. https://doi.org/10.1111/dmcn.12038.

Well, L., Jaeger, A., Kehrer-Sawatzki, H., Farschtschi, S., Avanesov, M., Sauer, M., De Sousa, M. T., Bannas, P., Derlin, T., Adam, G., Mautner, V. F., & Salamon, J. M. (2020). The effect of pregnancy on growth-dynamics of neurofibromas in neurofibromatosis type 1. *PloS One*, 15(4), e0232031. https://doi.org/10.1371/journal.pone.0232031.

Wientroub, S. & Grill, F. (2000). Congenital pseudarthrosis of the tibia: Part 1. *Journal of Pediatric Orthopedics B*, 9(1), 1–2.

Section V

Malformations of Brain and Spine

21 Spina Bifida

Jasmine G. Hammer and Carolyn K. Cassill

Introduction

Spina bifida (SB) is a congenital neural tube defect (NTD) of the central nervous system (CNS). From a historical perspective, identification and treatment of SB has come a long way. Prior to 1960, the survival rate for those diagnosed with SB was between 10% and 12%, and treatment was not typically available until 2 years of age. With medical advancements, both the evaluation and treatment of SB has significantly improved. Although SB remains one of the most common birth defects in the United States (approximately 2500 cases annually; Morley et al., 2020), studies estimate that since the addition of mandatory folic acid supplementation in 1998 there has been an approximately 50% reduction in the incidence of NTDs like SB (Code of Federal Regulations Title 21, Food and Drug Administration (FDA), 2023). This has been bolstered by early detection and intervention, oftentimes in utero (Sacco et al., 2019).

SB is typically classified into one of three categories with myelomeningocele being the most severe form of SB, SB with meningocele being the rarest form, and SB occulta being the most common and least severe form (Hassan et al., 2022). The prevalence of SB is 1 in every 2875 births in the United States (approximately 1278 per year). Those who are affected by SB are often at risk for challenges with motor function, reduced or absent sensation in lower extremities, bowel and bladder dysfunction, as well as neurological differences. Together these medical sequelae result in a myriad of difficulties across the lifespan, impacting developmental, educational, occupational, and day-to-day functioning.

Development of NTD

In order to understand defects in neural tube development associated with SB, it is important to understand the processes involved in embryonic development of the CNS (Purves et al., 2012). After fertilization of an egg cell, cells repeatedly multiply until a single layer of cells known as the blastula forms. The next phase is gastrulation, during which the blastula

DOI: 10.4324/9781032703923-26

reorganizes by folding itself to form three layers: the ectoderm (outer layer), mesoderm (middle layer), and endoderm (inner layer). During this stage a transient structure called the notochord also develops, which marks the midline of the developing embryo and is important for subsequent differentiation. The cells of the ectoderm above the notochord (neuroectoderm) later develop into the nervous system, while the remainder of the ectoderm later develops into the epidermis. The neuroectoderm then thickens until it forms the neural plate. Between 16 and 26 days after fertilization, the lateral edges of the neural plate come together and fuse to form the neural tube in a process known as primary neurulation. At the end of primary neurulation, the dorsal aspect of the neural tube (anterior or rostral neuropore) closes to form the neural crest, which later differentiates into the brain and ventricles (Purves et al.). Between days 45–53 of gestation, the caudal portion of the neural tube (caudal neuropore) fuses during secondary neurulation, forming the base of the spinal cord.

NTD encompass a broad category of disorders that occur when the neural tube fails to close. Failure of the anterior neuropore typically results in anencephaly (parts of brain and skull fail to form) and failure of the caudal neuropore typically results in SB (Ravi et al., 2021). NTDs are divided into two groups known as open and closed defects. Open defects involve external protrusions of neural tissue and are typically associated with greater clinical impairment (Avagliano et al., 2019). Closed defects occur when the spinal lesion is covered by skin, meaning neural tissue is not directly exposed and as such less clinical impairment is expected. If the neural tube fails to close at any point, abnormalities in the development of the vertebra leave the spinal cord vulnerable to injury resulting in SB.

Prenatal Identification of SB

Early identification of NTD has been crucial to providing timely treatment and support for those identified with SB and their families. SB can be identified prenatally with a routine screening through ultrasound at 18–22 weeks. Features found on imaging can include abnormalities of the skull (shape) and the cerebral ventricles (e.g., ventriculomegaly-enlargement of the ventricles) (Gotha et al., 2020). Additional differences include abnormalities in the posterior fossa, cerebellar herniation, saccular or cystic lesions, and incomplete closure of the posterior verbal arches or lower extremities of the fetus (Gotha). Often differences are identified during the first trimester and further confirmation is recommended later in gestation. Notably, early screening for SB might not be completed at each prenatal visit, which can result in delayed identification.

Once SB is identified, the mother is referred to a specialist for further evaluation (amniocentesis, neurosonography, or MRI) to confirm the diagnosis. Continued care is often recommended throughout pregnancy. Delivery is often uncomplicated, though 15% to 20% of pregnancies end with premature birth for those with SB (Gotha et al., 2020). Additionally, those with open defects are at risk for the presence of high levels of amniotic fluid, which has a caustic effect, placing the fetus at risk for prolonged exposure to neurotoxins in neural tissues as well as hydrocephalus and nerve loss (Avagliano et al., 2019).

SB starts in embryonic development but is characterized by misclosure of the vertebral arches of the spine. The three most common types of SB are SB occulta, SB with meningocele, and SB with myelomeningocele (Centers for Disease Control and Prevention [CDC], 2023). SB occulta is a closed NTD where a small gap in the spine is present; nothing protrudes from it because the gap is covered by skin. This is considered the mildest type of SB; there are limited to no symptoms observed, and it is not typically associated with significant disabilities (CDC, 2023; National Institute of Neurological Disorders and Stroke, 2023). SB with meningocele is an open NTD where the meninges protrude from openings in the vertebra to form a sac of cerebrospinal fluid (CSF), but the spinal cord remains intact and within the spine. Symptoms that may be observed are lower extremity weakness, and bowel/bladder differences. SB with myelomeningocele is considered the most severe, as part of the spinal cord protrudes into the sac of CSF formed by the protruding meninges, which is often associated with more severe disabilities.

SB most commonly occurs in the lumbosacral spine, with second highest incidence in the cervical spine, and lowest incidence in the thoracic spine (Yiğit et al., 2024). When describing SB, the CDC recommends specifying the location (e.g., cervical, thoracic, lumbosacral) and size of the lesion, as well as the covering (e.g., closed, or open), content (e.g., meningocele, meningocele and spinal cord), and associated anomalies (e.g., hydrocephalus) (Centers for Disease Control and Prevention, 2021).

Associated Genetic, Nutritional, and Medical Comorbidities

Information is limited about genetic contributions related to SB due to the lack of recurrent patterns attributable to a genetic profile. Notably, few incidences of SB have been associated with a specific genetic variant (Gotha et al., 2020). However, via animal studies and human research, several genes have been identified and associated with SB, including the VANGL1 gene, VANGL2 gene, FUZ gene, the CELSR1 gene, and the TBXT gene (Bartsch et al., 2012; Hassan et al., 2022; Lei et al., 2014). Chromosomal anomalies have also been related to SB, such as Trisomy 13 and 18 (Goetzinger et al., 2008; Greene et al., 2009). While there are several isolated genes associated with SB, a combination of several genes contribute to the development of SB. In addition to genetic predispositions, environmental factors are also believed to be contributing or causal factors.

From a nutritional perspective, folate has been strongly associated with NTDs. Folates can be found organically (greens and fruits) as well as synthesized pharmacologically. Folates are not organically formed by humans and must be obtained through diet. It is often recommended for those that are pregnant to take a daily prenatal vitamin with at least 400 mcg of folic acid to decrease the risk of NTD failure (CDC). Research is unclear as to the exact mechanism, but repair of DNA during growth of the neuroepithelium is considered a strong contributor. There are additional factors that may cause neural tube deficits even when taking folate supplements, such as health and diet of the pregnant person. Specifically, research has suggested that maternal consumption of alcohol and caffeine can disrupt the creation of the neural tube (Hassan et al., 2022).

As indicated above, risk factors associated with SB can include environmental factors that have a teratogenic effect, or in other words, impact the production of the neural tube during the embryonic stage. These factors can include nutritional intake during pregnancy, the pregnant person's history of diabetes and obesity, as well as environmental factors including hyperemia and fever (Hassan et al., 2022). For example, hyperglycemia and hyperinsulinemia levels associated with diabetes can result in disruption of the neuroepithelium and neural plate. Research has identified that antiepileptic drugs prescribed during pregnancy can impact embryonic development. Notably, valproate has been found to have the most severe impact compared to other commonly prescribed antiepileptic drugs (e.g., carbamazepine, lamotrigine) (Weston, et al., 2016).

It is critical to acknowledge that resources for pregnant people to obtain the appropriate care may not be accessible for all. Risk factors include, but are not limited to, socioeconomic status, social support, food availability, transportation challenges, access to medical care, and medical literacy. Additionally, disruptions in neural tube development occur very early in pregnancy meaning that an individual may not be aware of the pregnancy, which might impact the timely delivery of intervention or care.

Epidemiology

One of the greatest factors reducing the prevalence of SB is the fortification of grains and cereals with folic acid. This change was approved by the Federal Drug Administration (FDA) in 1996 (Centers for Disease Control and Prevention, 2004; Code of Federal Regulations Title 21, FDA, 2023). The CDC (2004) reported a 31% decline in SB following this mandate, though after this initial decline the rates of SB have remained relatively stable. This pattern has been observed in other countries as well, with reliable decreases in the number of births affected by SB in countries with voluntary or mandatory folic acid supplementation compared to countries without. Decreased rates were observed across race/ethnicity, though the effectiveness of folic acid supplementation appears to be moderated by several sociodemographic factors.

The prevalence of SB remains highest amongst Hispanic births followed by Non-Hispanic White births, with the lowest rate occurring amongst non-Hispanic Black births (Canfield et al., 2014). Less favorable outcomes are associated with individuals diagnosed with SB who identify as male, non-Hispanic Black, and patients without health insurance (Schechter et al., 2015). Review of lifespan tables in 2020 estimated that about 55% of people with SB identify as male. The ability to access treatment, such as fetal surgery, is also dependent on race and ethnic background as well as insurance status; non-Hispanic Whites with commercial insurance have the greatest access to care (Foy et al., 2021).

Although SB is typically thought of as a disorder of early development in young children, as of 2020 approximately 66% of individuals with SB were adults (age 30–80) while approximately 33% were children and young adults (age 0–29) (Briggs, 2022). With more than 75% of people living to adulthood, a lifespan approach is necessary for providing appropriate care (Mukherjee & Pasulka, 2017).

Characteristics and Symptoms

The presentation of SB is broad as symptom type and severity is dependent on size, type, and location of lesion (CDC, 2023; NIH, 2023). All nerves below the lesion are typically affected. SB occulta is typically asymptomatic, though research has demonstrated higher rates of back pain and enuresis compared to populations without NTD (Wenhao et al., 2021). Several brain abnormalities are associated with SB including ventriculomegaly, hydrocephalus, Chiari malformation-Type II (see Chapter 22), abnormal development of the corpus callosum, and anomalies in gyrification. Hydrocephalus resulting in ventriculomegaly can condense the parietal lobe, while Chiari malformation-Type II condenses the cerebellum and brainstem. Hydrocephalus is especially prevalent in SB with myelomeningocele, with 70% to 85% of children requiring placement of a shunt. The standard treatment is surgical placement of a ventriculoperitoneal (VP) shunt (Norkett et al., 2016), though this introduces the risk of shunt malfunction which is dangerous and requires immediate medical attention. Those with VP shunt placement are also at increased risk for seizure.

Secondary complications include tethered cord, neurogenic bladder and bowel, urinary tract infection (UTI), sleep apnea, skin breakdown, and chronic pain. Tethered cord syndrome occurs when the spinal cord is erroneously attached to the surrounding tissue in the spine which can limit mobility. Tethered cord can be corrected with a surgical procedure known as tethered cord release. Neurogenic bowel and bladder occur when nerves that innervate the bowel and bladder from the sacral spine are damaged resulting in reduced sensation and muscle control. The presence of neurogenic bladder and associated treatments (e.g., urethral catheter) increase the risk for UTI and kidney damage (Fairchild et al., 2023). While the mechanism remains unknown, up to 42% of individuals with SB struggle with sleep-related breathing disorders such as sleep apnea (Gunnett et al., 2023). Reduced mobility and the use of orthotics and/or mobility aids increase the risk of skin breakdown and irritation (Morley et al., 2020). Unfortunately, individuals with SB also have a high prevalence of chronic pain (Peterson, Haapala et al., 2021).

Neuropsychological Implications

In light of the neurological impact that can be associated with SB, neuropsychological evaluations are critical to document neurocognitive functioning and guide treatment, interventions, and support for individuals with SB. Additionally, evaluations ensure close monitoring of other neurocognitive differences often associated with SB, such as seizures and hydrocephalus. The following section will further outline neurodevelopmental deficits that are associated with SB. It is critical to note that a clinician should carefully monitor motor functioning of those with SB. In addition, cultural considerations that can alter the neurocognitive profile should also be accounted for such as race/ethnicity and language status.

Intellectual Functioning

Cognitive functioning between individuals is highly variable, although meningocele/myelomeningocele, hydrocephalus, Chiari malformation-Type II, and an abnormal corpus callosum are associated with lower cognitive functioning overall (Lindquist et al., 2022). In the case of myelomeningocele in monolingual people, verbal skills are typically stronger than visuospatial skills. The ability to process information and form connections can be impacted by reduced interhemispheric communication related to agenesis of the corpus callosum (Fletcher & Juranek, 2020).

Verbal and Language Functioning

Tasks that measure vocabulary, grammar, and word recognition are often a relative strength for those with SB (Queally et al., 2020). While language skills are often intact, those with SB can face challenges with reading, reading comprehension, and pragmatic language (Fletcher et al., 2002). In contrast to those who are monolingual English-speakers, those with SB who are multilingual or learning English, often demonstrate relative weaknesses within this area.

Visuospatial Skills

Visuospatial skills are especially impacted when hydrocephalus is present, as associated ventriculomegaly puts increased pressure on the parietal lobe

(Lindquist et al., 2022). This disrupts the dorsal pathway which projects from the primary visual cortex to the parietal lobe, also known as the "where" pathway. This can impact mental rotation and understanding of spatial relationships. Additional challenges associated with the parietal lobe include constructing and integrating information and "seeing the big picture," resulting in difficulties with reading comprehension and application of knowledge to novel problems. Visuospatial skills can be further impacted by difficulties with motor coordination, so motor-free visuospatial tasks are recommended.

Attention/Executive Functioning

Attention difficulties related to SB can be differentiated from ADHD by the absence of impulsivity and hyperactivity, reduced arousal and reaction time, and difficulty switching attention (Lindquist et al., 2022). Common weaknesses include processing speed and automaticity. Executive dysfunction is typically not frontally mediated and is instead associated with impaired development of the midbrain structures, the cerebellum, and posterior pathways needed for stimulus orientation (Queally et al., 2020). Voluntary attention such as inhibition and attention regulation are typically preserved; however, individuals with SB often meet criteria for the inattentive subtype of ADHD.

Memory/Learning

Individuals with hydrocephalus secondary to SB are often at risk for challenges with memory. While aspects of language and vocabulary recall associated with the temporal lobe are largely intact, research suggests that those with SB may have challenges with prospective memory and episodic memory. Notably, when looking at visual memory it is important to assess an individual's motor functioning, as several popular visual memory tasks (e.g., Rey Complex Figure, Wechsler Memory Scale) have a visual motor component. Without this consideration, observed weakness could be conflated due to motor challenges rather than an isolated memory deficit. Thus, it is important that clinicians consider using visual memory tasks that do not have a motor component such as Objects and Places from the Children and Adolescent Memory Profile (ChAMP; Sherman & Brooks, 2015) as well as Picture Memory from the Wide Range Assessment of Memory and Learning, Third Edition (WRAML-3; Adams & Sheslow, 2021).

Motor Functioning

Consistent with CNS impact, those with SB are at increased risk for challenges with motor functioning. These challenges can include gross and fine motor control (e.g., speeded dexterity, and single-hand or bilateral coordination), which can impact writing skills, manipulation of classroom materials and navigation of the environment. Individuals with SB may also demonstrate challenges on other neurocognitive tasks that have a motor component, such as construction or spatial arrangement tasks. For example, when using visual motor processing speed and visual construction tasks (e.g., WISC-V Block Design, KABC-II Triangles), evaluators may need to accommodate for testing or consider a measure with limited to no motor demands.

Academic Functioning

As outlined above, those with SB are at risk for challenges with visuospatial, working memory, processing speed, and motor functioning. From a model of patterns of strengths and weaknesses, these challenges are often associated with deficits in mathematics, reading, and writing. Thus, those with SB may be at increased risk for specific learning disabilities. It is not uncommon for those with attention deficits to also experience secondary challenges with academic functioning.

Emotional/Behavioral Functioning

People of all ages with SB have a high rate of comorbid psychiatric disorders (Peterson, Lin, et al., 2021). Parents of children and adolescents with SB report that their children experience increased psychosocial stress with higher rates of internalization, social challenges, and delayed independence and achievement of developmental milestones. Psychosocial functioning is further impacted by chronic pain and fatigue, which are also associated with high psychiatric comorbidity (Peterson, Haapala et al., 2021; Sattoe & Hilberink, 2023). Comorbidities such as depression and anxiety can exacerbate existing neurocognitive difficulties such as attention and executive function and further impede development of independence. Careful assessment of mood, fatigue, and pain is a necessary part of neuropsychological evaluation of SB to monitor psychosocial health and assess the impact of psychological sequelae on evaluation results. Children often do not have the language or vocabulary to express what they are feeling or experiencing. For younger children or those with developmental delays, pain may be expressed through disruptive behavior. Older children might be able to verbally communicate their experiences but may still be prone to increased irritability and lowered frustration tolerance.

The concept of disability is typically thought of as something that can be observed; however, many of the differences that someone with SB experiences can be considered an "invisible disability" or not apparent to the casual observer. Children with SB who have perceived deficits associated with their condition endorsed a lower quality of life. The more complex the presentation of SB and associated symptoms (e.g., hydrocephalus, shunt treatment, bowel impairment), the more impacted their quality of life becomes (Rocque et al., 2015). In addition to the complications associated with a complex medical history, those with SB are at risk for physical differences that impact their ability to conduct day-to-day tasks, such as mobility in their homes or interactions with peers.

Cultural Considerations

Cultural differences can include but are not limited to race/ethnicity, language differences, socioeconomic status, and the identification of having a disability. As indicated above, those with SB often present with visuospatial differences, challenges with attention, and motor differences. In contrast, those from a bilingual background often have visual reasoning skills as their relative strength, with scores on language constructs being lower than expected. When interpreting and providing evaluations for those with SB, it is important to consider how these cultural factors will impact their performance and neurocognitive profile.

Implications for School

The following section addresses implications for the schools and special education considerations related to the IDEA and Section 504 of the Rehabilitation Act of 1973. It is essential that school teams are aware of needs due to SB, such as physical differences, medical conditions associated with SB, pain, and fatigue, as well as neurocognitive deficits that can impact learning, emotional/behavioral functioning, and opportunities to access an appropriate education. Those with SB will likely qualify for modifications and accommodations through the IDEA or Section 504. Children and adolescents with SB often meet criteria for Other Health Impairment/Disability (OHI/OHD), Orthopedic Impairment (OI), or Specific Learning Disability (SLD).

The level of support and services can vary depending on the severity of symptoms associated with SB. For those with a less severe presentation, students may not require modifications to their education; however, students with more severe presentations, such as myelomeningocele, may require more one-on-one instruction or need a more restrictive environment to provide services.

School-Based Interventions/Accommodations

Common accommodations for those with SB include extra time on assignments, taking tests in a distraction-free environment, and other supports to aid with attention challenges. Additional motor accommodations can include not penalizing a student for messy handwriting and assistive technology such as voice-to-text dictation. In terms of gross motor or mobility differences, those with SB can benefit from adaptive physical education, access to an elevator, and extra passing time between classes. As indicated above, the modification of services can vary, but can include small group academic instruction, direct services, as well as emotional behavioral support from a mental health provider. Given frequent medical appointments, those with SB may benefit from modification to their attendance requirement or homework/make-up work policies. Lastly, there should be consideration regarding fatigue and pain for the student, such as a modified number of assignments or modifying an academic schedule to have challenging classes in the morning.

Those with SB may benefit from an Individualized Health Care Plan (IHP) to ensure that the educational team is aware of health concerns. An IHP provides an established plan to support the student in the case of possible seizures, bowel/bladder dysfunction, signs of a VP shunt malfunction (signs of a shunt malfunction can include sudden behavioral changes, vomiting/nausea, and dizziness) or fatigue and pain.

Resources

Spina Bifida Association: https://www.spinabifidaassociation.org/

Spina Bifida Resource Network: https://thesbrn.org/

Centers of Disease Control and Prevention has free material about Spina Bifida: https://www.cdc.gov/ncbddd/spinabifida/freematerials.html

References

Adams, W. & Sheslow, D. (2021). *Wide range assessment of memory and learning* (3rd ed.). Pearson.

Avagliano, L., Massa, V., George, T. M., Qureshy, S., Bulfamante, G., & Finnell, R. H. (2019). Overview on Neural tube defects: From development to physical characteristics. *Birth Defects Research*, 111(19), 1455–1467. https://doi.org/10.1002/bdr2.1380.

Bartsch, O., Kirmes, I., Thiede, A., Lechno, S., Gocan, H., Florian, I. S., Haaf, T., Zechner, U., Sabova, L., & Horn, F. (2012). Novel VANGL1 gene mutations in 144 Slovakian, Romanian and German patients with neural tube defects. *Molecular Syndromology*, 3(2), 76–81. https://doi.org/10.1159/000339668.

Briggs, V. G. (2022). Population estimates of people with spina bifida in the United States in 2020. *medRxiv*. https://doi.org/10.1101/2022.02.03.22268639.

Canfield, M. A., Mai, C. T., Wang, Y., O'Halloran, A., Marengo, L. K., Olney, R. S., Borger, C. L., Rutkowski, R., Fornoff, J., Irwin, N., Copeland, G., Flood, T. J., Meyer, R. E., Rickard, R., Alverson, C. J., Sweatlock, J., & Kirby, R. S. (2014). The association between race/ethnicity and major birth defects in the United States, 1999–2007. *American Journal of Public Health*, 104(9), e14–e23. https://doi.org/10.2105/AJPH.2014.302098.

Centers for Disease Control and Prevention (2004). Spina bifida and anencephaly before and after folic acid mandate—United States, 1995–1996 and 1999–2000. *MMWR. Morbidity and Mortality Weekly Report*, 53(17), 362–365. https://pubmed.ncbi.nlm.nih.gov/15129193/.

Centers for Disease Control and Prevention (2021, March 11). *Spina bifida*. Retrieved June 24, 2024 from https://www.cdc.gov/ncbddd/birthdefects/surveillancemanual/quick-reference-handbook/spinaBifida.html.

Centers for Disease Control and Prevention (2023, October 4). *What is spina bifida?* Retrieved July 7, 2024 from https://www.cdc.gov/ncbddd/spinabifida/facts.html.

Fairchild, R. J., Aksenov, L. I., Hobbs, K. T., Krischak, M. K., Kaplan, S. J., Purves, J. T., Wiener, J. S., & Routh, J. C. (2023). Medical management of neurogenic bladder in patients with spina bifida: A scoping review. *Journal of Pediatric Urology*, 19(1), 55–63. https://doi.org/10.1016/j.jpurol.2022.10.016.

Fletcher, J. M., Barnes, M., & Dennis, M. (2002). Language development in children with spina bifida. *Seminars in Pediatric Neurology*, 9(3), 201–208. https://doi.org/10.1053/spen.2002.35500.

Fletcher, J. M. & Juranek, J. (2020). Spina bifida myelomeningocele: the brain and neuropsychological outcomes. *Clinical Psychology and Special Education*, 9, 1–14. doi:10/17759/cpse.2020090301.

Food and Drug Administration (2023). *Code of Federal Regulations Title 21*. Retrieved July 24, 2024 from https://www.accessdata.fda.gov/scripts/cdrh/cfdocs/cfcfr/ cfrsearch.cfm?fr=101.79.

Foy, A. B., Sawin, K. J., Derflinger, T., Heffelfinger, A. K., Koop, J. I., Cohen, S. S., & Sherburne, E. C. (2021). Sociodemographic disparities in fetal surgery for myelomeningocele: A single-center retrospective review. *Journal of Neurosurgery: Pediatrics*, 29(4), 366–370. https://doi.org/10.3171/2021.7.PEDS20836.

Goetzinger, K. R., Stamilio, D. M., Dicke, J. M., Macones, G. A., & Odibo, A. O. (2008). Evaluating the incidence and likelihood ratios for chromosomal abnormalities in fetuses with common central nervous system malformations. *American Journal of Obstetrics and Gynecology*, 199(3), 285e1–6. https://doi.org/10.1016/j.ajog.2008.06.100.

Gotha, L., Pruthi, V., Abbasi, N., et al. (2020). Fetal spina bifida: What we tell the parents. *Prenatal Diagnosis*, 40, 1499–1507. https://doi.org/10.1002/pd.5802.

Greene, N. D., Stanier, P., & Copp, A. J. (2009). Genetics of human neural tube defects. *Human Molecular Genetics, 18*(R2), R113–R129. https://doi.org/10.1093/hmg/ddp347.

Gunnett, M., Rocque, B. G., Nourani, A., & Beltran-Ale, G. (2023). Impact of spina bifida on sleep quality: Current insights. *Nature and Science of Sleep*, 15, 967–978. https://doi.org/10.2147/NSS.S401269.

Hassan, A. S., Du, Y. L., Lee, S. Y., Wang, A., & Farmer, D. L. (2022). Spina bifida: A review of the genetics, pathophysiology, and emerging cellular therapies. *Journal of Developmental Biology*, 10(2), 22. https://doi.org/10.3390/jdb10020022.

Lei, Y., Zhu, H., Yang, W., Ross, M. E., Shaw, G. M., & Finnell, R. H. (2014). Identification of novel CELSR1 mutations in spina bifida. *PloS one*, 9(3), e92207. https://doi.org/10.1371/journal.pone.0092207.

Lindquist, B., Jacobsson, H., Strinnholm, M., & Peny-Dahlstrand, M. (2022). A scoping review of cognition in spina bifida and its consequences for activity and participation throughout life. *Acta Paediatrica*, 111(9), 1682–1694. https://doi.org/10.1111/apa.16420.

Morley, C. P., Struwe, S., Pratte, M. A., Clayton, G. H., Wilson, P. E., Dicianno, B. E., Formica, M. K., Schad, L. A., Thibadeau, J., & Turk, M. A. (2020). Survey of U.S. adults with spina bifida. *Disability and Health Journal*, 13(2), 100833. https://doi.org/10.1016/j.dhjo.2019.100833.

Mukherjee, S. & Pasulka, J. (2017). Care for adults with spina bifida: Current state and future directions. *Topics in Spinal Cord Injury Rehabilitation*, 23(2), 155–167. https://doi.org/10.1310/sci2302-155.

National Institute of Neurological Disorders and Stroke (2023). *Spina bifida*. Retrieved July 25, 2024 from https://www.ninds.nih.gov/health-information/disorders/spina-bifida.

Norkett, W., McLone, D. G., & Bowman, R. (2016). Current management strategies of hydrocephalus in the child with open spina bifida. *Topics in Spinal Cord Injury Rehabilitation*, 22(4), 241–246. https://doi.org/10.1310/sci2204-241.

Peterson, M. D., Haapala, H., Kamdar, N., Lin, P., & Hurvitz, E. A. (2021). Pain phenotypes among adults living with cerebral palsy and spina bifida. *Pain*, 162 (10), 2532–2538. https://doi.org/10.1097/j.pain.0000000000002240.

Peterson, M. D., Lin, P., Kamdar, N., Mahmoudi, E., Marsack-Topolewski, C. N., Haapala, H., Muraszko, K., & Hurvitz, E. A. (2021). Psychological morbidity among adults with cerebral palsy and spina bifida. *Psychological Medicine*, 51 (4), 694–701. https://doi.org/10.1017/S0033291720001981.

Purves, D., Augustine, G. J., Fitzpatrick, D., Hall, W. C., LaManita, A.-S., & White, L. E. (Eds). (2012). *Neuroscience* (5th ed., pp. xix,820). Sinauer Associates.

Queally, J. T., Barnes, M. A., Castillo, H., Castillo, J., & Fletcher, J. M. (2020). Neuropsychological care guidelines for people with spina bifida. *Journal of Pediatric Rehabilitation Medicine*, 13(4), 663–673. https://doi.org/10.3233/PRM-200761.

Ravi, K. S., Divasha, Hassan, S. B., Pasi, R., Mittra, S., & Kumar, R. (2021). Neural tube defects: Different types and brief review of neurulation process and its clinical implication. *Journal of Family Medicine and Primary Care*, 10(12), 4383–4390. https://doi.org/10.4103/jfmpc.jfmpc_904_21.

Rocque, B. G., Bishop, E. R., Scogin, M. A., Hopson, B. D., Arynchyna, A. A., Boddiford, C. J., Shannon, C. N., & Blount, J. P. (2015). Assessing health-related quality of life in children with spina bifida. *Journal of Neurosurgery: Pediatrics*, 15(2), 144–149. https://doi.org/10.3171/2014.10.PEDS1441.

Sacco, A., Ushakov, F., Thompson, D., Peebles, D., Pandya, P., De Coppi, P., Wimalasundera, R., Attilakos, G., David, A. L., & Deprest, J. (2019). Fetal surgery for open spina bifida. *The Obstetrician & Gynaecologist*, 21(4), 271–282. https://doi.org/10.1111/tog.12603.

Sattoe, J. N. & Hilberink, S. R. (2023). Impairments and comorbidities in adults with cerebral palsy and spina bifida: A meta-analysis. *Frontiers in Neurology*, 14, 1122061. https://www.frontiersin.org/journals/neurology/articles/10.3389/fneur.2023.1122061.

Schechter, M. S., Liu, T., Soe, M., Swanson, M., Ward, E., & Thibadeau, J. (2015). Sociodemographic attributes and spina bifida outcomes. *Pediatrics*, 135(4), e957–e964. https://doi.org/10.1542/peds.2014-2576.

Sherman, E. M. S. & Brooks, B. L. (2015). *Child and adolescent memory profile*. PAR, Inc.

Wenhao, L., Zhencheng, X., Dong, C., Song, J., Zhang, L., Zhou, J., Wang, Y., Yi, P., Yang, F., Tang, X., & Tan, M. (2021). Distribution and imaging characteristics of spina bifida occulta in young people with low back pain. *Journal of Orthopaedic Surgery and Research*, 16, 1–8. https://doi.org/10.1186/s13018-021-02285-w.

Weston, J., Bromley, R., Jackson, C. F., Adab, N., Clayton-Smith, J., Greenhalgh, J., Hounsome, J., McKay, A. J., Tudur Smith, C., & Marson, A. G. (2016). Monotherapy treatment of epilepsy in pregnancy: Congenital malformation outcomes in the child. *The Cochrane Database of Systematic Reviews*, 11(11), CD010224. https://doi.org/10.1002/14651858.CD010224.pub2.

Yiğit, H., Güler, H., Yılmaz, H., Gümü, Ü. Ö., Karaman, Z. F., & Güneş, T. (2024). Effect of cervical and lumbosacral spina bifida cystica on volumes of intracranial structures in children. *Child's Nervous System*, 40(2), 527–535. https://doi.org/10.1007/s00381-023-06153-2.

22 Chiari Malformation

Cortney Bindrich and Ruba Hamad

Introduction

Chiari malformation (CM) is a neurological condition in which there are structural defects in the cerebellum and brainstem (National Institute of Neurological Disorders [NINDS], n.d.) wherein part of the cerebellum extends below the foramen magnum and into the upper spinal canal. Structurally the base of the skull (called the posterior fossa) is where the cerebellum is located. The cerebellum is composed of two halves and a central connecting vermis. The cerebellum sits above the 4th ventricle (filled with cerebral spinal fluid), which is located in front of the cerebellum but behind the brainstem. These structures are just above the foramen magnum, the largest opening at the base of the skull where the spinal cord enters and connects to the brain stem. CM results when the lower part of the brain pushes down into the spinal canal.

The incidence of symptomatic CM is about 1 in 1000 live births and tends to be more prevalent in females; however, about 1 in 100 meet radiological criteria for CM-I (Sadler et al., 2020). CM is considered to be a congenital disorder (i.e., present at birth), but in rare cases, it can be acquired usually as the result of a neurological insult. There is no singular definitive cause for congenital CM (McClugage & Oakes, 2019). Four subtypes of CM are typically identified, with Types I and II being the most common.

Chiari malformation-Type I is the most frequently occurring form and is typically caused by structural defects in the brain and spinal cord that occur during fetal development. It is sometimes called "primary" Chiari malformation (NINDS, n.d.) and commonly presents in pediatric patients with headache, neck or back pain, memory deficits, and non-specific neurological symptoms. Although CM-I is present at birth, the individual may be asymptomatic, or symptoms may not manifest until later childhood or even adulthood. Almost one quarter of individuals with CM-I exhibit no signs or symptoms of the disorder (McClugage & Oakes, 2019). In CM-I, only a small amount of brain tissue (usually the cerebellar tonsils) extrudes into the spinal canal, but it puts pressure on the brainstem and spinal cord and may obstruct the flow of cerebral spinal fluid (CSF). About 25% to 50% of individuals with CM-I have signs that the bones of the skull and spine did not

DOI: 10.4324/9781032703923-27

properly develop in utero. For instance, the cervical vertebrae (usually C^1) may not be completely formed or may be fused to the base of the skull, or the skull itself may be underdeveloped and too small. Additionally, 30% to 50% display compression of the spine into the base of the skull, resulting in compression of the brain stem.

Chiari malformation-Type II (CM-II; previously called Arnold Chiari formation) involves more pronounced abnormalities and is often associated with other congenital anomalies, such as spina bifida (NINDS, n.d.. CM-II has been described as a "migration" of the brain stem, cerebellum, and fourth ventricle through the foramen magnum with a displacement of the spinal cord (Hiremath et al., 2020). This is thought to be a result of the non-closure of the neuropore's caudal end, leading to the exit of cerebrospinal fluid (CSF) from the central nervous system (CNS). The absence of CSF leaves the CNS without a supportive structure for neurodevelopment, resulting in the disorganized development of the CNS, which then results in abnormalities (Hiremath). CM-II is related to the myelomeningocele type of spina bifida and is often identified prenatally via ultrasound or soon after birth. It can be mitigated for some individuals with an in-utero procedure to close the neural tube defect when identified early. (See Chapter 21 for information on spina bifida). CM-II is the type most associated with hydrocephalus. A common problem with CM-II is that there is too much fluid on the brain, which causes the pressure in the brain to increase and the skull bones to expand beyond normal size.

Chiari malformation-Type III (CM-III) typically results in more significant symptomology as the majority of the cerebellum and brain stem herniate into the spinal canal. Indicators of this form of CM appear in infancy and can cause debilitating and life-threatening complications. Babies with CM-III who survive (CM-III is associated with high mortality) have many of the same symptoms as those with CM-II but can also have additional acute neurological defects such as seizures and more severe mental and/or physical delays (NINDS, n.d.).

Chiari malformation-Type IV (CM-IV) is the rarest and most severe form. CM-IV involves an incomplete or underdeveloped cerebellum (a condition known as cerebellar hypoplasia). In this form of CM, the cerebellum is in its normal position, but parts of it are missing, and portions of the skull and spinal cord may be visible (Kennedy Krieger, 2020). Most neonates born with CM-IV do not survive infancy.

Characteristics and Symptoms of CM

The symptoms of CM are quite variable, and some individuals with CM may not show any symptoms at all (Garciá et al., 2023). Additionally, presenting symptoms may change for some individuals, depending on the compression of the tissue and nerves and on the buildup of CSF pressure. Most symptoms of CM can be classified into 3 groups: (1) symptoms related to CSF obstruction; (2) symptoms related to the brainstem or cerebellar compression; and (3) symptoms related to spinal cord dysfunction or syringomyelia (McClugage & Oakes, 2019). Pediatric patients are more likely to present with signs of brainstem dysfunction. Symptoms may include severe headache and neck pain (particularly occipital headaches), hearing or balance problems, muscle weakness or numbness (such as loss of pain and temperature sensation in the arms and hands), dizziness, difficulty swallowing or speaking (slurred speech), vomiting, ringing in the ears, curvature of the spine, insomnia or sleep apnea, problems with coordination or fine motor skills (spasticity and drop attacks), excessive drooling, difficulty eating and an inability to gain weight (NINDS, n.d.). Abnormalities impacting the eyes can also affect individuals with CM, including double vision (diplopia), abnormal sensitivity to light (photophobia), blurred vision, involuntary eye movements (nystagmus) and pain behind the eyes. Overall, the most common symptom is headaches, defined by intense pressure in the back of the head, which is aggravated by exercise, strain, coughing, sneezing, or laughing. In very young children, trouble swallowing is usually the most frequent symptom.

As previously noted, CM-II is commonly accompanied by myelomeningocele and usually results in partial or complete paralysis below the spinal opening. CM-II can cause a variety of symptoms, which can impact each individual differently. Symptoms, in addition to those listed above for CM-I, may include light sensitivity, ringing and pressure in the ears, balance issues, brain fog, and a profound mental health effect (Garciá et al., 2023). In some cases, neuropsychiatric manifestations may include impulsiveness, disinhibition, lability, agitation, panic, anhedonia, dysphoria, anxiety, and depression. Personality changes sometimes seen in children and adolescents with CM may include the flattening or blunting of affect, disinhibited behaviors (i.e. over-familiarity, flamboyance, impulsivity), or obsessive-compulsive behaviors. Some children may experience trouble swallowing, chronic cough, gagging, reflux, and hoarseness, and adolescents may exhibit scoliosis (Garcia). In infants, parents have observed seizures, developmental delays, and head banging.

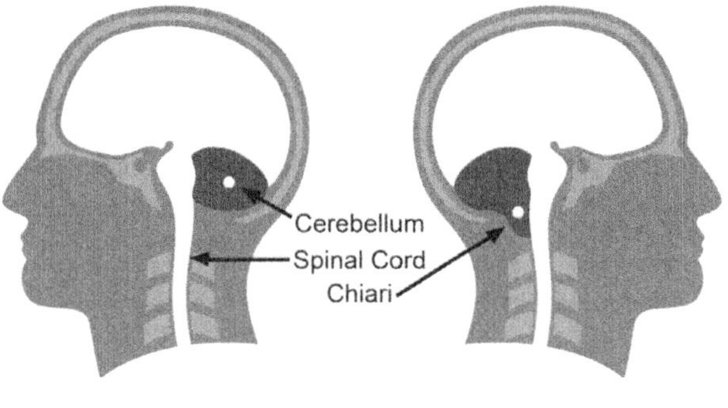

Figure 22.1
Source: Adapted from Conquer Chiari, n.d.

Neuropsychological Profile and Implications

The neuropsychological impact of CM includes cognitive impairments, motor dysfunction, sensory abnormalities, speech and swallowing difficulties, behavioral and emotional challenges, and educational implications.

Cognitive Functioning

Our understanding of the cerebellum, its role, and its functions has changed dramatically in the last 10 years. Clinical research has found that the cerebellum is more interconnected with cortical areas than previously thought and, thus, more related to cognitive functioning, especially in five major areas: executive functions, memory consolidation, spatial cognition, language, and personality. When cognitive functioning is affected, it appears to impact attention, executive functions, visual–spatial abilities, episodic memory, and processing speed the most. Evidence for significant neuropsychological dysfunction in patients with CM-I is scarce. Almotairi and colleagues (2020) noted that individuals with CM-I who underwent neuropsychological evaluations generally demonstrated cognitive functioning within the normal range; however, individuals with CM-II, III, and IV tend to experience more severe cognitive difficulties including problems with attention, memory, and executive functions. Individuals with CM-II have been found to perform significantly lower than normative individuals (Vinck, et al. 2006). Cognitive abilities often predict academic success (Nesayan et al., 2019) and the cognitive impairments experienced from CM can affect academic performance, daily activities, and overall quality of life. Difficulties with processing auditory information and language usage; visual perception, sensory integration, and handwriting (dysgraphia) or math reasoning; and challenges with inattention, distractibility, and organization are common (Kennedy Krieger, n.d.). Children with CM-II most often experience learning difficulties related to language, concentration, and organization (Conquer Chiari, 2006). Individuals with CM-III and CM-IV tend to have very severe cognitive deficits and often meet the criteria for intellectual disability (ID).

A confounding factor in addressing the neurocognitive sequelae of CM is that the surgery used to treat some incidences of CM can also contribute to neurocognitive deficits, such as problems with attention (inattentiveness and distractibility), problems with memory (both visual and verbal), problems with executive functioning (planning and task completion), problems with information processing and processing speed, problems with visual–spatial tasks, and problems with auditory processing (Garciá et al., 2023).

Motor Functioning

The cerebellum plays a crucial role in motor coordination and control, and it is often highly impacted by CM. Motor dysfunction may present itself as problems with balance, coordination, fine motor skills, and muscle strength (Salman et al. 2016). These challenges can affect activities such as walking, writing, and other fine and gross motor tasks. Clinical myelopathy (sensory/autonomic disorders, motor weakness) can result from direct compression of the cervical spinal cord by the herniated cerebellar tonsils or can be due to the presence of a syrinx, reported in association with CM-I in 35% to 75% of pediatric patients (Ciaramitaro et al., 2019). Syrinx (syringomyelia) is a fluid-filled cyst that forms within the spinal cord. The cyst fills with CSF, swells, and puts pressure on the spinal cord, affecting neuromuscular functions and resulting in limb weakness or difficulty walking or breathing.

Speech

The brainstem controls vital functions including swallowing, breathing, and speaking. Although clinical evidence suggests speech may be affected in terms of articulation, fluency, or voice modulation (Conquer Chiari, n. d.), the research on cognitive symptoms such as verbal fluency is scant. Generally, a child with CM may display hoarseness, trouble speaking, or problems with verbal fluency (dysarthria), swallowing/choking difficulties (dysphagia), and sometimes difficulty breathing (dyspnea). In young children with CM-I, oropharyngeal dysfunction, namely dysphagia, reflux, and dyspnea, are common presenting symptoms (Hazkani et al., 2023).

Mental Health

Individuals with chronic health issues are at a higher risk of being diagnosed with a mental illness (Lázaro et al., 2018) and individuals with CM are no exception. These individuals experience challenges most of their peers do not, and this, along with pain and the impact of neurological deficits, can contribute to emotional and behavioral challenges. Individuals with CM may experience mood disorders, anxiety, and difficulties coping with the demands of their condition. A 2018 study by Lazaro and colleagues found that when assessed for anxiety and depression, individuals with CM, regardless of type, exhibited significantly higher scores in the area of anxiety.

Diagnosis of CM

CM-1 can often go undetected due to its frequent benign presentation. Clinical diagnosis of CM is based upon identification of characteristic symptoms, a detailed patient history, a thorough clinical evaluation, and a neurological exam. Imaging techniques may include magnetic resonance imaging (MRI), cine MRI (a type of MRI sequence acquired to capture motion) and plain X-rays. An MRI can reveal excess CSF and loss of neural tissue. A cine MRI is like a traditional MRI but can be used to measure and assess CSF flow. A plain X-ray can reveal skeletal malformations such as skull defects, abnormalities of cervical vertebrae or abnormal curvature or abnormal motion of the spine. Computed tomography (CT) scans may be helpful in clarifying congenital bony abnormalities at the skull base. Additional tests assess other complications associated with a CM, for example, a swallowing test to assess how well someone can drink fluids or swallow thickened food, or sleep studies to detect sleep disorders potentially associated with CM.

Treatment Approaches for CM

Treatment of CM is directed toward the specific symptoms that are unique to each individual. Treatment may require the coordinated efforts of a team of specialists such as pediatricians, neurosurgeons, neurologists, eye specialists (ophthalmologists), and other healthcare or educational professionals. Treatment procedures and interventions may vary depending upon numerous factors such as disease progression, the presence or absence of certain symptoms, the relationship of the malformation to the main physical symptoms, the impact of symptoms on the overall quality of life, an individual's age and general health, and/or other elements. There is no universal, agreed-upon therapy or treatment regimen (Spazzapan et al., 2021).

Generally, individuals who are asymptomatic are not treated but are regularly monitored to see whether the disorder progresses. If mild symptoms are present, such as neck pain or headaches, conservative treatment such as pain medications, massage therapy, or a reduction in activities, particularly those involving heavy lifting or straining, might be recommended. Physical therapy may be tried in some cases.

Symptomatic CM is most often treated by surgery. There are no specific criteria or objective tests that can be used to determine when to undergo surgery or the best procedures to choose. The most common surgery is known as posterior fossa decompression (Spazzapan et al., 2021). With this procedure, a surgeon creates room by removing small pieces of bone in the back of the skull, thereby enlarging the foramen magnum. This relieves pressure and reduces compression on the brainstem and may allow the cerebellar tonsils to move back to a more normal position. Surgical treatment of CM has variable results; some individuals experience significant improvement, whereas others may have symptoms that persist including residual pain, muscle weakness, and loss of sensation.

Individuals with hydrocephalus may be treated by the implantation of a tube (shunt) to drain excessive cerebrospinal fluid away from the skull and brain to another part of the body where the CSF can be absorbed. In some cases, shunts may relieve CSF pressure and improve symptoms. The procedure is often an endoscopic ventriculostomy (EVT) where CSF is drained from the 3rd ventricle or via retroperitoneal shunting (shunt from the ventricles into the peritoneal cavity).

A myelomeningocele, which is usually associated with CM-II, also requires surgical repair. Syringomyelia usually does not require direct treatment. In most cases, syringomyelia improves on its own after surgery to correct a Chiari malformation because the normal flow of cerebrospinal fluid is restored. However, the presence of syringomyelia is the most important criterion for determining the necessity of surgery in asymptomatic children. The size and location of the cyst determines the neurological sequelae experienced by the individual; for instance, if centrally located, it is more likely to see sensory disturbances, but if posteriorly located, the primary presentation may be burning pain (McClugage & Oakes, 2019). Occasionally, if the spinal cord is abnormally attached or fused to the skull, an untethering procedure will be implemented.

Educational Considerations

Not all children with CM will meet the criteria for service under the Individuals with Disabilities Education Act (IDEA), but most (unless they are asymptomatic) will qualify for accommodations under Section 504 of the Rehabilitation Act of 1973 (Oró, 2012). The IDEA classification that is most relevant is likely to be Other Health Impairment (OHI), although some children my qualify under other categories such as Intellectual Disability (ID) or Orthopedic Impairment (OI). Regardless of whether it is an IEP or 504 Accommodation Plan, children with CM should have an Individual Health Plan (IHP) in place that outlines how their health condition is to be managed in the school setting.

When serving a student who is diagnosed with CM, it is important to keep in mind the neuropsychological implications of the diagnosis. Children with CM may face challenges in the educational setting due to cognitive, motor, social, and emotional difficulties. These factors can impact academic achievement, and individuals may require special accommodation or educational support. Additionally, when considering the cognitive and academic impacts on individuals with CM, it is important to acknowledge that these impacts can be a result of many factors, such as chronic pain, medications, depression, and unrelated conditions (Conquer Chiari, n.d.). It is important to address the whole child and consider their unique experiences and needs. For example, a child with CM may not be able to bend over without becoming lightheaded; may not be able to lift objects without a resulting headache; may not be able to stand or sit for any length of time or be able to walk even a short distance without fatigue or pain; may not be able to engage in strenuous activities such as recess, PE, or sports; and may have difficulties in noisy environments with attention and concentration (Oró, 2012).

Assessment and Support

The majority of pediatric and school psychologists will not be assessing children and adolescents to diagnose CM; however, assessment may be required by such professionals in order to determine eligibility for school services and to provide recommendations for effective and useful interventions, modifications, or accommodations. In such cases, because of the neurological nature of this disorder, a comprehensive neuropsychological evaluation will likely be warranted. Critical to this process will be the pediatric professional's expertise. For instance, ensuring that the multidisciplinary team is aware of the neuropsychological implications of CM will allow for a clear understanding of what testing to administer and what to expect as far as strengths and areas in need of support. Given that a significant portion of children with CM-I are asymptomatic or demonstrate mild diffuse symptoms, a perceptive school psychologist who is knowledgeable regarding CM may hear of a child experiencing headaches, frequent neck and back pain, and diffuse neurological symptoms and rather than attribute these issues to anxiety or something behavioral, may suggest parents consult a neurologist to rule out the possibility of CM. As mentioned earlier, individuals with CM are at higher risk of displaying symptoms of depression and anxiety. Living with a chronic illness is a unique stressor that can have great impacts on emotional and behavioral functioning. It will be important to not only evaluate these areas but also continue to monitor for any signs or symptoms of mental illness.

Given the motor difficulties associated with the diagnosis, some motor and sensory assessments may be conducted by occupational or physical therapists. It is important that psychologists are aware of motor and sensory symptoms of CM, observe and note how they impact assessment and learning, and assure appropriate accommodations during testing.

In school settings, children with CM often need accommodations to support their learning and well-being. Since CM can affect everything from physical coordination to cognitive abilities, accommodations might include things like extra breaks, help with writing tasks, or adjusted workloads. Some children may need modified physical education activities, especially if they experience pain or fatigue. It's also important to consider challenges with attention, memory, or processing speed, which can impact classroom performance. Schools typically develop an IEP (Individualized Education Program) or a 504 Plan to ensure these students get the support they need, adjusting their school day so they can succeed academically and are supported sufficiently.

In order to best support a student with this condition, a team effort with frequent consultation and collaboration is important. The team may consist of the parents, medical team, out-of-school therapeutic services, teachers, special education professionals, and administrators. Clear communication, consistency, and understanding of the student's current symptoms will allow for the best provision of services.

Summary

Chiari Malformation (CM) is a neurological condition where part of the brain, specifically the cerebellum, pushes down into the spinal canal. CM can be present from birth or, in rare cases, can develop later due to a brain or spinal injury. There are four types of CM, with Type I and Type II being the most common. Symptoms vary widely and can include headaches, neck pain, balance issues, and cognitive difficulties. Diagnosis is usually made with imaging tests like MRIs, and treatment often involves surgery to relieve pressure on the brain and spinal cord. School-based assessment, intervention, and support is unique to the individual based on the presenting characteristics and concerns. An excellent resource is Oró (2012) *Taking Chiari to School: A Guide for Parents.*

Resources

Designed for Children/Adolescents

Bandaids & Blackboards (www.lehman.cuny.edu)

Center for Pediatric Pain (www.itdoesnthavetohurt.ca)

Designed for Parents and Professionals

Oró, S. (2012) Taking Chiari to School: A Guide for Parents. C & S Parent Education Foundation (conquerchiari.org).

American Syringomeyelia and Chiari Alliance Project (ASAP.org)

C & S Patient Education Foundation (conquerchiari.org)

Bobby Jones Chiari and Syringomyelia Foundation (bobbyjonescsf.org)

American Association of Neurological Surgeons (www.aans.org/patients/conditions-treatments/chiari-malformation/)

References

Almotairi, F. S., Hellström, P., Skoglund, T., Nilsson, Å. L., & Tisell, M. (2020). Chiari I malformation: Neuropsychological functions and quality of life. *Acta Neurochirurgica*, 162(7), 1575–1582. https://doi.org/10.1007/s00701-019-03897-2.

Ciaramitaro, P., Ferraris, M., Massaro, F., & Garbossa, D. (2019). Clinical diagnosis–part I: What is really caused by Chiari I? *Child's Nervous System*, 35(10), 1673–1679. https://doi.org/10.1007/s00381-019-04206-z.

Conquer Chiari (2006). *Pediatric/08.06: Chiari related memory and learning problems.* Retrieved February 1, 2024 from www.conquerchiari.org/library/index/click/175.

Conquer Chiari (n.d.). *Conquer Chiari.* Retrieved February 1, 2024 from https://www.conquerchiari.org/index.asp.

Garciá, M., Amayra, I., Perez, M., Salguiero, M, Martínez, O., Lopez-Paz, J., & Allen, P. (2023). Cognition in Chiari malformation Type I: An update of a systemic review. *Neuropsychology Review*, 34, 1–22. doi:10.1007/s11065-023-09622-2.

Hazkani, I., Voyles, C., Reddy, K., Alazraki, A. & Raol, N. (2023). The prevalence of Chiari malformation among children with persistent dysphagia. *American Journal of Otolaryngology*, 44(4), 103887. https://doi.org/10.1016/j.amjoto.2023.103887.

Hiremath, S. B., Fitsiori, A., Boto, J., Torres, C., Zakhari, N., Dietemann, J.-L., Meling, T. R., & Vargas, M. I. (2020). The perplexity surrounding Chiari malformations – Are we any wiser now? *American Journal of Neuroradiology*, 41 (11), 1975–1981. https://doi.org/10.3174/ajnr.A6743.

Kennedy Krieger (2020) *Chiari malformation fact sheet*. Retrieved August 25, 2024 from www.kennedykrieger.org/sites/default/files/library/Chiari%20Malformation %20factsheet%202020.pdf.

Kennedy Krieger (n.d.) *Chiari malformation*. Retrieved August 28, 2024 from www.kennedykrieger.org/sites/default/files/library/documents/community/specia lized-health-needs-interagency-collaboration-shnic/factsheets-medical-condi tions/Chiari%20Malformation_0.pdf.

Lázaro, E., García, M., Amayra, I., López-Paz, J.-F., Martínez, O., Pérez, M., Berrocoso, S., Al Rashaida, M., Fernández, P., Rodríguez, A., Jometón, A., & Ruiz, B. (2018). Anxiety and depression in Chiari malformation. *Journal of Integrative Neuroscience*, 17(4), 343–348. https://doi.org/10.31083/j.jin.2018.04.0414.

McClugage, S. G. & Oakes, W. J. (2019). The Chiari I Malformation. *Journal of Neurosurgery*, 24(3), 217–226. https://doi.org/10.3171/2019.5.PEDS18382.

National Institute of Neurological Disorders and Stroke. (NINDS, n.d.). *Chiari malformations information page*. Retrieved August 25, 2024 from https://www.ninds.nih.gov/health-information/disorders/chiari-malformations.

Nesayan, A., Amani, M., & Asadi Gandomani, R. (2019). Cognitive profile of children and its relationship with academic performance. *Basic and Clinical Neuroscience*, 10(2), 165–174. doi:10.32598/bcn.9.10.230.

Oró, S. (2012) *Taking Chiari to school: A guide for parents*. C & S Parent Education Foundation. Retrieved August 15, 2024 from conquerchiari.org.

Sadler, B., Kuensting, T., Strahle, J., Park, T. S., Smythe, M., Limbrick, D. D., Dobbs, M., Hallor, G., & Gurnett, C. A. (2020). Prevelance and impact of underlying diagnosis and comorbidities of Chiari I malformation. *Pediatric Neurology*, 106, 32–37. https://doi.org/10.1016/j.pediatrneurol.2019.12.005.

Salman, M. S. & Tsai, P. (2016). The role of the pediatric cerebellum in motor functions, cognition, and behavior: A clinical perspective. *Neuroimaging Clinics of North America*, 26(3), 317–329. doi:10.1016/j.nic.2016.03.003.

Spazzapan, P., Bosnjak, R., Prestor, B., & Velnar, T. (2021). Chiari malformation in children: An overview. *World Journal of Clinical Cases*, 9(4), 764–773. doi:10.12998/wjcc.v9.i4.764.

Vinck, A., Maassen, B., Mullaart, R., & Rotteveel, J. (2006). Arnold-Chiari-II malformation and cognitive functioning in spina bifida. *Journal of Neurology & Neurosurgy Psychiatry*, 77(9), 1083–1086. https://doi.org/10.1136/jnnp.2005.075887.

23 Cerebral Palsy

Heather Roberts and Angela Shierk

Introduction

William Little first defined cerebral palsy (CP) in 1843, describing spasticity and an injury that occurred during birth. (Pietrzak et al., 2016). Over the years, the definition has evolved to include scientific discoveries and medical advances. Currently, the most widely accepted definition of CP is delineated by Rosenbaum and colleagues (2007):

> Cerebral palsy (CP) describes a group of permanent disorders of the development of movement and posture, causing activity limitation, that are attributed to non-progressive disturbances that occurred in the developing fetal or infant brain. The motor disorders of cerebral palsy are often accompanied by disturbances of sensation, perception, cognition, communication, and behavior, by epilepsy, and by secondary musculoskeletal problems.
>
> (p. 9)

CP is caused by damage to or abnormalities inside the developing brain that disrupt the brain's ability to control movement and maintain posture and balance. CP occurs in 2 to 3 per 1000 live births in the USA and that rate has been stable for decades.

Risk Factors and Etiology

Cerebral palsy is an umbrella term describing multiple heterogeneous presentations. As such, there are many risk factors and etiologies associated with CP, and uncovering the root cause can be complex. Historically, it was thought that CP only developed during the perinatal period and was primarily the result of brain injury or asphyxia during birth. However, current research has demonstrated that damage to the brain can occur during prenatal, perinatal, or postnatal periods (Reddihough & Collins, 2003). Recent evidence has also found genetic and predisposing risk factors. (Sadowska et al., 2020). For example, Lewis and colleagues (2021)

DOI: 10.4324/9781032703923-28

report that genetic etiology is a notable contributor to the development of CP, potentially through both disrupted brain development and dysregulated responses to risk factors. A small number of recurrent genes with strong evidence of pathogenicity have been described. Still, the most common cause of CP is prematurity, which is discussed in Chapter 3. Please see Table 23.1 for causes of cerebral palsy divided by the different natal periods.

Risk factors for CP can be categorized based on when they occur: antenatal (before birth), perinatal (around the time of birth), and postnatal (after birth). The majority of the risk (70%–80%) occurs during the antenatal period. During this time, factors such as premature birth, low birth weight, infections within the womb, multiple pregnancies (like twins or triplets), and pregnancy complications can increase the risk. Premature birth, especially before 37 weeks or with a birth weight under 2.5 kilograms, is a significant risk factor for periventricular leukomalacia (PVL), the leading cause of CP. Careful obstetrical management, including the treatment of conditions like preeclampsia and preterm labor, can help lower the risk of CP (van Lieshout et al., 2017). Risk factors during the perinatal period, which account for about 10% of CP diagnoses, typically involve birth asphyxiation or complications during delivery. The remaining risk factors, which occur postnatally, are often due to non-accidental injury, head trauma, meningitis, or cardiopulmonary arrest (Sadowska et al., 2020).

Clinical Presentation

A variety of tools exist to describe the diverse presentations of children with CP. These tools classify children based on their primary motor type (spasticity, dyskinesia, chorea, and athetosis), functional status, and severity. When classified by the primary motor type, the descriptions generally describe the child's muscle tone. Hypertonia is defined as abnormally increased resistance to externally imposed movement on a

Table 23.1 Possible Causes of Cerebral Palsy Based on Different Natal Periods

Prenatal Causes	*Perinatal Causes*	*Postnatal Causes*
Congenital brain malformations	Hypoxic ischemic encephalopathy (HIE)	Hypoxic ischemic encephalopathy (HIE)
Genetic factors	Kernicterus (bilirubin encephalopathy)	Intraventricular hemorrhage (IVH)
Intrauterine infections	Periventricular leukomalacia (PVL)	Stroke
Intrauterine stroke	Prematurity	
	Stroke	

joint. It may be caused by (1) spasticity, (2) dystonia, (3) rigidity, or (4) a combination. The majority of children with CP present with spasticity or a combination of spasticity and dystonia. Spasticity is a type of CP where muscles are unusually tight and resistant to stretching. This means that the more quickly you try to stretch these muscles, the harder it becomes to move them. Dystonia is a movement disorder where muscles contract in a way that causes unusual, often repetitive movements or postures. These movements usually involve twisting and can be shaky. Dystonia often gets worse with voluntary actions and can cause extra muscle activity in nearby areas.

CP is also described according to the body parts affected by the impaired neurological signals to the motor and sensory nerves that produce impaired movements in the extremities. The distribution of impairment may be referred to as "quadriplegia" when all four limbs are impaired; "triplegia" when three limbs are affected (usually both legs and one arm, or more rarely one leg and both arms); "diplegia" is identified when there is symmetrical stiffness, weakness or lack of mobility on both sides of the body, usually in the lower extremities; and "unilateral or hemiplegia" refers to CP affecting the arm and leg on the same side of the body. Thirty-six percent of children with CP will present with a unilateral difference (Stanley et al., 2000).

Clinical Implications

Impaired signals may lead to the child presenting with a variety of symptoms: (1) lack of muscle coordination; (2) stiff or tight muscles and exaggerated reflexes; (3) weakness in one or more arms or legs; (4) walking on toes, crouched, or scissor gait; (5) variations in muscle tone, either too stiff or too floppy; (6) excessive drooling or difficulties swallowing or speaking; (7) shaking or random involuntary movements; and (8) delays in reaching motor skill milestones.

Current Classification Systems

Due to the heterogeneity and variability in presentation and function, researchers developed four central classification systems to help distinguish the function and activity limitations children demonstrate. The four central systems include tools for gross motor skills, manual abilities, communication, and feeding abilities, (Paulson & Vargus-Adams, 2017). All four classification systems utilize a five-level system, with Level I describing the least severe impairment and Level V describing the most severe. Determination of level is based on performance of everyday activities with an emphasis on usual performance and not capacity performance.

Gross Motor Function Classification System (GMFCS)

The GMFCS was developed to standardize how clinicians and researchers classify gross motor functions of children with CP (Palisano et al., 1997). Children at Level I ambulate typically whereas children at Level V require a wheelchair pushed by a caregiver. In 2007, the GMFCS was expanded to include more definitive age bands: (1) before age 2, (2) 2 to 4 years, (3) age 4 to 6, (4) between ages 6 and 12, and (5) between ages 12 and 18. The use of more specific age ranges gives a clearer and more accurate picture of how a child's movement abilities might change as they grow. By breaking it down into detailed age bands, it helps in understanding and tracking a child's motor skills development more precisely at different stages of their life. This way, parents and doctors can better plan treatments and set realistic goals based on the child's age and abilities. (Palisano et al., 2007).

Manual Ability Classification System (MACS)

People with CP encounter challenges every day when using their hands during play and self-care activities. The hand is used for nearly all activities of daily living: dressing, bathing, eating, and playing. The Manual Abilities Classification System (MACS) describes how children aged 4 to 18 years with CP use their hands during activities of daily living (Eliasson et al., 2006). The classification system reflects the typical performance of the child's hand use throughout the day rather than "their best effort". There are five different levels to the classification system. Level I is the least involved, and children perform activities quite typically. Level V is the most severe, with children having no hand function and, therefore, must rely on others for all care. The Mini-MACS was developed for children 1 to 4 years of age and works similarly to the MACS (Eliasson et al., 2017). The clinician or parent rates how well the child does handling toys or objects. (Eliasson et al.).

Communication Function Classification System (CFCS)

The CFCS classifies children aged 4 to 18 years with CP based on how they communicate during their typical day (Hidecker et al., 2011). The tool can be used for clinical purposes to inform targeted intervention and support research purposes. Clinicians use this system to better understand a child's communication needs and challenges. By knowing the specific level a child is at, they can create more effective communication strategies and choose appropriate tools or therapies to help the child express themselves better. It helps ensure that each child gets the right support for their unique needs. (Barty et al., 2016).

Eating and Drinking Ability Classification System (EDACS)

The EDACS describes the eating and drinking ability of children with CP aged three years and older (Sellers et al., 2014). Impairments from CP may include challenges with bringing food and drink to the mouth. This tool allows clinicians and researchers to better recognize and differentiate the eating and drinking abilities of children with CP.

Early Detection and Assessment for Diagnosis

In 2017, an international committee published guidelines to support early accurate detection and diagnosis of CP (Novak et al., 2017). Before developing the Early Detection Guidelines, CP was typically diagnosed around 12 to 24 months of age (American Academy for Cerebral Palsy and Developmental Medicine [AACPDM] Care Pathway Team, 2020). With the implementation of these new guidelines, children can be diagnosed as early as three months of age. Two algorithms or pathways are recommended for early detection based on the child's age (Novak et al.). The "Newborn Detected Risks" pathway is used for infants under the age of 5 months, and the "Infant Detected Risks" pathway should be used with infants over the age of 5 months.

The "Newborn Detected Risks" pathway uses Prechtl's General Movements Assessment (GM), and magnetic resonance imaging (MRI) to identify damage to the motor areas and to accurately predict CP (AACPDM). Combining neuroimaging, plus abnormal motor function classified as "absent fidgety" on the GM has a sensitivity and specificity value of 97.86% and 99.22%, respectively (Morgan et al., 2019). For infants born at full-term with brain abnormalities, an MRI is recommended to be administered within the first week of life (AACPDM). Overall, using this pathway of the early detection guidelines enables early diagnosis of cerebral palsy at 12 weeks of age with over 95% accuracy.

For infants older than 5 months, the "Infant Detected Risks" pathway is recommended. This pathway includes the Hammersmith Infant Neurological Exam (HINE; Ljungblad et al., 2022), MRI scans, and the Developmental Assessment of Youth and Children (DAYC-2; Voress & Maddox, 2013). The Alberta Infant Motor Scale (AIMS; Piper & Darrah, 1994) or the Neuro Sensory Motor Development Assessment (NSMDA, 2009) can also be used to assess motor function in this pathway. If a child scores lower than 73 on the HINE (at 6, 9, or 12 months) and has an abnormal MRI indicating damage to the motor area, these results accurately predict cerebral palsy 90% of the time (Novak et al., 2017).

There are scenarios when obtaining an MRI of the brain is unsafe or not affordable. Alternative assessments can be used to determine if a CP diagnosis is warranted. These alternative assessments include the HINE, the Test of Infant Motor Performance (TIMP; Campbell, 2012), the

DAYC-2, and the Motor Assessment for Infants (MAI; Chandler et al., 1980). Although these assessments are not as predictively accurate as the recommended pathways, they are safer and more universally accessible (Novak et al., 2017).

Descriptions of Tests and Assessments in the Early Detection Guidelines

Magnetic resonance imaging (MRI) uses a magnetic field to create pictures of internal organs, bones, and muscles. It is a non-invasive way of assessing what is internally happening within people (American Academy of Family Physicians, 2023). An MRI can determine if there is abnormal activity or development within the brain. For example, for a child where CP is suspected, a scan of the brain could determine if there is abnormal brain development or damage to the motor area(s).

Pretchl's General Movements Assessment is a non-invasive early observational assessment used to identify neurological deviations (Glass et al., 2021). It involves a video of the baby lying on their back while they are awake, calm, and alert. The assessment can be completed from birth up to 20 weeks of age (corrected age). In the Newborn pathway, this is the most effective gross motor assessment (AACPDM Care Pathway Team, 2020). The Hammersmith Infant Neurological Exam (HINE) is a standardized exam designed for infants within the adjusted age range of 2 to 24 months. This exam investigates nerve function, reflexes, motor movements, posture, and tone to evaluate for movement disorders (Maitre et al., 2016).

The Development Assessment of Youth and Children, 2nd Edition (DAYC-2; Voress & Maddox, 2013) is an observational and parent report that assesses cognition, communication, socioemotional development, physical development, and adaptive behavior. The assessment can be administered by clinicians within the fields of psychology, education, speech–language pathology, occupational therapy, social work, counseling, or in a field closely related to the intended use of the assessment.

The Alberta Infant Motor Scale (AIMS; Piper & Darrah, 1994) is a performance-based scale that measures an infant's risk for motor delay and the attainment of motor milestones. Childcare professionals who have knowledge of normal motor development can utilize this assessment tool. The assessor observes the child's motor performance in prone, supine, sitting, and standing positions. This tool is suitable to use with children 0–18 months or until the child can walk independently (Eliks & Gajewska, 2022).

The Neuro Sensory Motor Development Assessment (NSMDA) is a standardized assessment used by therapists to assess the motor development of children between the ages of 1 month and 6 years. The test records areas of concern and abnormal or dysfunctional components of movement. The Test of Infant Motor Performance (TIMP; Campbell, 2012) assesses functional motor behavior in early infancy. This assessment is appropriate for infants 34 weeks post-conception to 4 months post-term. The assessment focuses on postural and selective control of movement needed for functional motor performance. The Movement Assessment of Infants (MAI; Chandler et al., 1980) targets infants in the first year of life born at a low birth weight. When administering this assessment, the clinician will test muscle tone, primitive reflexes, automatic reactions, and volitional movement.

Overall, the Early Detection Guidelines provide a systematic process for clinicians to test, examine, and assess children at a young age who present with risk factors for CP. The use of these recommended pathways allows for an earlier diagnosis and provides the opportunity for children and families to receive early intervention at a very young age optimizing neuroplasticity and promoting positive outcomes.

Members of the Care Team

For a child and their family who receive the diagnosis of CP or are identified to be at risk for developing CP, a component of delivering the diagnosis is to provide support, education, and initiate intervention for the child (Novak et al., 2017). Intervention for a child with CP often includes a team of clinicians from multiple disciplines (Krigger, 2006). Key professionals who may be a member of the child's care team include a primary care physician, physiatrist, orthopedic surgeon, neurologist, physical or occupational therapist, speech language pathologist, therapeutic recreational specialist, psychologist, audiologist, ophthalmologist, dietician, special education teacher, diagnostician, assistive technology specialist, and orthotist.

Services in the Educational Setting

Educational interventions, modifications or accommodations for children with cerebral palsy (CP) are essential for optimizing their functional abilities and ensuring an inclusive learning environment. The Individuals with Disabilities Education Act (IDEA) mandates that all children with disabilities receive a free appropriate public education (FAPE). Under IDEA, special education services are provided to children with disabilities from birth through age 21. Children with CP may qualify for these services under the classification of Orthopedic Impairment (OI), which refers to a severe orthopedic condition that negatively impacts the child's educational performance. The process for securing these services involves an Individualized Education Program (IEP) committee, which evaluates the child's needs based on comprehensive assessment data, including documentation from a licensed physician confirming the CP diagnosis.

These services are offered at no cost to the family through the local public school system. They may include special education, related services such as occupational, physical, and speech therapy, adaptive equipment, and supplementary aids and services. For students who do not require an IEP but may still need specific accommodations, a Section 504 Plan can be requested. Section 504 accommodations are designed to ensure equal access and may include provisions such as an elevator pass for students who need to access upper floors, early dismissal from class to navigate hallways without crowds, or alternative response methods like speech-to-text technology.

Overview of Treatment Planning

Assessments and interventions for youth with CP are often guided by the International Classification of Functioning, Disability, and Health Framework (ICF) (WHO, 2001). The ICF is a bio-psycho-social model that includes the domains of body function and structure, activity and participation, and the environment. Each of these domains are important to assess when working with a child with CP. A comprehensive summary of assessment tools across the ICF domains for youth with CP can be found on the National Institute of Neurological Disorders and Strokes (NINDS) Cerebral Palsy Common Data Elements (CP-CDE) website at https://commondataelements.ninds.nih.gov/cerebral%20palsy.

The CP-CDE project was initiated in 2016 as a collaborative effort between NINDS and AACPDM with the aim of providing a resource for researchers and clinicians to collect similar data points when conducting research or providing care (Schiariti et al., 2018). The assessment tools are categorized in the following outcome and endpoint categories: functional outcomes, motor function, participation, cognitive and emotional status, quality of life/patient reported outcomes, spasticity/movement, pain, visual–spatial processing, executive functioning, trunk control/balance, social-emotional functioning, memory, family, and environment, as well as speech, language, and communication. On the website, each assessment tool is accompanied with a Notice of Copyright (NOC) form that provides an overview of the assessment, psychometric properties of the assessment, and information on where to obtain the assessment.

After a comprehensive evaluation is completed, clinicians should share the results of the evaluation with the child/family and collaboratively set goals for intervention. Clinicians can use the "F-Words" framework to discuss and prioritize goal setting when working with the child and their family (Rosenbaum & Gorter, 2012). The "F-Words" include function, family, fitness, fun, friends, and future. The use of this framework can help youth with CP and their families use a broader perspective to frame what is meaningful and important in their lives, and then develop goals based on these priorities. Once goals are established, the child/family and the clinical team continues to work together to identify barriers and areas in need of improvement that would support goal attainment. When selecting which interventions to use, it is important to select interventions that are evidence based and target problem areas that are specific to the child's goals. Using a goal-driven approach to care provides an opportunity for shared decision-making and collaboration between the child/family and the clinical team (Mastos et al., 2007). The clinical team often needs to collaborate and work together to provide multiple interventions simultaneously to wholistically provide care that addresses all components needed for goal attainment.

Based on a systematic review of interventions for CP conducted by Novak et al. (2020), 33 evidence-based interventions were given a "green light" classification across the categories of motor, early intervention, tone, contracture alignment, pain, sleep, pulmonary, mealtime, drooling, and oral health, communication, cognition, self-care/function, and parent outcomes. A "green light" classification signifies to a clinician that there is adequate evidence to implement the intervention. An additional 134 interventions were classified as "yellow light" positive interventions across the same categories. A "yellow light" positive classification signifies that there is some evidence, and that the clinician should probably implement the intervention, but outcomes and the response of the child should be closely monitored.

The most common interventions that should be considered standard of care for youth with CP include: (1) casting for improving ankle range of motion for weight bearing and/or walking; (2) hip surveillance for maintaining hip joint integrity; (3) bimanual training, constraint-induced movement therapy, context-focused therapy, goal-directed/functional training, and/or home programs for improving motor activities or self-care function; (4) BoNT, diazepam, or selective dorsal rhizotomy for spasticity management; (5) fitness training for aerobic fitness; (6) pressure care for reducing the risk of ulcers; (7) bisphosphonates for improving bone mineral density; and (8) anticonvulsants for managing seizures (Novak et al., 2013). The majority of evidence-based interventions focus on the body function/structure and activity domains of the ICF, and there is a need for developing and testing additional interventions focused on participation and the environment. The diagnosis of CP is very heterogenous, and it is imperative to complete a comprehensive evaluation utilizing assessment across ICF domains, collaborate with the child/family to set intervention goals, and collaboratively work with a clinical team to develop and implement an individualized intervention plan.

Conclusion

CP is the most prevalent childhood-onset physical disability that varies in etiology and severity. Clinicians need to understand the risk factors for CP, the etiologies of CP, the associated impairments that may be present in addition to the motor disorders, the variability of the severity of the impairments and how they impact daily skills, as well as the strengths, abilities, and goals of individuals with CP and their families. Early detection and diagnosis are a key component of optimizing recovery in the early stage of life, and continued medical care, education, support, and resources through childhood and adulthood are necessary for maximizing potential and ensuring a positive quality of life. Because each individual with CP has their own unique needs and abilities, using a collaborative goal-directed approach is essential to providing optimal care for individuals with CP.

Resources, Organizations, and Websites

American Academy of Cerebral Palsy and Developmental Medicine (AACPDM) www.aacpdm.org

Assess Child www.assesschild.com

CanChild https://canchild.ca

Cerebral Palsy Foundation www.yourcpf.org

CP Teaching www.cpteaching.com

GoMove https://gomove.org/en

Manual Ability Classifications System www.macs.nu

NINDS Common Data Elements – Cerebral Palsy https://commondataelements.ninds.nih.gov/cerebral%20palsy

Queensland Cerebral Palsy and Rehabilitation Research Centre https://qcprrc.centre.uq.edu.au/

References

American Academy of Cerebral Palsy and Developmental Medicine (AACPDM) Care Pathway Team (2020, May). *Early Detection of Cerebral Palsy*. Retrieved June 14, 2024, from https://www.aacpdm.org/publications/care-pathways/early-detection-of-cerebral-palsy.

American Academy of Family Physicians (2023, May 5). Magnetic resonance imaging (MRI). *Family Doctor*. Retrieved June 14, 2024, from https://familydoctor.org/magnetic-resonance-imaging-mri/.

Barty, E., Caynes, K., & Johnston, L. M. (2016). Development and reliability of the Functional Communication Classification System for children with cerebral palsy. *Developmental Medicine and Child Neurology*, 58(10), 1036–1041. https://doi.org/10.1111/dmcn.13124.

Campbell, S. K. (2012). *The test of infant motor performance: Test user's manual version 3.0*. Chicago: Infant Motor Performance Scales, LLC.

Centers for Disease Control and Prevention (CDC) (2023, October 6). *Tracking Methods for Cerebral Palsy*. Retrieved June 14, 2024, from https://archive.cdc.gov/www_cdc_gov/ncbddd/cp/research.html.

Chandler, L. S., Andrews, M. S., & Swanson, M. W., (1980). *Movement assessment of infants: A manual.* Rolling Bay, Washington: MAI.

Eliasson, A.C., Krumlinde Sundholm, L., Rösblad, B., Beckung, E., Arner, M., Öhrvall, A.M., & Rosenbaum, P. (2006). The Manual Ability Classification System (MACS) for children with cerebral palsy: Scale development and evidence of validity and reliability. *Developmental Medicine and Child Neurology*, 48(7), 549–554. https://doi.org/10.1017/S0012162206001162.

Eliasson, A. C., Ullenhag, A., Wahlström, U., & Krumlinde-Sundholm, L. (2017). Mini-MACS: Development of the Manual Ability Classification System for children younger than 4 years of age with signs of cerebral palsy. *Developmental Medicine and Child Neurology*, 59(1), 72–78. https://doi.org/10.1111/dmcn.13162.

Eliks, M. & Gajewska, E. (2022). The Alberta infant motor scale: A tool for the assessment of motor aspects of neurodevelopment in infancy and early childhood. *Frontiers in Neurology*, 13, 927502. doi:10.3389/fneur.2022.927502.

Glass, H. C., Li, Y., Gardner, M., Barkovich, A. J., Novak, I., McCulloch, C. E., & Rogers, E. E. (2021). Early identification of cerebral palsy using neonatal MRI and General Movements Assessment in a cohort of high-risk term neonates. *Pediatric Neurology*, 118, 20–25. https://doi.org/10.1016/j.pediatrneurol.2021.02.003.

Hidecker, M. J., Paneth, N., Rosenbaum, P. L., Kent, R. D., Lillie, J., Eulenberg, J. B., Chester, K., Jr, Johnson, B., Michalsen, L., Evatt, M., & Taylor, K. (2011). Developing and validating the Communication Function Classification System for individuals with cerebral palsy. *Developmental Medicine and Child Neurology*, 53(8), 704–710. http://dx.doi.org/10.1111/j.1469-8749.2011.04035.x.

Krigger, K.W. (2006). Cerebral palsy: An overview. *American Family Physician*, 73 (1), 91–100.

Lewis, S. A., Shetty, S., Wilson, B. A., Huang, A. J., Jin, S. C., Smithers-Sheedy, H., Fahey, M. C., & Kruer, M. C. (2021, Jan) Insights from genetic studies of cerebral palsy. *Frontiers in Neurology*, 11, 625428. doi:10.3389/fneur.2020.625428.

Ljungblad U. W., Paulsen, H., Tangeraas, T., & Evensen, K., (2022, May) Reference material for Hammersmith Infant Neurologic Examination Scores based on healthy, term infants age 3–7 months. *Journal of Pediatrics*, 244, 79–85.e12. doi:10.1016/j.jpeds.2022.01.032.

Maitre, N., Chorna, O., Romeo, D., & Guzzetta, A. (2016). Implementation of the Hammersmith Infant Neurological Examination in a high-risk infant follow-up program. *Pediatric Neurology*, 65, 31–38. https://doi.org/10.1016/j.pediatrneurol.2016.09.010.

Mastos, M., Miller, K., Eliasson, A.C., & Imms, C. (2007). Goal-directed training: Linking theories of treatment to clinical practice for improved functional activities in daily life. *Clinical Rehabilitation*, 21(1), 47–55. https://doi.org/10.1177/0269215506073494.

Morgan, C., Romeo, D. M., Chorna, O., Novak, I., Galea, C., Del Secco, S., & Guzzetta, A. (2019).The pooled diagnostic accuracy of neuroimaging, general movements, and neurological examination for diagnosing cerebral palsy early in high-risk infants: A case control study. *Journal of Clinical Medicine*, 8(11), 1879. doi:10.3390/jcm8111879.

Novak, I., McIntyre, S., Morgan, C., Campbell, L., Dark, L., Morton, N., Stumbles, E., Wilson, S. A., & Goldsmith, S. (2013). A systematic review of interventions for children with cerebral palsy: State of the evidence. *Developmental Medicine and Child Neurology*, 55(10), 885–910. https://doi.org/10.1111/dmcn.12246.

Novak, I., Morgan, C., Adde, L., Blackman, J., Boyd, R. N., Brunstrom-Hernandez, J., Cioni, G., Damiano, D., Darrah, J., Eliasson, A. C., de Vries, L.S., Einspieler, C., Fahey, M., Fehlings, D., Ferriero, D. M., Fetters, L., Fiori, S., Forssberg, H., Gordon, A. M., … Badawi, N. (2017). Early, accurate diagnosis and early intervention in cerebral palsy: Advances in diagnosis and treatment. *JAMA Pediatrics*, 171(9), 897–907. doi:10.1001/jamapediatrics.2017.1689.

Novak, I., Morgan, C., Fahey, M., Finch-Edmondson, M., Galea, C., Hines, A., Langdon, K., McNamara, M., Paton, M. C. B., Popat, H., Shore, B., Khamis, A., Stanton, E., Finemore, O. P., Tricks, A., te Velde, A., Dark, L., Morton, N., & Badawi, N. (2020). State of the evidence traffic lights 2019: Systematic review of interventions for preventing and treating children with cerebral palsy. *Current Neurology and Neuroscience Reports*, 20(3), 1–21. https://doi.org/10.1007/s11910-020-1022-z.

NSMDA (2009). *NSMDA physiotherapy assessment for infants and young children*. Retrieved June 14, 2024 from https://www.nsmda.com.au/about.html#%3A~%3Atext%3DTraining%20in%20use%20of%20the%2Can.

Palisano, R., Rosenbaum, P., Bartlett, D., & Livingston, M. (2007). *Gross Motor Classification System Expanded and Revised*. https://canchild.ca/system/tenon/assets/attachments/000/000/058/original/GMFCS-ER_English.pdf.

Palisano, R., Rosenbaum, P., Walter, S., Russell, D., Wood, E., & Galuppi, B. (1997). Development and reliability of a system to classify gross motor function in children with cerebral palsy. *Developmental Medicine and Child Neurology*, 39 (4), 214–223. https://doi.org/10.1111/j.1469-8749.1997.tb07414.x.

Paulson, A. & Vargus-Adams, J. (2017). Overview of four functional classification systems commonly used in cerebral palsy. *Children (Basel, Switzerland)*, 4(4), 30. https://doi.org/10.3390/children4040030.

Pietrzak, K., Gryzbowski, A., & Kaczmarczyk, J. (2016). William John Little (1810–1894). *Journal of Neurology*, 263, 1047–1049. https://doi.org/10.1007/s00415-015-7890-5.

Piper, M. C. & Darrah, J. (1994) *Motor assessment of developing infant*. Philadelphia, PA: Saunders.

Reddihough D. S. & Collins K. J. (2003). The epidemiology and causes of cerebral palsy. *Australian Journal of Physiotherapy*, 49(1), 7–12. https://doi.org/10.1016/S0004-9514(14)60183–60185.

Rosenbaum, P. & Gorter, J.W. (2012). The "F-words" in childhood disability: I swear this is how we should think! *Child: Care, Health and Development*, 38, 457–463. https://doi.org/10.1111/j.1365-2214.2011.01338.x.

Rosenbaum, P., Paneth, N., Leviton, A., Goldstein, M., Bax, M., Damiano, D., Bernard, D., & Jacobsson, B. (2007). A report: The definition and classification of cerebral palsy. April 2006. *Developmental Medicine and Child Neurology*, 109 (suppl 109), 8–14.

Sadowska, M., Sarecka-Hujar, B., & Kopyta, I. (2020). Cerebral palsy: Current opinions on definition, epidemiology, risk factors, classification, and treatment options. *Neuropsychiatric Disease and Treatment*, 16, 1505–1518. https://doi.org/10.2147/NDT.S235165.

Schiariti, V., Fowler, E., Brandenburg, J. E., Levey, E., Mcintyre, S., Sukal-Moulton, T., Ramey, S. L., Rose, J., Sienko, S., Vogtle, L., Feldman, R. S., & Koeing, J. I. (2018). A common data language for clinical research studies: The National Institute of Neurological Disorders and Stroke, and American Academy for

Cerebral Palsy and Developmental Medicine cerebral palsy common data elements version 1.0 recommendations. *Developmental Medicine & Child Neurology*, 60(10), 976–986. https://doi.org/10.1111/dmcn.13723.

Sellers, D., Mandy, A., Pennington, L., Hankins, M., & Morris, C. (2014). Development and reliability of a system to classify the eating and drinking ability of people with cerebral palsy. *Developmental Medicine and Child Neurology*, 56(3), 245–251. https://doi.org/10.1111/dmcn.12352.

Stanley, F. J., Blair, E., & Alberman, E. (2000). Cerebral palsies; Epidemiology and causal pathways. *Clinics in Developmental Medicine*, 151.

van Lieshout, P., Candundo, H., Martino, R., Shin, S., & Barakat-Haddad, C. (2017). Onset factors in cerebral palsy: A systematic review. *Neurotoxicology*, 61, 47–53. https://doi.org/10.1016/j.neuro.2016.03.021.

Voress, J. K. & Maddox, T. (2013). *Developmental assessment of young children* (2nd ed.). Pro-Ed, Inc.

World Health Organization (WHO) (2001). *International classification of functioning, disability, and health* (ICF). WHO, Geneva (www.who.org).

24 Demyelinating Disorders

Ashley Nguyen-Martinez and Christa Hutaff-Lee

Introduction

Pediatric demyelinating disorders refers to immune-mediated diseases caused by demyelination of the central nervous system (CNS). This is thought to happen when the immune system mistakenly attacks the myelin on the brain and/or spinal cord. Myelin is an insulated sheath made up of proteins and fatty substances surrounding nerves that allows for transmission of electrical impulses. This chapter aims to discuss the intricate terrain of pediatric demyelinating disorders, including pediatric onset multiple sclerosis (POMS), acute disseminated encephalomyelitis (ADEM), neuromyelitis optica spectrum disorder (NMOSD), optic neuritis, and transverse myelitis (TM). Recent research has also focused on the role that myelin oligodendrocyte glycoprotein (MOG) plays in demyelinating diseases by understanding the unique contribution of MOG antibody disease (MOGAD). A review of epidemiology, genetic and environmental contributions, diagnostic criteria, clinical, medical, and neuropsychological manifestations, and treatment management strategies for each of the diseases is presented. The chapter ends by reviewing implications for school providers and providing relevant resources. It is important to note that research regarding the disease mechanisms and cognitive outcomes for immune-mediated demyelinating diseases is complicated and has advanced quickly in recent years. Readers are encouraged to consult with review articles in the reference section and online resources to ensure they have access to the most comprehensive, up-to-date information.

Pediatric-Onset Multiple Sclerosis (POMS)

Epidemiology and Genetic and Environmental Contributions

POMS occurs in approximately 2% to 5% of all individuals with MS (Ekmekci, 2017). Research examining prevalence rates of POMs indicates that the female–male ratio increased from 1.2:1 in children younger than 12 years old to 2.8:1 in children older than 12 years old (Jeong et al., 2019). This is a notable change from early research indicating higher

DOI: 10.4324/9781032703923-29

prevalence rates in males prior to onset of puberty. The onset of menarche has been thought to play a role in increasing the rate of POMs in those designated as female at birth (Jeong et al.). Previous research (Belman et al., 2016) has indicated a higher proportion of individuals with POMS who are of African American and Hispanic/Latinx descent. In addition, the study noted a high proportion of second-generation Americans (United States native-born children whose parents were foreign-born) were diagnosed with POMS.

While the precise etiology of POMS is not yet understood, researchers believe that POMS may stem from possible gene–environment interaction when the impact of environmental exposure on disease susceptibility depends on an individual's genetic predisposition. This has been thought to help explain the paradoxical situation where children with a strong genetic predisposition (family history) may still not develop the disease, while others who have less of a genetic risk may develop it. That said, ongoing research on gene studies in individuals with MS has identified an association between the HLA DRB1*1501 gene as a risk factor in both adult and pediatric MS (Gianfrancesco et al., 2018). Various environmental influences have also been identified as potential risk factors for triggering the disease, including certain infections (i.e., Epstein-Barr Virus), living further away from the equator, second-hand cigarette exposure, adolescent obesity, and low levels of vitamin D exposure (Huang et al., 2022).

Diagnosis

MS is considered to have a pediatric onset when symptoms occur prior to the age of 18, with typical age of symptom-onset after age 10 (Jakimovski et al., 2022). Similar to the adult MS population, the diagnosis of POMS is guided by the revised 2017 McDonald Criteria (Thompson et al., 2018), which proposes that an individual meets the criteria for a diagnosis of MS if there is clear evidence of damage to their CNS that is disseminated in time and in space. In other words, there must be damage that has occurred across different time points and in different areas of the CNS. Examination of lesion findings on magnetic resonance imaging (MRI) or the presence of oligoclonal bands in the cerebrospinal fluid collected during spinal taps are common biomarkers used for a MS diagnosis (Filippi et al., 2019). At the time of this chapter's publication, the 2024 revision of the McDonald Criteria was being published. The revised criteria will increase the sensitivity of diagnostic criteria.

Four types of MS have been identified in the adult population: clinically isolated syndrome (CIS), relapsing and remitting MS (RRMS), primary progressive MS, and secondary progressive MS. Individuals who are diagnosed with CIS are thought to exhibit symptoms that are consistent with MS, but they have not met the clinical threshold for the full diagnosis yet (e.g., have only had one episode of symptoms). In the RRMS type, individuals have met diagnostic criteria for POMS, and symptoms ("episodes") occur ("flare-ups") and are subsequently followed by periods of episode remission. There is emerging evidence that primary and secondary progressive MS patterns may not occur in the pediatric population.

Characteristics and Symptoms

Youth with POMS may present differently from one another, with symptomology dependent primarily on the lesion location and lesion burden. On MRI, areas most susceptible to lesions in POMS include the periventricular, cortical or juxtacortical infratentorial brain regions (especially the pons and the cerebellum) and the cervical areas of the spinal cord (Filippi et al., 2019). Lesion burden refers to the cumulative impact of brain lesions observed on MRI. A heavier lesion burden has been associated with greater disability progression in MS.

In general, youth with POMS present with symptoms that are similar to their adult counterparts. Neurological symptoms, such as vision issues (e. g., blurry vision, double vision, optic neuritis) and challenges with bladder control may occur in some youth. Optic neuritis is an inflammation of the optic nerve, which can impact visual abilities, as evidenced by color vision impairment, vision loss, reduced vision sensitivity, and at times pain with eye movement. In addition, sensory symptoms are also common and include paresthesia (i.e., tingling in the hands and feet), weakness in the limbs, loss of balance or coordination, dizziness, and fatigue. In certain severe untreated cases of MS, motor symptoms may be debilitating enough and can lead to paralysis, necessitating the use of wheelchairs. Youth may also present with cognitive or mood/emotional challenges that impact their overall functioning and well-being, as described below.

Medical/Neurological Implications

In comparison to adult-onset MS, youth with POMS may recover better after each relapse. This is thought to be related to neuroplasticity in the pediatric brain and a better rate of myelin repair in youth. That said, providers should be aware that while there is a slower rate of progression toward disability in POMS, longer disease duration and an earlier age of onset have been associated with greater deterioration over time.

In terms of neurological implications, disease progression in POMS may lead to the gradual accumulation of neurological deficits over time, potentially affecting mobility, coordination, sensation, and cognitive function. Although the research is still novel, there have been studies that suggest that youth with POMS may present with reduced brain volume (Bartels et al., 2019; Fuentes et al., 2012; Kerbrat et al., 2012). More disease activity has also been associated with severe brain volume loss (Bartels et al.).

Fatigue is a common symptom in youth, and studies have proposed that at least half of youth with POMS report at least mild levels of fatigue, with a subset experiencing severe fatigue that may impact daily functioning in the home, school, and social settings. Fatigue has been significantly associated with the female gender and depression and can often impact overall quality of life (Storm Van's Gravesande et al., 2019).

Neuropsychological Implications

Approximately one-third of all individuals with POMS display cognitive impairments (MacAllister et al., 2005). Given this, routine screening for cognitive changes in this population has been implemented as part of the standard of care for youth with POMS to detect disease activity, assess treatment effects, and evaluate for the progression of cognitive problems. Cognitive impairment in these children is thought to be due to the demyelinating nature of this disorder, influencing processes like attention, emerging executive functioning skills, and processing speed. In general, youth with POMS are at a higher risk of being diagnosed with attention-deficit/hyperactivity disorder (ADHD). In addition, damage to aspects of visual and motor functions in youth with POMS may contribute to difficulties with visuospatial, fine motor, and visual-motor skills (Tan et al., 2018). Verbal and nonverbal/visual memory weaknesses have also been implicated in this population, although the rate at which this occurs varies across studies and is thought to be partially related to disease duration as well as background characteristics (e.g., socioeconomic status, parental education; Fuentes et al., 2012).

Unlike adult-onset MS, youth with POMS may also report greater challenges in both simple and complex language-based skills, including vocabulary, receptive language, naming, and verbal learning, as well as in language functions more reliant on speed or fluency (Tan et al., 2018). In addition, studies with healthy age-matched controls show that youth with POMS demonstrate lower group means on measures of intellectual quotients (IQ; Tan et al.). The likely difference in comparison to adult cases in terms of language performance is thought to be attributed to the role of development on language, such that the onset of MS may disrupt critical language acquisition processes in children, leading to delays or disruption, whereas these skills are already established in adults.

Researchers have also started to examine factors that shield against cognitive decline in youth with POMS. Higher overall IQ has been identified as a protective factor, with the findings highlighting the potential safeguarding influence of cognitive reserve against neuropsychological decline in youth with POMS (Portaccio et al., 2021). In addition, early diagnosis, and initiation of disease-modifying therapies (DMTs; discussed further below) can help manage disease activity and inflammation, decreasing the risk of cognitive decline. Psychosocial factors such as emotional well-being and social support also play a role in contributing to better cognitive outcomes and overall quality of life, which are discussed further below. A number of targeted batteries have been developed for monitoring potential disease progression in individuals with POMS, although there is not yet a consensus regarding a universal testing battery. Readers are encouraged to read the review article by Oreja-Guevara and colleagues (2019) for more information.

Treatment

Medical Procedures and Pharmacology

Initial neurological symptoms and any subsequent relapses are often treated with high-dose intravenous (IV) steroids followed by disease modifying therapies (DMT). There are several oral DMT treatments for MS in adults; however, research investigating their efficacy in the pediatric population is still ongoing. Most individuals with POMS are currently treated with IV DMTs via infusions every 4 to 6 months. Vitamin D has also been found to be lower in individuals with POMS, and treatment often includes supplemental vitamin D. Improved outcomes have been associated with physical exercise and well-balanced diets. Research is currently investigating treatment with stem-cell transplants.

Acute Disseminated Encephalomyelitis (ADEM)

Epidemiology and Genetic and Environmental Contributions

ADEM is a demyelinating disease affecting the brain, optic nerves, and spinal cord. The exact cause of ADEM is unknown, but it is thought to the result of an environmental trigger. A majority of diagnoses occur after a bacterial or viral infection, although the exact cause is not always identified (Paolilo et al., 2020). ADEM typically affects children with a mean age of onset around 5 to 8 years. There is an estimated 0.07 to 0.9 per 100,000 children affected by ADEM each year. ADEM occurs more often in individuals assigned male at birth, with a male-to-female ratio of 1.3 to 1, and occurs equally in all ethnic groups. ADEM presents as an acute episode of encephalopathy leading to neurological symptoms that can vary depending on the area of the CNS involved. As described in the POMS section above, individuals can present with vision impairment as well as motor and sensory changes. In addition to physical and neurological symptoms, mental status changes (e.g., irritability, confusion, psychosis) are required for a diagnosis of ADEM.

Diagnosis

The International Pediatric Multiple Sclerosis Study Group developed criteria for a clinical diagnosis of ADEM that includes the presence of polyfocal CNS involvement and demyelinating lesions noted on neuroimaging. Neuroimaging results in individuals with ADEM are typically reported to reveal single lesions that vary in size and location, multiple lesions involving the white matter in the periventricular and subcortical regions of the brain, or grey matter involvement of the subcortical cortex. Less frequently occurring lesions in the spinal cord or cerebellum may also be described (Codjia et al., 2019). To distinguish it from POMS, a diagnosis of ADEM also requires the presence of encephalopathy (Krupp et al., 2013). Most episodes of ADEM occur as a single episode (monophasic), although multiphasic episodes have been defined as a second episode of demyelination occurring three months after the first episode. A subset of individuals with multiphasic ADEM have been found to have anti-MOG antibodies.

Medical/Neurological Implications

ADEM symptoms tend to progress rapidly and often require hospitalization for neurological symptoms, including changes in mental status, motor or sensory changes, or other physical symptoms (e.g., confusion, paraparesis, apraxia, aphasia, seizures, etc.). While many of these symptoms can be resolved with treatment, some individuals experience more permanent impairments.

Neuropsychological Implications

Research into cognitive outcomes of children has indicated an increased risk for neurocognitive difficulties in approximately 15% to 22% of children with ADEM (Tan et al., 2018). Attention and processing speed are often the most affected areas. It is important to consider the age of onset when determining an individual's unique risk for neurocognitive deficits. For example, a provider may need to consider the age of symptom onset and potential disruption to development (e.g., involvement of language areas of the brain during key language development ages). Alternatively, it is also important to consider the risk of a child "growing into" deficits. It is well-established that children who experience neurological insults during early development may not present with evidence of cognitive impairment until they are older. This is especially true for later developing cognitive skills such as attention or executive functioning skills.

Treatment

Medical Procedures and Pharmacology

Initial treatment involves intravenous (IV) acyclovir and antibiotics and immunosuppression with high-dose IV glucocorticoids. Some individuals require IV immunoglobulin, plasma exchange, or cyclophosphamide.

Neuromyelitis Optica Spectrum Disorder (NMOSD) or Neuromyelitis Optica

Epidemiology and Genetic and Environmental Contributions

NMOSD, previously known as Devic's disease, is an autoimmune and inflammatory disorder that primarily affects the optic nerves and spinal cord. NMOSD is more prevalent in individuals assigned female at birth, with a median age of onset around 40 years of age. While NMOSD primarily affects adults, approximately 5% of the diagnoses are thought to occur in the pediatric population. NMOSD is also more likely to be diagnosed in individuals from African American or Asian backgrounds. Individuals from diverse backgrounds are at greater risk for earlier diagnosis and increased disease severity. While NMOSD does not typically involve the brain or brainstem, a percentage of individuals will experience involvement in these areas, with those from diverse backgrounds being at high risk for brain/brainstem involvement. Approximately 40% of individuals with NMOSD are thought to carry a genetic risk for the disease associated with FCGR3A gene involvement (Mahaweni et al., 2018).

NMOSD was initially thought to be a rare form of MS as the progressive nature of the neurological symptoms often overlaps with MS; however, NMOSD is now considered a unique diagnosis. A percentage of individuals with NMOSD are initially misdiagnosed with MS due to the overlapping presentation of symptoms.

Diagnosis

In 2015, a diagnostic consensus for NMOSD was developed, outlining the core clinical characteristics and antibody testing necessary for diagnosis (Wingerchuk et al., 2015). Individuals with NMOSD tend to be more significantly affected during the initial and subsequent relapses due to the severity of the neurological involvement and the limited ability of the CNS to recover from neuronal involvement. Individuals with recurrent episodes may experience permanent visual loss, motor involvement including paralysis, bladder dysfunction, respiratory issues, and neuropathic pain.

Medical/Neurological Implications

Aquaporin 4 (AQP4) is a protein in astrocytes that helps regulate water flow to support neuronal function. In most individuals with NMOSD, the immune system develops AQP4 autoantibodies that target AQP4, resulting in damage to neurons and loss of function. A smaller percentage of individuals with NMOSD do not present with these antibodies. Initial neurological symptoms involve changes in vision and motor skills. Individuals with NMOSD experience repeated episodes of neurological insult, resulting in progressive symptoms that can advance over time.

Neuropsychological Implications

Many of the cognitive outcome studies for individuals with NMOSD have involved adults. One pediatric study found an increased risk for difficulties with fine and gross motor skills in approximately half of the sample (Tan et al., 2018). Additionally, vulnerabilities in working memory and aspects of executive functioning (e.g., verbal fluency) were also noted. Individuals in the study were also reported to be at increased risk for internalizing symptoms, including anxiety, depression, and social withdrawal.

Treatment

Medical Procedures and Pharmacology

First-line treatment for NMOSD involves high-dose intravenous steroids. Other potential treatments, including plasma exchange (PLEX), immunoadsorption, and intravenous immunoglobulins (IVIG) therapy, are often used to treat acute attacks. Several other potential treatments are under investigation. Also, many oral or intravenous medications are available to prevent relapse for individuals with NMOSD. Please see the review article by Chan and Lee (2021) for more detailed information.

Transverse Myelitis (TM)

TM is caused by inflammation involving the spinal cord resulting in motor and sensory changes. It can be caused by infections, vascular disorders, parasites, or inflammatory disorders. TM can also be caused by other demyelinating disorders.

Epidemiology and Genetic and Environmental Contributions

About 1400 cases of TM are diagnosed each year, with an estimated 20% occurring in individuals under 18. A recently described potential variant of myelitis, acute flaccid myelitis (AFM), has been identified in children.

AFM presents in children with neurological symptoms including rapid onset of muscle weakness, decreased reflexes, difficulty swallowing, and reduced eye-movement. AFM has been identified in conjunction with the enterovirus D68 (Greenberg et al., 2021).

Diagnosis

TM and AFM are diagnosed through the identification of a lesion in the spinal cord on neuroimaging and medical examination involving blood tests or lumbar punctures to identify potential infectious causes.

Medical/Neurological Implications

Inflammation of the spinal cord can result in motor changes such as paralysis and muscle weakness. Changes in sensation can also result in pain or changes in touch and temperature perception. Individuals with TM are also at increased risk for bladder and bowel dysfunction.

Neuropsychological Implications

Although TM is thought to primarily affect the spinal cord, research has shown an increased risk for neurocognitive and psychiatric concerns. One study found a higher rate of cognitive difficulties, including reduced attention, fluency, and working memory, despite controlling for medication side effects and potential cognitive effects of mental health challenges (e.g., adjustment difficulties, depression, anxiety, and self-esteem issues).

Treatment

Medical Procedures and Pharmacology

Like many of the demyelinating diseases described above, treatment for TM focuses on reducing inflammation in the spinal cord through the use of high-dose intravenous (IV) corticosteroid drugs. Additionally, some individuals will benefit from PLEX therapy (plasmapheresis) and/or IVIG. If needed, treatment for infections may require antiviral medications. Depending on symptom severity, some individuals require pain management strategies.

Psychological Implications of Demyelinating Diseases

Individuals with demyelinating disorders should be screened for mental health symptoms. Depending on the severity of the initial symptoms, individuals may experience symptoms of anxiety or depression. Additionally, fatigue, either directly related to neurological symptoms or secondary to mental health symptoms, can significantly interfere with an individual's ability to participate in everyday life. Evidence-based therapeutic interventions for mood-related concerns are encouraged, with a focus on effective coping strategies. It is also important to consider the effects on the individual and family systems when there is a chronic medical condition diagnosed in early childhood or adolescence. A percentage of individuals may benefit from medication to treat co-occurring psychiatric or attentional disorders.

Implications for the School

It is recommended that individuals with demyelinating diseases be considered for formal academic modifications, accommodations, and/or school-based interventions as needed. During the initial onset of symptoms, individuals will benefit from the quick implementation of academic support. Individuals with demyelinating disorders are often hospitalized for 1 to 2 weeks for treatment after their initial presentation of neurological symptoms. Upon their return, accommodations for fatigue, such as partial school days or increased opportunities for break, should be considered. School personnel are encouraged to implement academic accommodations quickly to support an individual during hospitalization and reduce anxiety related to missed academic work. Due to medically related absences, this may include modifying work expectations or the consideration of waiving some academic expectations. During the initial return to school after hospitalization, an individual will benefit from continuation of academic accommodations for lingering cognitive concerns as well as intervention for any continued neurological symptoms (e.g., academic, speech–language, occupational, or physical therapies). Long-term cognitive outcomes for individuals with demyelinating disorders vary significantly, with a subset of individuals requiring ongoing support due to lingering cognitive difficulties.

Additionally, several disorders are associated with an increased risk for recurrent episodes of neurological symptoms or relapse (e.g., POMS, ADEM). Outside of the acute disease period, individuals with demyelinating diseases often require close medical follow-up. Many individuals will benefit from an additional number of excused absences due to medically related appointments (e.g., medical appointments, MRIs, infusions). Having an established 504 Accommodation Plan, even if an individual is doing well academically, provides a framework for any necessary accommodation during a potentially difficult time for a family. School teams are also encouraged to consider assisting with prioritizing or modifying expectations for make-up work during medically related absences. The most common cognitive vulnerabilities for individuals with demyelinating diseases include attention, executive functioning, and processing speed; however, individuals may not meet formal criteria for a diagnosis of attention-deficit/hyperactivity disorder (ADHD) as defined by the

Diagnostic and Statistical Manual of Mental Disorders, 5th Edition (DSM-5)/*International Classification of Diseases*, 11th Revision (ICD-11). Regardless, they often benefit from accommodations through a 504 Accommodation Plan to support their academic success. Other potential neurological symptoms, including fine/gross motor skills or visual impairments, do not improve with treatment. If related cognitive, motor, vision, or communication deficits are severe enough, school teams would be encouraged to consider formal special educational support through an Individualized Education Program (IEP) under the classification of Other Health Impairment to provide school-based occupational, physical, speech–language, or vision therapies. A subset of individuals may meet criteria for specific learning disabilities in reading, written language, or mathematics, and may benefit from associated interventions and accommodations through an IEP or multi-tiered support system.

Resources

POMS

- The National Multiple Sclerosis Society: www.nationalmssociety.org/
- Rocky Mountain MS Center: www.mscenter.org
- Multiple Sclerosis Association of America: www.mymsaa.org/
- Oscar the MS Monkey: www.mroscarmonkey.org/

ADEM/NMOSD/TM

- The Siegel Rare Neuroimmune Association (SRNA): www.wearesrna.org

References

Bartels, F., Nobis, K., Cooper, G., Wendel, E., Cleaveland, R., Bajer-Kornek, B., Blaschek, A., Schimmel, M., Blankenburg, M., Baumann, M., Karenfort, M., Finke, C., & Rostásy, K. (2019). Childhood multiple sclerosis is associated with reduced brain volumes at first clinical presentation and brain growth failure. *Multiple Sclerosis Journal*, 25(7), 927–936. https://doi.org/10.1177/1352458519829698.

Belman, A. L., Krupp, L. B., Olsen, C. S., Rose, J. W., Aaen, G., Benson, L., Chitnis, T., Gorman, M., Graves, J., Harris, Y., Lotze, T., Ness, J., Rodriguez, M., Tillema, J-M., Waubant, E., Weinstock-Guttman, B., Casper, T. C., & US Network of Pediatric MS Centers (2016). Characteristics of children and adolescents with multiple sclerosis. *Pediatrics*, 138(1), e20160120. https://doi.org/10.1542/peds.2016-0120.

Chan, K-H. & Lee, C-Y. (2021). Treatment of neuromyelitis optica spectrum disorders. *International Journal of Molecular Sciences*, 22(16), 8638. doi:10.3390/ijms22168638.

Codjia, P., Ayrignac, X., Carra-Dalliere, C., Cohen, M., Charif, M., Lippi, A., Collongues, N., Corti, L., De Seze, J., Lebrun, C., Vukusic, S., Durand-Dubief,

F., Labauge, P., SFSEP, & OFSEP (2019). Multiple sclerosis with atypical MRI presentation: Results of a nationwide multicenter study in 57 consecutive cases. *Multiple Sclerosis and Related Disorders*, 28, 109–116. https://doi.org/10.1016/j.msard.2018.12.022.

Ekmekci, O. (2017). Pediatric multiple sclerosis and cognition: A review of clinical, neuropsychologic, and neuroradiologic features. *Behavioral Neurology*, 2017(1), 1463570. https://doi.org/10.1155/2017/1463570.

Filippi, M., Preziosa, P., Banwell, B. L., Barkhof, F., Ciccarelli, O., De Stefano, N., Geurts, J. J. G., Paul, F., Riech, D. S., Toosy, A. T., Traboulsee, A., Wattjes, M. P., Yousry, T. A., Gass, A., Lubetzki, C., Weinhenker, B. G., & Rocca, M. A. (2019). Assessment of lesions on magnetic resonance imaging in multiple sclerosis: Practical guidelines. *Brain*, 142(7), 1858–1875. https://doi.org/10.1093/brain/awz144.

Fuentes, A., Collins, D. L., Garcia-Lorenzo, D., Sled, J. G., Narayanan, S., Arnold, D. L., Banwell, B. L., & Till, C. (2012). Memory performance and normalized regional brain volumes in patients with pediatric-onset multiple sclerosis. *Journal of the International Neuropsychological Society*, 18(3), 471–480. doi:10.1017/S1355617711001913.

Gianfrancesco, M. A., Stridh, P., Shao, X., Rhead, B., Graves, J. S., Chitnis, T., Waldman, A., Lotze, T., Schreiner, T., Beiman, A., Greenberg, B., Weinstock-Guttman, B., Aaen, G., Tillema, J. M., Hart, J., Caillier, S., Ness, J., Harris, Y., Rubin, J., … & Network of Pediatric Multiple Sclerosis Centers (2018). Genetic risk factors for pediatric-onset multiple sclerosis. *Multiple Sclerosis Journal*, 24 (14), 1825–1834. doi:10.1177/1352458517733551.

Greenberg, B., Plumb, P., Cutter, G., Dean, J., Desena, A., Hopkins, S., Krishnan, C., Pardo, C., Recio, A., Schreiner, T., Yeh, E. A., & McCreary, M. (2021). Acute flaccid myelitis: long-term outcomes recorded in the CAPTURE study compared with paediatric transverse myelitis. *BMJ Neurology*, 3(1), e000127. doi:10.1136/bmjno-2021-000127.

Huang, J., Kockum, I., & Stridh, P. (2022). Trends in the environmental risks associated with earlier onset in multiple sclerosis. *Multiple Sclerosis and Related Disorders*, 68, 104250. https://doi.org/10.1016/j.msard.2022.104250.

Jakimovski, D., Awan, S., Eckert, S. P., Farooq, O., & Weinstock-Guttman, B. (2022). Multiple sclerosis in children: Differential diagnosis, prognosis, and disease-modifying treatment. *CNS Drugs*, 36(1), 45–59. https://doi.org/10.1007/s40263-021-00887-w.

Jeong, A., Oleske, D. M., & Holman, J. (2019). Epidemiology of pediatric-onset multiple sclerosis: A systematic review of the literature. *Journal of Child Neurology*, 34(12), 705–712. https://doi.org/10.1177/0883073819845827.

Kerbrat, A., Aubert-Broche, B., Fonov, V., Narayanan, S., Sled, J. G., Arnold, D. A., Banwell, B., & Collins, D. L. (2012). Reduced head and brain size for age and disproportionately smaller thalami in child-onset MS. *Neurology*, 78(3), 194–201. https://doi.org/10.1212/WNL.0b013e318240799a.

Krupp, L. B., Tardieu, M., Amato, M. P., Banwell, B., Chitnis, T., Dale, R. C., Ghezzi, A., Hintzen, R., Kornberg, A., Pohl, D., Rostasy, K., Tenembaum, S., Wassmer, E., & International PediatricMultiple SclerosisStudy Group Criteria for Pediatric Multiple Sclerosis and Immune-Mediated CentralNervous System-Demyelinating Disorders (2013) Revisions to the 2007 definitions. *Multiple Sclerosis Journal*, 19(10), 1261–1267. https://doi.org/10.1177/1352458513484547.

MacAllister, W. S., Belman, A. L., Milazzo, M., Weisbrot, D. M., Christodoulou, C., Scherl, W. F., Preston, T. E., Cianciulli, C., & Krupp, L. B. (2005). Cognitive functioning in children and adolescents with multiple sclerosis. *Neurology*, 64(8), 1422–1425. doi:10.1212/01.WNL.0000158474.24191.BC.

Mahaweni, N. M., Olieslagers, T. I., Rivas, I. O., Molenbroeck, S. J. J., Groeneweg, M., Bos, G. M. J., Tilanus, M. G. J., Voorter C. E. M., & Wieten, L. (2018). A comprehensive overview of FCGR3A gene variability by full-length gene sequencing including the identification of V158F polymorphism. *Nature*, 8(1), 15983. doi:10.1038/s41598-018-34258-1.

Oreja-Guevara, C., Ayuso Blanco, T., Brieva Ruiz, L., Hernández Pérez, M. Á., Meca-Lallana, V., & Ramió-Torrentà, L. (2019). Cognitive dysfunctions and assessments in multiple sclerosis. *Frontiers in Neurolology*, 10, 581. doi:10.3389/fneur.2019.00581.

Paolilo R. B., Deiva, K., Neuteboom, R., Rostásy, K., & Lim, M. (2020) Acute disseminated encephalomyelitis: Current perspectives. *Children*, 7(11), 210. https://doi.org/10.3390/children7110210.

Portaccio, E., De Meo, E., Bellinvia, A., & Amato, M. P. (2021). Cognitive issues in pediatric multiple sclerosis. *Brain Sciences*, 11(4), 442. https://doi.org/10.3390/brainsci11040442.

Storm Van's Gravesande, K., Blaschek, A., Calabrese, P., Rostásy, K., Huppke, P., Kessler J. J., Kalbe, E., Mall, V., & MUSICADO Study Group (2019). Fatigue and depression predict health-related quality of life in patients with pediatric-onset multiple sclerosis. *Multiple Sclerosis and Related Disorders*, 36, 101368. https://doi.org/10.1016/j.msard.2019.08.010.

Tan, A., Hague, C., Greenberg, B. M., & Harder, L. (2018). Neuropsychological outcomes of pediatric demyelinating diseases: A review. *Child Neuropsychology*, 24(5), 575–597. https://doi.org/10.1080/09297049.2017.1339785.

Thompson, A. J., Banwell, B. L., Barkhof, F., Carroll, W. M., Coetzee, T., Comi, G., Correale, J., Fazekas, F., Filippi, M., Freedman, M. S., Fujihara, K., Galetta, S. L., Hartung, H. P., Kappos, L., Lublin, F. D., Marrie, R. A., Miller, A. E., Miller, D. H., Montalban, X., ... Cohen, J. A. (2018). Diagnosis of multiple sclerosis: 2017 revisions of the McDonald criteria. *The Lancet. Neurology*, 17(2), 162–173. https://doi.org/10.1016/S1474-4422(17)30470–30472.

Wingerchuk, D. M., Banwell, B., Bennett, J. L., Cabre, P., Carroll, W., Chitnis, T., de Seze, J., Fuijhara, K., Greenberg, B., Jacob, A., Jarius, A., Lana-Peixoto, M., Levy, M., Simon, J. H., Tenembaum, S., Traboulsee, A. L., Waters, P., Wellik, K. E., & Weinshenker, B. G. (2015). International consensus diagnostic criteria for neuromyelitis optica spectrum disorders. *Neurology*, 85(2), 177–189. https://doi.org/10.1212/WNL.0000000000001729.

Index

Note: Locators in **bold** refer to tables.